Death, Dying, and Grief

Yan Z. Ciupak • Douglas C. Smith

Death, Dying, and Grief

Theories, Tools, and Cases

Springer

Yan Z. Ciupak
Department of Sociology and Anthropology
and Grief Support Specialist Certificate
Program, Continuing Education and
Workforce Development Department
Northern Michigan University
Marquette, MI, USA

Douglas C. Smith
Grief Support Specialist Certificate Program
Northern Michigan University
Marquette, MI, USA

ISBN 978-3-031-88466-5 ISBN 978-3-031-88467-2 (eBook)
https://doi.org/10.1007/978-3-031-88467-2

This Springer imprint is published by the registered company Springer Nature Switzerland AG
The registered company address is: Gewerbestrasse 11, 6330 Cham, Switzerland

In memory of my father, Zhiling Zhao, and my grandparents.
In celebration of my family: Brian, Andrew, Alex, and Bella.
With gratitude to my loved ones in China and around the world.
Dedicated to all beings for their liberation from suffering and
In honor of all endeavors to enable healing.
—Yan

In memory of my daughters, Kristin and Maren. For my family who gave love and created such joy in my life: my wife, Tara, stepchildren, Conley, Eann, Gwen, and son Joshua.
—Doug

Foreword

It was in the second decade of the twentieth century, that humankind rediscovered death. It was not that death disappeared for a while, nor was it because it was a topic unbroached and unspoken. In fact, it was well addressed in varied literary endeavors, religious texts and literature, and other human endeavors. It was just not addressed by the scientific community outside of medicine. It was generally ignored in the emerging disciplines of the social sciences. Sociology and psychology tended to give it little focus outside of Durkheim's seminal study of suicide, first published in 1897. Even in this book, suicide was incidental to Durkheim's primary focus on showing that even the most personal behaviors were deeply influenced by societal factors. The ultimate importance of Durheim's book on suicide (Durkheim, 1951) was not to offer suicide prevention or postvention but rather to establish the discipline of sociology.

One could persuasively argue the Freud's (1917) classic essay, *Mourning and Melancholia,* that attempted to differentiate typical grief from depression, is the beginning of the social scientific study of death. Throughout the next four decades, a variety of books and articles were published. Perhaps, one of the most significant was Lindemann's (1944) study of the symptomatology of grief based on a number of groups including the survivors of persons who died in a Boston disaster when the Coconut Grove, a nightclub, caught fire, killing near 500 patrons. Yet, it was the publication of Kübler Ross' (1969) *On Death and Dying* that engaged the interest of the population and led to a increased interest in this now emerging field called thanatology—or the study of death.

The time was right. Much of the Western world was undergoing a significant demographic shift. Due to new antibiotics, the threat of acute diseases diminished. New therapies allowed people to live longer with chronic diseases. Life is not only extended—death did as well. New technologies have allowed medicine to keep older persons alive much longer by sustaining nurturance, hydration, and even respiration through technological means. This prolongation of death has created new strains for medical staff, new ethical issues, and new forms of care, which all have served to increase public awareness of and interest in the discussion and organization of dying and death. Unlike prior times when death either came suddenly or after a brief illness, people were *dying.*

This was a time of war and conflict and as the century continued and the new century began humans had to cope with new threats to existence such as the proliferation of nuclear weapons, acts of terrorist, natural disasters, and the emergence of new diseases such as AIDS and COVID-19.

Though the notion of dying stages was largely discarded by thanatological scholars, Kübler-Ross' work was important heuristically (Corr, 1993; Doka & Tucci, 2011). It spanned a number of social movements including the Death Awareness Movement that led to the development of studies, educational programs and course, journals, and professional associations such as ADEC (The Association for Death Education and Counseling) and IWG (The International Work Group on Death, Dying and Bereavement). It also spurred the development of the hospice movement, one of the most successful social movements of the last decade of the Twentieth Century as the first hospice opened, St. Christopher's outside of London in 1967 would become a model for the development of literally thousands of hospices and palliative care movements across the globe.

The result has been that in the last 60 years, we have learned much about death, dying, and grief.

The great value of Yan Ciupak and Douglas Smith's *Death, Dying and Grief: Theories, Tools, and Cases* is that it offers a concise summary of what we have learned in those years. Readers will not only enjoy a rich distillation of the field, but one buttressed by activities for self-reflection, tools for support, and rich case studies that translate concepts and theories into situations oft encountered in the dying and bereaved.

Senior Vice President for Grief Programs, Kenneth J. Doka
The Hospice Foundation of America
Washington, DC, USA

References

Corr, C. (1993). Coping with dying: Lessons that we should learn and not learn from the work of Elizabeth Kubler-Ross. *Death Studies, 117*, 69–83.

Doka, K., & Tucci, A., (Eds.). (2011). *Beyond Kübler-Ross: New perspectives on death, dying, and Bereavement*. The Hospice Foundation of America.

Durkheim, E. (1951). *Suicide: A study in sociology*. Free Press.

Freud, S. (1917/1957). Mourning and melancholia. *Standard edition* (V. XIV). Hogarth.

Kubler-Ross, E. (1969). *On death & dying*. MacMillan.

Lindenmann, E. (1944). Symptomatology and management of acute grief. *American Journal of Psychology, 101*, 141–148.

Preface

This book was born out of love, grief, and the continuing bonds that connect us beyond the veil of life and death.

While teaching courses on death, dying, and grief and co-leading the Grief Support Specialist Certificate Program that I founded with Doug, we recognized a growing need. There were excellent books offering comprehensive knowledge, but many professionals found them insufficient to guide practical application. In contrast, practitioner handbooks with valuable tools often lack systematic coverage of foundational theories. Moreover, many of these resources are confined to mental health practitioners and therapists, yet grief support extends far beyond the closed doors of therapy sessions. First responders, healthcare providers, educators, and countless others encounter grief—whether by supporting others or navigating their own—every day.

Grief is not simply an individual emotional experience; it is a deeply multifaceted process influenced by psychological, sociological, and cultural dimensions. Far from being limited to private struggles, death and grief operate as a social and relational phenomenon shaped by the intersections of personal experience and broader societal structures. These structures are multi-dimensional, such as gender, race, class, family dynamics, care systems, cultural norms, and the political and economic environment of the time. Recognizing this complexity, I often discussed with Doug and others how the field could benefit from a comprehensive resource that integrates these perspectives—sociological, psychological, and multicultural—while bridging the gap between theory and practical tools. The development of modern academic disciplines has brought valuable depth. Yet, it often imposes constructed boundaries that fragment the holistic pursuit of authentic knowledge, much like the parable of the blind people and the elephant, where each person perceives only a part of the whole. Recognizing this, we felt compelled to address the topics of death, dying, and grief in their totality, reflecting the intrinsic psychosocial and spiritual dimensions of human existence.

That is undoubtedly an ambitious endeavor. One day, I said to Doug, "Let's create a book that combines my theories and scholarship with the tools and case studies you've developed through all these years of clinical practice!" In our training program, Doug was lovingly nicknamed the "toolbox," while I am known as the "bookworm." Together, a bookworm with a toolbox should be able to craft something meaningful and useful!

However, academic life is a double-edged sword, with both exciting opportunities and relentless demands. Squeezed between heavy committee work, teaching, and existing scholarly projects, my progress in this endeavor was painfully slow. Meanwhile, Doug's heart condition was steadily declining.

One day in December 2023, I finally carved out a weekend to draft the book proposal. As I excitedly sent the draft to Doug, I noticed an email from him in my inbox. In it, he thanked me for our friendship and collaboration and shared the news that he had just started hospice care.

The email hit me like a blow. A surge of emotions swept over me: shock, sadness, anxiety, and an overwhelming sense of guilt.

Doug was not only a cherished colleague but also a mentor and a dear friend. He introduced me to the field of thanatology, offering steadfast support and guidance. Whether navigating a media presence or co-founding our training program at my institution, Doug was just a phone call away, ready with encouragement and insights. I couldn't imagine continuing the project without him. Yet, the most overwhelming emotion I felt was guilt and regret—knowing that his health had been declining, why had I put off this work for so long?

Anticipatory grief is hard, but it can also spark extraordinary strength and motivation. I found myself rising before 6 am and staying up past midnight, squeezing in writing amidst the packed demands of teaching, committee work, and family responsibilities. I was racing against time, knowing that Doug didn't have much left.

Each response from him was a gift, filled with his characteristic encouragement and unwavering cheerleading. However, every email carried the lingering fear that it might be his last. I felt relief when I completed all the chapters (Part III) of the materials he provided, and by July, I had nearly finished the first draft. Doug's clarity and calmness never wavered, which I heard remained until his very last moments and amazed even his doctors. Doug's last email was sent at 1:46 pm on July 7th, less than 3 days before his passing. He told me that his health had taken a dramatic downturn in the last couple of days and thanked me for all I've been doing.

If the first half of the year working on the book was fuelled by anticipatory grief, the second half was instrumental in processing that grief. Carrying forward our shared commitment to alleviating suffering and empowering those who help others, continuing work on the project became a bond that transcended his physical absence. It was a bittersweet experience—editing the cases he shared and the tools he developed vividly brought him to life in my mind. I could almost see his smile, radiating warmth and offering solace even to the most troubled hearts.

I saw again the gentle, humble man who viewed everyone as Jesus, a Buddha. His profound humility toward those he served, combined with his authenticity and willingness to reveal his deepest vulnerabilities and wounds, embodied the essence of what made him a "wounded healer" that he used to call himself. I know there are many such compassionate healers out there—quietly, tirelessly, transforming lives.

This book is for them.

When All is Done
In the quiet cadence as a meal concludes,
Does the nourishment linger, or does it elude?
As a book wraps up, does the author fade,
Or does it resonate like a serenade?
With the setting sun, do the day's gifts recede,
Or in their twilight dance, do they intercede?
Why, then, should I, at life's twilight, harbor doubt?
When each chapter closes, can it not reveal
A story of worth, a legacy concealed?
Guide me to uncover the nourishment I've bestowed,
Reveal the seeds of kindness in the world I have sown.
Help me grasp the ripples of hope I have shared,
When the melody of life feels out of tune.
Embracing the circle of life, let my heart find its home.
A legacy woven in kind intention wherever I may roam.
For love is the aroma that lingers in the air,
A symphony of connection, a fabric exquisite and rare.
In the still moments, and the tales I've spun,
May this legacy be one that forever runs.
And as compassion weaves through the fabric of time,
A soft whisper in hearts, a rhythm and rhyme.
So, let me release any wounds I still bear,
Let me not question the worth of my share.
Remember the trials from which I was spared,
Cherish grace and kindness, which is always there.
For in the legacy I leave and the experiences I've had,
I discover the true measure of a life beyond compare—
A wounded healer, forever mending the world with love and care.

Now, the book is complete, undoubtedly with imperfection. The work must continue through trial and error. May we honor the shared vulnerability of humanity and enable inherent connection and healing power within us and beyond. May suffering be alleviated. May every heart and every corner of the world find peace, compassion, healing, and hope.

Organization of the Book

This book is structured into five major parts, each progressively building on foundational knowledge, theoretical insights, and practical tools and cases. Together, these sections aim to provide a comprehensive guide integrating multidisciplinary perspectives for understanding and supporting death, dying, and grief.

Part I: An Integrative Understanding of Death, Dying, and Grief

Part I lays the foundation for understanding death, dying, and grief from an integrated psychological, sociological, and multicultural perspective. Chapter 1 discusses the recent Spiral Model of Grieving and Healing, a framework adopted for the book. It explores the motivations and benefits of studying death, dying, and grief, emphasizing the socially embedded nature of these experiences. It provides a historical overview of the death awareness movement, revealing the central themes of contemporary development: diversity and autonomy. The positive and negative aspects of death and grief in the contemporary digital age are also explored.

Chapter 2 examines the multi-dimensional nature of culture, the interplay between the self and culture, and the intersectionality of various cultural and social elements. The distinctions and connections among cultural awareness, humility, and competency are examined, providing theoretical and practical guidance for culturally responsive care.

Part II Theories and Concepts in Loss, Grief, and Dying

Part II delves into the theoretical foundations and complexities of loss, death, and grief. Chapter 3 examines different types of losses, such as primary, secondary, ambiguous, and disenfranchised grief, as well as prolonged grief disorder. These frameworks help contextualize the diverse and multifaceted nature of grief. Chapter 4 provides an overview of classical and contemporary grief models, from stage-based theories to task-oriented frameworks and the dual process model, culminating in the recent Spiral Model of Grieving and Healing. Chapter 5 shifts the focus to the end-of-life experience, discussing the trajectories of dying, such as sudden death, terminal illness, and prolonged frailty. It offers principles for compassionate, person-centered care, highlighting the World Health Organization's pillars of physical, emotional, social, and spiritual support. Ethical considerations, such as advance care planning and medically assisted death, are also discussed.

Part III: Principles and Practices in End-of-Life and Grief Support

Part III introduces key principles and competencies for effective end-of-life and grief support. Chapter 6 outlines professional competencies, drawing on guidelines from major organizations and introducing the 4A4C competency framework as an overarching framework to guide end-of-life and grief support and healing. Chapter 7 focuses on assessment and care planning, offering tools for palliative and bereavement contexts. Chapter 8 provides holistic psychosocial care plan models for professionals to guide their practices to offer person-centered support.

Part IV: Supporting Psychosocial Needs in End-of-Life and Grieving

Part IV includes practical tools for addressing the psychosocial needs of individuals and families. Chapters 9 and 10 introduce exercises such as life review, legacy building, humor, and guided visualization, providing care providers with a wide range of interventions for holistic support. Case studies are included throughout the chapters to illustrate the real-world application of these tools, offering concrete examples to enhance understanding.

Part V: Supporting Spiritual Needs in End-of-Life and Grieving
Part V focuses on the often-overlooked spiritual dimensions of grief and end-of-life care. Chapters 11 through 13 present integrative spiritual tools, such as mindfulness practices, spiritual storytelling, and contemplative exercises, which draw from multicultural resources designed to nurture spiritual well-being. These chapters offer professionals concrete strategies, tools, and examples to address the spiritual needs of the dying and the bereaved, emphasizing the transformative power of meaning-making and connection.

This book explores multidisciplinary perspectives and practical tools to provide a comprehensive guide for understanding and supporting experiences of death, dying, and grief. Each part can be independent but builds on the previous parts. Whether through social-cultural understanding, psychosocial care, or spiritual support, the book invites readers to engage deeply with the complexities of loss and to find ways to foster healing, connection, and hope. Overall, it serves as a companion for those dedicated to walking alongside others through life's most difficult and transformative moments.

Marquette, MI, USA
November 22, 2024

Yan Z. Ciupak

Acknowledgments

Like any human endeavor, this book's fruition results from collective inspiration and effort. I thank my colleagues, students, family, and friends for their support throughout this journey.

I am honored by the encouragement and endorsement of esteemed experts, including Dr. Kenneth J. Doka, who contributed to the foreword. Special thanks to Dr. Ira Byock, Dr. Gerry Cox, Dr. Neil Thompson, Dr. Robert Neimeyer, Dr. Harold Smith, and Dr. Andy Ho for their support.

I am grateful to my home institution, Northern Michigan University, for its Reassigned Time Award, Curriculum Development Award, and other grants, as well as to my dean, Dr. Robert Winn, for his consistent support of faculty scholarship. Professor Daric Christian helped with digitalizing two important graphics. Professors Alex Stoner, Alan McEvoy, Dr. LaMart Hightower read a foundational chapter. Dr. Jonathan Johnson, Professor of Creative Writing at Eastern Washington University, and Tim DeMarte, Professor of English, shared their insights on some poetry in the book.

My spiritual teachers, Jetsunma Tenzin Palmo, Swami Omkarananda, and Swami Sankarananda, offered grounding wisdom that shaped the Buddhist and Vedanta-related content. Neuroscientist Dr. Shikah Goodwin and clinical psychologist Dr. Debra Smith provided invaluable expertise and support. Friends from Dr. Gabor Maté's Compassionate Inquiry circle, particularly June, offered input and encouragement.

Special thanks to Tara Potter, my coauthor's wife, for her timely assistance in matters related to the book after Doug's passing.

This book began as a response to requests from my students and the Grief Support Specialist Certificate participants. I thank my student assistant, Caden, for assisting with the preparation of the manuscript from beginning to completion and MSW student, Alyssa Brown, for her meticulous attention to reference checks. I also appreciate the involvement and feedback of students in my Winter and Fall 2024 death, dying, and grief classes, whose inputs and feedback enriched early drafts.

I deeply value the efficient communication and diligent work of Springer editors Janet Kim, Kausalya Boobalan, and the production team, as well as the anonymous reviewers who recognized this book's potential contribution to the field.

My heartfelt gratitude goes to my family in China and the United States. My parents and brother have given immense love and made countless sacrifices. My in-law family provided consistent emotional support. 15-year-old Andrew was instrumental in digitizing the graphics, while 12-year-old Bella took charge of family dinners during the months of my intensive writing. Alex's daily practice of Chinese provided comfort to my immigration-related grief, and my husband, Brian, has been a steadfast anchor for our family.

To all who are on the journey of healing, both for themselves and others, I hope this book serves as a supportive companion.

Yan

Competing Interests The authors have no competing interests to declare that are relevant to the content of this manuscript.

Endorsements

"The great value of Yan Ciupak and Douglas Smith's book is that it offers a concise summary of what we have learned in the past decades. Readers will not only enjoy a rich distillation of the field but one buttressed by activities for self-reflection, tools for support, and rich case studies that translate concepts and theories into situations often encountered in the dying and bereaved."

—Kenneth J. Doka, PhD, *Senior Vice President for Grief Programs, The Hospice Foundation of America*

"Ciupak and Smith have effectively integrated recognized theoretical frameworks and empiric evidence into straightforward and practical caring models, therapeutic exercises and plans for care that can be tailored to the unique history, and personal preferences of each patient or client.

This highly readable book is a resource for professional caregivers, academicians, students, and anyone wishing to delve into the human experiences of illness, dying, and grieving.

The authors' integrative model is broad in scope and profound in depth, yet the clinical applications they offer are straightforward and accessible."

—Ira Byock, MD, Palliative Care Physician, Emeritus Professor, *Dartmouth Geisel School of Medicine, author of Dying Well and The Best Care Possible*

"For many years now I have been making the case for a more holistic approach to death, dying and bereavement that incorporates a sociological dimension to complement the psychological understandings. I was therefore delighted to see that this book adopts this wider approach in recognizing the significance of social factors in shaping people's experiences of loss. Add this to the rich insights brought from years of experience in supporting dying and grieving individuals and you have an invaluable resource that will be a very worthwhile addition to the literature."

—Neil Thompson, Ph.D., Author and educator

“Yan Ciupak and Doug Smith have put together an excellent, practical book that is destined to become one of the more important books in the field. As a sociologist, I am impressed with the awareness of the impact of social processes and social institutions on grief and bereavement. Grief and bereavement are not simply matters for psychologists or counselors to analyze and support those who are grieving, but they also require an understanding of the social forces that enhance or make grieving more difficult. The authors also offer models for aiding the grieving and bereaved with spiritual, ethical, and systematic models for assessing and supporting the grieving and bereaved. The book presents a compassionate, caring framework for working with the grieving and bereaved. It offers important tools for anyone working in the field.”

—Gerry Cox, Ph.D., *University of Wisconsin-La Crosse*

“This heartfelt book fills a gap in grief studies by bridging theory to practical, creative tools for professionals to use in their work with the bereaved. The case examples and multicultural perspectives allow for an understanding of the breadth of individual experiences with death. I have implemented many of these mindfulness exercises and rituals in my practice and found that they empower clients to gain insight, concretize memories, as well as promote creative healing and integration of loss. Well done!”

—Molly Tomony, LPC, MA, ATR-BC, Licensed Professional Counselor and Art Therapist

“This book is approachable, well informed and grounded in the process of helping professionals assist people with loss of a loved one. The authors provide prime examples which encourages practitioners to engage in critical thinking and further explores the complexities surrounding death and dying. The authors examine cultural issues and challenge us to consider different points of views from a diversified population.”

—LaMart Hightower, Ph.D., LMSW, *Department of Social Work, Northern Michigan University*

Contents

Part I An Integrative Understanding of Death, Dying, and Grief

1 Death and Grief Studies 3
1.1 Understanding Death, Dying, and Grief 3
1.2 Why Study Death and Grief? 6
1.2.1 Fostering Acceptance and Resilience 7
1.2.2 Psychological and Emotional Benefits 7
1.2.3 Cultivating Empathy and Awareness 8
1.2.4 Improving Caregiving and Professional Competence 8
1.3 Personal and Professional 8
1.3.1 Therapeutic Alliance and the Self as an Instrument 9
1.4 Forms of Death and Grief Education 12
1.5 Need for Integrative Training 13
1.6 Death Attitudes and Encounters 14
1.6.1 Death Attitudes 14
1.6.2 Death Encounters 15
1.6.3 Impact of Death Attitudes 16
1.7 The Death Awareness Movement 17
1.7.1 Modern Death Awareness Movement 17
1.7.2 Early Influences and Pioneers 17
1.7.3 Organizations, Journals, and Formal Education 19
1.8 Diversity and Autonomy: Contemporary Development 19
1.9 Death and Grief in Digital Age 22
1.9.1 Benefits of Digital Support 23
1.9.2 Challenges of Digital Grief 23
1.9.3 Cyberthanatology 24
1.10 Concluding Reflections 25
References 25

2 Culture in End-of-Life and Grief Support . . . 29
2.1 What Is Culture . . . 29
2.1.1 Cultural Significance of Rituals . . . 30
2.1.2 Multidimensions of Cultural Diversity . . . 31
2.2 Culturally Responsive Policies and Practices . . . 34
2.3 Culture Awareness, Competence, and Humility . . . 35
2.3.1 Cultural Awareness . . . 35
2.3.2 Cultural Competence: Definition and Dimensions . . . 37
2.3.3 Cultural Humility . . . 41
2.3.4 Integrating Cultural Awareness, Humility, and Competence . . . 43
2.4 Practical Guidelines for Culturally Responsive Care . . . 44
2.5 Concluding Reflection . . . 46
References . . . 47

Part II Theories and Concepts in Loss, Grief, and Dying

3 Loss and Grief: Concepts and Types . . . 53
3.1 Introduction . . . 53
3.2 Primary and Secondary Loss . . . 56
3.3 Death-Related Loss and Nonfinite Loss . . . 57
3.4 Ambiguous Loss . . . 58
3.5 Traumatic Loss and Death . . . 60
3.5.1 Traumatic Loss & Assumptive Worlds . . . 60
3.5.2 Supporting Traumatic Loss: From Victims to Survivors . . . 61
3.5.3 Mechanisms for Supporting and Coping with Traumatic Loss . . . 62
3.5.4 Transitioning from Grief to Growth . . . 63
3.6 Anticipatory Grief . . . 63
3.7 Disenfranchised Grief . . . 65
3.8 Vicarious Grief . . . 67
3.9 Cumulative and Collective Loss and Grief . . . 70
3.10 Prolonged Grief Disorder/Complicated Grief . . . 71
3.10.1 Definition and Diagnostic Criteria: Overview . . . 71
3.10.2 ICD-11 Criteria for PGD . . . 72
3.10.3 DSM-5-TR Criteria for PGD . . . 74
3.10.4 Summary on ICD-11 and DSM-5-TR Criteria for PGD . . . 75
3.10.5 Boundary with Posttraumatic Stress Disorder and Depressive Episodes (ICD-11) . . . 75
3.10.6 Cultural and Developmental Considerations . . . 76
3.10.7 Concerns and Challenges . . . 77
3.10.8 Practical Tips for Professionals and Practitioners . . . 78
3.11 Concluding Reflection . . . 79
References . . . 80

4 Grieving Process Models and Theories 83
4.1 Introduction 83
4.2 Classical Perspectives and Models 84
4.2.1 Freud's "Grief Work" 84
4.2.2 Kübler-Ross's Stage Theory 86
4.3 Worden's Task Model of Mourning 88
4.4 Dual Process Model 89
4.5 Grieving Styles 92
4.6 Meaning Reconstruction 92
4.7 Continuing Bonds 95
4.8 Five Critical Variables that Influence the Grieving Experience 97
4.9 Spiral Model of Grieving and Healing 101
4.10 Concluding Reflection 102
References 103

5 Dying and End-of-Life Care 105
5.1 Introduction 105
5.2 End-of-Life Trajectories 106
5.2.1 Terminal Decline Approach to EOL Trajectories 106
5.2.2 Primary Cause Approach 107
5.2.3 Integrating Care Strategies 109
5.3 Theoretical Frameworks: Stage and Tasks 110
5.3.1 Stage Model: Cautions and Lesson 110
5.3.2 Corr's Task-Based Model 112
5.4 Four Pillars of Holistic End-of-Life Care (WHO) 113
5.5 Major Types of End-of-Life Care 114
5.6 Global Development of End-of-Life Care 118
5.7 Advance Care Planning and Decision-Making 119
5.7.1 Introduction 119
5.7.2 Living Wills & Durable Power of Attorney 120
5.7.3 Importance of Advance Care Planning 121
5.7.4 Challenges and Strategies 121
5.7.5 What to Do Once You Have an Advance Directive 122
5.8 Medically Assisted Death: Debate and Current State 122
5.8.1 Legalization and Practices in the United States 123
5.8.2 International Perspectives on Physician-Assisted Death . . . 123
5.8.3 Active vs. Passive Euthanasia 124
5.8.4 Physician-Assisted Death Debates 125
5.9 Navigating the Complexities of EOL Care: Ethical and Legal Considerations 127
5.9.1 Overview 127
5.9.2 End-of-Life Decision-Making for Families 129
5.9.3 Professionals' Roles in End-of-Life Care 130
5.9.4 Conclusion on Ethical and Legal Complexity 135
5.10 Concluding Reflection 135
References 135

Part III Principles and Practices in End-of-Life and Grief Support

6 Competencies and Principles in End-of-Life and Grief Support 141
6.1 Introduction 141
6.2 Grief Support, Counseling, and Therapy 143
6.2.1 Grief Counseling vs. Grief Therapy 143
6.2.2 Principles and Goals of Grief Counseling 144
6.2.3 Couple and Family Counseling 146
6.2.4 Grief Counseling and Therapy Techniques 148
6.3 End-of-Life Support 151
6.4 Ethics and Guidelines 152
6.5 4A4C Competency Framework in End-of-Life and Grief Support 153
6.5.1 Awareness 155
6.5.2 Acceptance 156
6.5.3 Affirmation 156
6.5.4 Actualization 156
6.5.5 Compassion 157
6.5.6 Connection 157
6.5.7 Composure 158
6.5.8 Commitment 159
6.5.9 Summary 159
6.6 Communication in End-of-Life and Grief Support 160
6.6.1 Nature of Communication 161
6.6.2 Validating and Invalidating Statements 162
6.6.3 Effective Communication Strategies in End-of-Life and Grief Support 163
6.7 Self-Care for Professionals and Prevention of Compassion Fatigue 164
6.7.1 Understanding Compassion Fatigue and Vicarious Grief 165
6.7.2 Warning Signs and Prevention Strategies 166
6.7.3 Self-Care and Resilience 166
6.7.4 Integrating Compassion and "Skillful Means" for Sustainable Support 168
6.8 Concluding Reflection 169
References 170

7 Assessments and Care Plans in End-of-Life and Grief Support 175
7.1 Introduction: Strength-Based Approach 175
7.2 Assessments in Hospice and Palliative Care 176
7.3 Bereavement Assessment 177
7.4 Strength-Based Assessments 178
7.4.1 Case Example: The Preacher 179
7.4.2 Case Example: The Dancer 180
7.4.3 Case Example: Discovering Jane's Inner Peace 180

7.4.4 Tool: Assessing Personal Strength, Peace, and Security 181
7.4.5 Tool: Glue of My Life 182
7.4.6 Case Example: Gertrude 182
7.4.7 Case Example: Scott's Strength 183
7.4.8 Case Example: Using Some Detective Work 183
7.4.9 Tool: Psychosocial Comfort Assessment Form 184
7.5 Family Strength Assessment 185
7.6 Grieving Style Assessment 186
7.6.1 Case Example: Wally's and Djuna's Grieving Styles 187
7.7 Physical Dimension Assessment 188
7.8 Developing Personalized Care Plans 189
7.8.1 Allowing Our Roles to Be Defined 189
7.9 One Question Care Plan for End-of-Life 192
7.9.1 Case Example: The Fishing Trip 193
7.9.2 Case Example: Trevor's Campfire 194
7.9.3 Case Example: One Last Christmas 195
7.10 One Question Care Plans for Grieving 195
7.10.1 Case Example: Kayak Trip 195
7.10.2 Case Example: Personalized Ritual and Spaces 197
7.10.3 Tool: Self-Care Plan for a Grieving Person 197
7.10.4 Tool: From "I Need" to "I Can Get" 198
7.10.5 Tool: My Ideal Death Story 199
7.11 Games and Activities to Start the Conversation 200
7.12 Tool: Guided Imagery/Visualization: The Medicine Man 200
7.13 Concluding Reflection 201
References 202

8 Holistic Psychosocial Care Plans 203
8.1 Holistic Psychosocial Care (HPC): An Integrative Approach 203
8.1.1 Overview of the Three HPC Plans 203
8.1.2 Implementation Guidelines 204
8.1.3 4A4C and Honor the Spiral Journey 205
8.2 Systematic Care Plan A: Relationship Peaks and Valleys 206
8.2.1 Step One: Processing Grief 207
8.2.2 Step Two: Relationship Complexity Mapping 209
8.2.3 Step Three: 5,4,3,2,1—Recovery Has Begun 211
8.3 Systematic Care Plan B: Continuing Treasure 212
8.3.1 Step One: Honor Treasured Moments 213
8.3.2 Step Two: Giving Forgiveness 213
8.3.3 Step Three: Continuing Bonds 214
8.4 Systematic Care Plan C: Acceptance and Carrying On 215
8.4.1 Step One: Accepting the Reality of the Loss 217
8.4.2 Step Two: Working Through the Pain 217
8.4.3 Step Three: Filling Gaps 218

8.4.4 Step Four: Carrying on with Life . . . 218
8.5 Finish the Unfinished Business Letter . . . 219
8.6 Affirmations . . . 221
8.6.1 Tips for Affirmations . . . 221
8.6.2 Sample Affirmations . . . 223
8.7 Monthly Review . . . 224
8.7.1 Step 1. Review and Reflection . . . 224
8.7.2 Step 2: Identify Area of Focus . . . 224
8.7.3 Step 3: Set SMART Goals . . . 225
8.8 Concluding Reflections . . . 226
References . . . 227

Part IV Supporting Psychosocial Needs in End-of-Life and Grieving

9 Psychosocial Support for End-of-Life Transition . . . 231
9.1 Introduction . . . 231
9.1.1 Emotions and Tasks in Terminal Illness . . . 231
9.1.2 Corr's Task-Based Model . . . 232
9.2 Five Essential Themes for Supporting Dying Individuals . . . 233
9.3 Honoring and Facilitating Final Wishes . . . 234
9.3.1 Case Example: Smelling of a Horse . . . 234
9.3.2 Case Example: Werther's Candy and a Beer . . . 235
9.3.3 Case Example: Just One Little Pill . . . 235
9.4 Emotional and Practical Support . . . 236
9.4.1 A Tool: The Imaginary Sledgehammer . . . 236
9.4.2 Case Example: Get Out of My Room . . . 237
9.4.3 Case Example: Susan's Release Room . . . 237
9.4.4 Case Example: Martha's Denial and Naughty Words . . . 238
9.4.5 Case Example: Sam's Defiant Clarity . . . 238
9.5 Respecting and Engaging with "Unresponsive" Patients . . . 239
9.5.1 Case Example: Richie's Response to Kind Words . . . 240
9.5.2 Case Example: Dottie's Son . . . 240
9.6 Life Review and Legacy Building . . . 241
9.6.1 Tool: A Simple Life Review . . . 241
9.6.2 Tool: Photographic Life Review . . . 242
9.6.3 Tool: Pass It On . . . 242
9.6.4 Tool: Leaving a Message . . . 243
9.6.5 Tool: A Tribute . . . 243
9.6.6 Case Example: Linda's Healing Journey . . . 244
9.7 Healing Power of Touch . . . 245
9.7.1 Case Example: Candy's Touching Moment . . . 245
9.7.2 Case Example: A Loving Family's Final Touch . . . 246
9.7.3 Case Example: Role Modeling Touch . . . 246
9.7.4 Case Example: The Final Touch . . . 246
9.8 Humor and Joy in Care . . . 247

9.8.1 Tool: Smiling and Laughing Permitted Here 248
9.8.2 Tool: A Funny Life Review 248
9.8.3 Tool: Funny Videos 248
9.8.4 Willy's Dance 249
9.9 Cognitive and Spiritual Shift 249
9.9.1 Tool: Eliminating Self-Blaming Over Illness 250
9.9.2 Tool: The Grass Could Have Been Browner 251
9.9.3 A Tool: Positive Affirmations 251
9.9.4 Tool: Empowerment by Care 252
9.9.5 Guided Visualization/Imagery: Dialog with Death 253
9.9.6 Guided Imagery: My Funeral 254
9.9.7 Case Example: Amanda's Breakthrough 256
9.10 Autonomy and Control at End-of-Life 256
9.10.1 Jonathan's Pain Management 257
9.10.2 Case Example: Elmer's Empowerment in Pain Relief 257
9.10.3 Case Example: Conflicting Wishes 257
9.11 Love and Connection 258
9.11.1 Tool: Activities and Games for End-of-Life Conversations 258
9.11.2 Tool: Coupons 259
9.11.3 Tool: Sharing Dreams 259
9.11.4 A Tool: Giveaway Ceremony/Party 260
9.11.5 Tool: Family Litany as Death Is Near 260
9.11.6 Case Example: Priscilla's Birthday Party 261
9.11.7 Case Example: Carlo's Wedding Anniversary 261
9.11.8 Case Example: Christopher's Last Bath 262
9.12 Concluding Reflection 262
References 263

10 Psychosocial Support for Grieving 265
10.1 Introduction: Navigating the Complexities of Grief 265
10.2 Relationship to Disease 266
10.3 Relationship to Depression 266
10.4 Relationship to Guilt 267
10.5 Forgiveness 268
10.6 Social-Emotional Tools 269
10.6.1 Forgiving the Deceased 269
10.6.2 From Guilt to Self-Forgiveness 270
10.6.3 Ritual of Self-Forgiveness 271
10.6.4 Forgiving Those Who Hurt Us 272
10.6.5 Grieving Diary 273
10.6.6 Memory Book 273
10.6.7 Memory Collage 274
10.6.8 Memorial Quilt 274

10.6.9 Memory Jar 275
10.6.10 Service of Remembrance 276
10.6.11 Litany of Remembrance 276
10.6.12 Guided Visualization: Dialogue with the Lost One 277
10.6.13 Guided Visualization: Experiencing Unity 278
10.7 Cognitive Tools 280
10.7.1 Relationship Life Review 280
10.7.2 The Fun(ny) Times 281
10.7.3 Intentions 281
10.7.4 Opening Up to Wonder 281
10.7.5 Life-Giving Energy 282
10.8 Social-Behavioral Approaches 282
10.8.1 Creating a Buddy System 282
10.8.2 Being My Own Best Caregiver 283
10.8.3 Becoming Proactive with the Reactive 283
10.8.4 Commitment to Myself 284
10.9 Concluding Reflection 285
References 285

Part V Supporting Spiritual Needs in End-of-Life and Grieving

11 Spiritual Support for End-of-Life and Grieving 289
11.1 Introduction: Human's Search for Meaning 289
11.1.1 Spirituality and Religiosity 290
11.1.2 Spiritual Diversity 290
11.1.3 Spiritual Support in End-of-Life and Grieving 291
11.2 Spiritual Assessments 292
11.2.1 Consensus Report 292
11.2.2 Spiritual History Tools 293
11.2.3 Word Association 295
11.2.4 Spiritual Life Map 296
11.2.5 Exploratory Questions 297
11.2.6 Imagined Roles 297
11.2.7 Case Example: Spiritual Language (Narrated by Doug Smith) 298
11.2.8 Conclusion 299
11.3 Dynamic and Diverse Spiritual Exploration Tools 299
11.3.1 Supporting Spiritual Exploration 299
11.3.2 Cases Examples of Spiritual Exploration 301
11.4 The Wounded Healer: Reflection and Reconstruction Exercises 302
11.4.1 The Wounded Healer Resume 303
11.4.2 Reconstruct the Shattered Assumptive World 303
11.4.3 How Can I Use This 304
11.4.4 Refining Personal Philosophy 305

11.5 Self-Care Practices 306
11.5.1 Flexing Spiritual Muscle 306
11.5.2 Giving Thanks 307
11.5.3 Joy and Concerns Altar 307
11.5.4 Ritual of Radiant Living 308
11.5.5 Reward Yourself 309
11.6 Mindfulness and Contemplative Exercises 309
11.6.1 Mindfulness, Health, Spirituality 309
11.6.2 Dr. C's ABC Meditation 311
11.6.3 Mindful Senses 312
11.6.4 Mindful Tasting for Non-attachment 313
11.6.5 A Mindful Mirror Journey 315
11.6.6 Free-Expression Dance 315
11.6.7 Tonglen Practice (Sending and Receiving) 317
11.6.8 Guided Visualization and Yoga Nidra 318
11.6.9 Yoga Nidra (Complete Scheme) 321
11.6.10 Short Relaxation Script 1 324
11.6.11 Short Body Scan and Relaxation Script 2 325
11.6.12 Guided Mediation: Self-Inquiry 325
11.6.13 Guided Visualization: On Peace 326
11.7 Concluding Reflection 326
References 327

12 Spiritual Care for End-of-Life Transition 329
12.1 Introduction 329
12.2 Importance and Challenges 330
12.2.1 Significance of Spiritual Dimension in EOL Care 330
12.2.2 Challenges 331
12.3 End-of-Life Spiritual Care Guidelines 333
12.3.1 Consensus Report Model and Implementation 333
12.3.2 Formulation of a Spiritual Care Plan 334
12.3.3 Primary Spiritual Concerns at End of Life 334
12.4 Research-Informed End-of-Life Spiritual Care 335
12.5 Tools for End-of-Life Spiritual Exploration and Support 337
12.5.1 Spiritual Storytelling: My Spiritual Travelogue 338
12.5.2 Spiritual Life Map 339
12.5.3 Dream Journal 340
12.5.4 A Worthy Self/Fulfilled Life Letter 340
12.5.5 Meditation Exercises 342
12.5.6 Guided Visualization/Imagery Exercises 345
12.5.7 Prayers and Transcendental Conversations 349
12.6 Real-Life Cases 356
12.6.1 Case Example: New Assignments 356
12.6.2 Case Example: Jean's Unveiling Perspective 357
12.6.3 Case Example: A Special Visitor 357

12.6.4 Case Example: My Body Is Sick, But I Am Well 358
12.6.5 Case Example: Doug's Growing Awareness 359
12.7 Concluding Reflection 360
References.. 361

13 Spiritual Support Tools for Grieving.............................. 363
13.1 Spirituality and Religiosity 363
13.2 Spirituality in Grieving and Healing 364
13.3 Rituals and Other Spiritual Practices in Grief Therapy 365
13.4 Remembrance 366
13.4.1 Private Service of Remembrance.................. 366
13.4.2 Anniversary Service of Remembrance 367
13.4.3 Remembrance from Afar 367
13.5 Personal Spaces and Altars 368
13.5.1 Altar of Remembrance............................ 368
13.5.2 Memory Jar 369
13.6 Rituals and Symbolic Actions 369
13.6.1 The Ancient Stone Ceremony 370
13.6.2 A Farewell Ceremony 371
13.6.3 River of Life..................................... 372
13.7 Guided Visualization 373
13.7.1 Guided Visualization: Releasing Your Loved One...... 373
13.7.2 Guided Visualization: Healing the Heart 374
13.8 Affirmations and Journaling 375
13.8.1 A Bereaved Person's Spiritual Affirmations 375
13.8.2 Grief Journaling.................................. 376
13.8.3 Dream Journal 377
13.9 Holidays.. 377
13.9.1 Alternative Holiday Rituals 377
13.9.2 The First Christmas After a Death................. 378
13.9.3 The Holiday Tablecloth 378
13.10 Prayers and Remembrance.................................... 379
13.11 Inspirations from the World 379
13.11.1 Ngaben in Bali 380
13.11.2 Qingming Festival in China....................... 380
13.11.3 Tibetans at Anniversaries......................... 380
13.11.4 Obon Festival in Japan........................... 380
13.11.5 A Bowl for the Departed 381
13.12 Concluding Reflection 381
References.. 381

Epilogue 383

Index 385

About the Authors

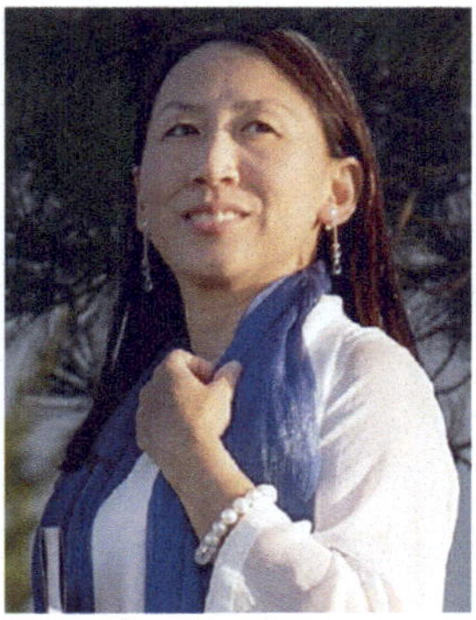

Yan Z. Ciupak, Ph.D., is an Associate Professor of Sociology at Northern Michigan University. She developed the university's first sociology and master of social work course on death, dying, and grief. She co-founded the Grief Support Specialist Certificate program, endorsed by the Association for Death Education and Counseling, the Department of Education, the National Association for Social Workers, and other professional associations. The U.S. National Center for Institutional Diversity (NCID) awarded her the title "Diversity Scholar" in recognition of her contribution to institutional diversity. Her extensive portfolio includes national and international publications, academic presentations, media appearances, and keynote speeches. She is known for her integrative and multicultural approach to death and grief education. In addition to her academic endeavors, Dr. Ciupak is a meditation teacher and certified yoga instructor. She advocates for mindfulness-based contemplative practices to foster a holistic and compassionate culture.

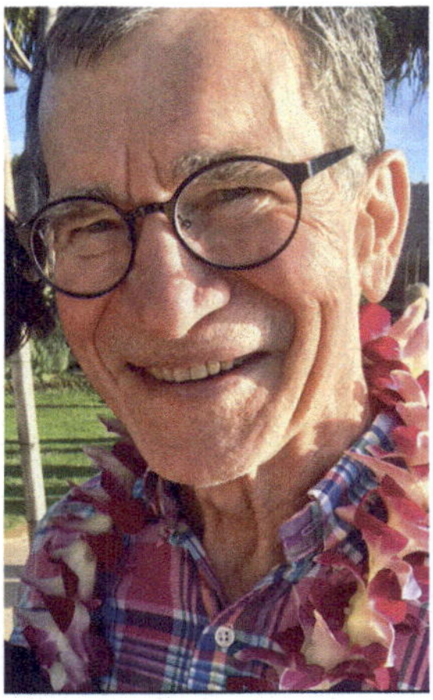

(Doug C. Smith, 1947–2024)

Douglas C. Smith had master's degrees in three different healthcare disciplines (M.Div., MA, MS), giving him a holistic approach to healthcare. He was a lead instructor at Northern Michigan University's Grief Support Specialist Certificate program. Before that, he was a dynamic trainer for social workers, psychotherapists, counselors, nurses, chaplains, physicians, and other healthcare professionals in meeting the various needs of dying and grieving, training, and workshops in all 50 states and all provinces in Canada. He authored eight books on those subjects and numerous articles. He is the author of *Caregiving: Hospice-Proven Techniques for Healing Body and Soul* (2004 Reprint by Wiley and 1997 by Macmillan) and *The Tao of Dying* (1994 by Caring Publications). In addition to working for several hospices in multiple capacities throughout his career, he also had much personal experience in grieving, having lost his parents, a brother, and two daughters to death.

List of Figures

Fig. 1.1 Spiral model of healing and grieving. Source: Ciupak (2025). Spiral Model of Grief and Healing (unpublished manuscript) 5
Fig. 2.1 Self and culture. Source: Based on Spiral Model of Grieving and Healing (Ciupak, 2025) 33
Fig. 4.1 Grieving styles 93
Fig. 6.1 4A4C 155

List of Tables

Table 1.1 Integrated frameworks for navigating grief and healing 6
Table 1.2 Formal vs. informal death and grief education 12
Table 3.1 Types of losses 55
Table 3.2 Types of grief 56
Table 3.3 Prolonged Grief Disorder (PGD) vs. common grief 72
Table 3.4 Comparison of PGD criteria by ICD-11 (2018) vs. DSM-5-TR (2022) 73
Table 4.1 Overview of Worden's tasks of mourning and support strategies 90
Table 4.2 Key activities of dual-process 91
Table 5.1 Dying trajectory and support 109
Table 5.2 Kübler-Ross's five-stage model for facing dying 110
Table 5.3 Comparison of curative care, palliative care, and hospice care 115
Table 5.4 Core philosophical concepts of hospice care 116
Table 5.5 Key organizational values for hospice providers 117
Table 5.6 National Association of Social Workers Standards for Palliative and End-of-Life Care 133
Table 6.1 Awareness, acceptance, affirmation, and actualization (4A) 160
Table 6.2 Compassion, connection, composure, and commitment (4C) 161
Table 8.1 SMART goal template 226

Part I
An Integrative Understanding of Death, Dying, and Grief

Chapter 1
Death and Grief Studies

1.1 Understanding Death, Dying, and Grief

An Integrated Sociological, Psychological, and Cultural Perspective
Death, dying, and grief are universal experiences deeply woven into private and public lives. Throughout history, communities have developed rich symbols, rituals, memorials, and other shared practices, honoring these profound experiences and strengthening communal bonds. However, the modern capitalist structure, driven by profit and efficiency alongside its individualistic ideology, has transformed these once collective events into privatized, institutionalized, and sometimes pathologized experiences. This shift has heightened death anxiety and isolated those who grieve.[1] Death has become constructed as a biological-medical event to be delayed or circumvented with technical interventions, and grief is often narrowly viewed as a "neuropsychological response to loss" (Bruce, 2007).

Grief is the *response to a loss, encompassing psychosocial, spiritual, and physical dimensions.*[2] *These micro-level aspects further reflect and interact with social, cultural, and historical dimensions.*

The profound ways social, political, and structural factors shape dying and grieving experiences are exemplified by the recent COVID-19 pandemic. During this period, ageism, ableism, xenophobia, gender gaps, regional disparities, and other local and global inequalities were exacerbated (Ramirez et al., 2022). Disruptions to normalcy and traditional mourning practices further isolated individuals from support networks, leading to a multifaceted collective experience of loss and grief (Kumar, 2023).

---

[1] Beck and Beck-Gernsheim's influential 2002 book discussed how individualization and privatization in modernity pushes communal events such as death and grief into a suppressed, private event, heightening anxiety and isolating people. Warraich (2017) critiqued the medicalization of death as a "technological phenomenon," emphasizing the need for a human-centered care.

[2] Refer to Chaps. 3 and 4 for more discussions about the various types and dimensions of grief.

Y. Z. Ciupak, D. C. Smith, *Death, Dying, and Grief*,
https://doi.org/10.1007/978-3-031-88467-2_1

Though deeply personal, death and grief are deeply influenced by societal systems and practices. Consider the following scenario:

> A 32-year-old mother was devastated when her partner died suddenly in an accident. Already juggling the demands of a low-wage job and caring for her children, she was now swept into a storm of grief and practical challenges. She found herself navigating legal hurdles, insurance claims, accident investigations, and funeral plans while trying to comfort her children. Without bereavement leave for hourly workers, any time off depended on her boss's goodwill. The exhaustion left her with no space to grieve for herself.

If the woman happens to be in a culture where public displays of mourning are expected, such as in certain parts of China, she might feel compelled to mourn visibly. Failure to do so may invite judgment and reduce much-needed social support. Conversely, in a Western setting, the pressure to quickly return to "normal" performance could push her to suppress her pain and act as though nothing had changed.

In both contexts, her grief experience is profoundly shaped by the interplay of gender, social class, legal systems, cultural practices, and social norms. Private experiences are inevitably influenced by and embody cultural and social structures. Drawing from the founding figure of sociology, Émile Durkheim, these "social facts"—patterns of thinking, feeling, and acting—influence individuals and shape their attitudes and actions through both tangible and intangible social influences. Death- and grief-related experiences are not limited to private emotions or family matters; they are woven into almost every domain of society: individual, communal, religious, economic, legal, and moral.

In today's culture, shaped by a capitalist economic framework, views on death and grief often lean toward "essentialist, individualistic." As Neimeyer et al. (2002) stated, *"This tendency to 'psychologize' grief is particularly evident in American culture, abetted by both genuine advances in psychological and medical research and an optimistic ethos that posits some form of counseling or psychotherapy as the appropriate response to a wide range of problems" (Neimeyer et al., 2002, p. 236).* Many scholars have advocated integrating sociological and cultural insights to enrich and expand the understanding of death, dying, and grief.

To address these needs, one of the authors recently proposed the "Spiral Model of Grieving and Healing" (Spiral Model), which integrates sociological, psychological, and cultural perspectives. The model presents grieving as a nonlinear, dynamic, and culturally embedded allostatic process aimed at healing and integration (Ciupak, 2025; see Fig. 1.1). Represented as a tornado-shaped spiral, the model depicts grief as an intertwined process of processing loss and restoring life and the self. The forces of grief and healing manifest in intrapersonal dimensions but interact with a complex web of social and cultural factors. These factors shape the grieving experience and either enable or hinder the journey toward healing. This process unfolds within a matrix of four interconnected dimensions:

(1) **Micro**: Biology, affect (pronounced *af-ekt*, meaning feelings or emotions), cognition, behavior, and spirituality.
(2) **Social identity and positioning**: Age, gender, sexual orientation, race/ethnicity, nationality/immigration status, socioeconomic class, ability, and marital status.

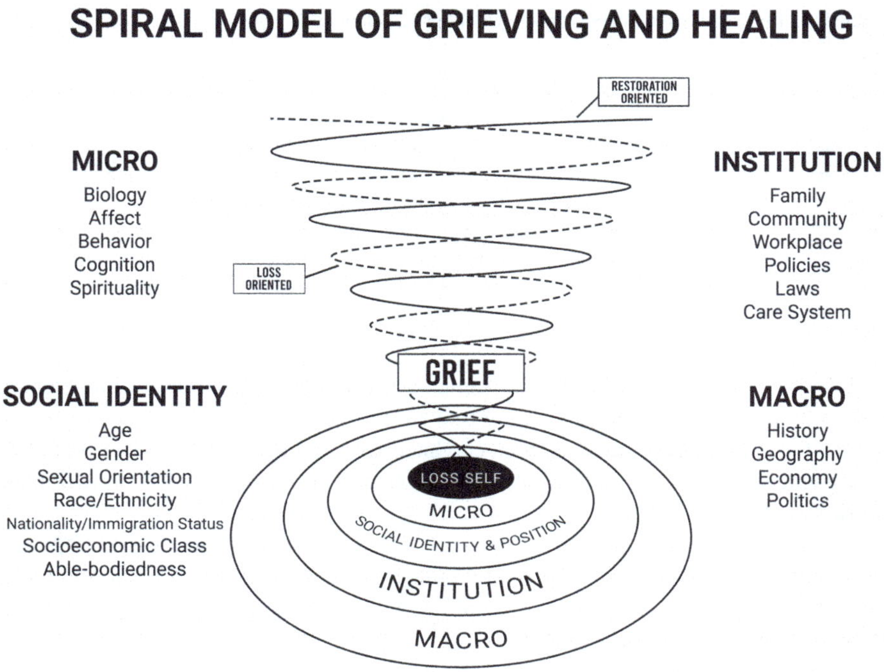

Fig. 1.1 Spiral model of healing and grieving. Source: Ciupak (2025). Spiral Model of Grief and Healing (unpublished manuscript)

(3) **Institutions and Systems**: Family, community, workplace, policies, law, and care systems (e.g., medical and end-of-life care).
(4) **Macro dimensions**: Historical, geographical, economic, and political contexts.

The Spiral Model promotes a balanced "middle-path" approach, moving beyond the passivity in phase-based models and overactive coping and intervention indicated by other models. This shift suggests four guiding principles for understanding grief, including anticipatory grief of those facing dying:

(1) Grief is nonlinear and dynamic, with diverse expressions.
(2) Grief holds the potential for growth and healing.
(3) Grief understanding and support should align with holistic and humanistic principles.
(4) Grief is embedded within sociocultural structures that shape lived experiences.

This book adopts this comprehensive conceptual framework, integrating sociological and psychological insights with a multicultural perspective. It encourages viewing death and grief not merely as biological events but as holistic human experiences, acknowledging the interconnected psychosocial and spiritual dimensions. Building on this foundation, the clinical application of the Spiral Model reflects a Holistic Psychosocial Care (HPC) approach to support grief and end-of-life transitions.

Table 1.1 Integrated frameworks for navigating grief and healing

Framework	Description
Spiral model of grieving and healing	A conceptual and theoretical model for understanding grieving and healing as a nonlinear, dynamic process embedded within multidimensional contexts, including micro, institutional, and macro levels
Holistic psychosocial care	A clinical application that honors the holistic dimensions of human experiences, addressing psychosocial and spiritual needs
4A4C	A competency model for professionals and a guiding tool for individuals, consisting of eight interconnected components: awareness, acceptance, affirmation, actualization (4A), and compassion, connection, composure, commitment (4C)

Complementing this, the 4A4C framework provides a structured competency model for professionals and a guiding tool for individuals. It comprises eight interconnected components: awareness, acceptance, affirmation, and actualization (4A), along with compassion, connection, composure, and commitment (4C). This framework is elaborated in Chap. 6.

Together, the Spiral conceptual framework, the Holistic Psychosocial application, and the 4A4C competency model create a cohesive roadmap for individuals and professionals to navigate the complexities of dying and grieving, fostering holistic healing and growth (Table 1.1).

This book is organized to guide readers through an integrative journey of understanding and applying end-of-life and grief support. Parts I and II establish the theoretical and conceptual foundations for understanding death, dying, and grief. Parts III, IV, and V focus on the practical application of Holistic Psychosocial Care (HPC), presenting principles, competencies, and tools—woven through theories and case studies—to address psychosocial and spiritual needs. These sections provide guidance for navigating the profound complexities of these human experiences with compassion and insight.

1.2 Why Study Death and Grief?

People who study death, dying, and grief are often asked, "Why are you so obsessed with such a depressing topic like death?" A concise response is, "Because it helps us live fully." As Kastenbaum (2004) famously stated, thanatology is "the study of life—with death left in" (p. 19). Life and death are commonly viewed as two separate events occurring at two ends, but when truly examined, living and dying are just two aspects of the same process. The end starts to evolve from the beginning. A swami once joked in a cemetery: since the tombstone shows one's birth year and death year with a dash in between, "Is life just a dash between the womb and tomb?"

Reflecting on death and grief often reveals profound insights into life and living. The title of Pema Chödrön's book *How We Live Is How We Die* (2022) succinctly captures the link between living and dying. Facing death with curiosity and openness transforms how we navigate uncertainty while living fully in the present. Recognizing life's finiteness inspires self-reflection, authenticity, and mindfulness, fostering compassion and connections. Examining death, dying, and grief enriches understanding and offers meaningful social, personal, and professional benefits.

1.2.1 Fostering Acceptance and Resilience

One of the essential benefits of discussing death and grief is that it fosters acceptance and resilience in the face of them. Death is an inevitable part of life, and avoiding the topic can hinder the ability to cope and increase anxiety. Research indicates that adults often avoid discussing death to protect children from painful emotions. However, this avoidance misses the opportunity of "teachable moments" (Havighurst, 1953) to facilitate understanding death and processing emotions. Studies have shown that discussing death in a sensitive and humanizing way helps even children move from denial to acceptance, aiding their grief process (Stylianou & Zembylas, 2018).

Effective communication about mortality and grief not only destigmatizes and demystifies these natural phenomena but also promotes healing. Normal grieving involves experiencing and expressing emotions such as anger and sadness, followed by reassessing and reorganizing one's narratives about the self and life. This process is crucial for personal growth and adaptation after loss. Open and honest communication about death and grief can facilitate this process and foster healthy awareness and coping strategies (Stylianou & Zembylas, 2018; Wong & Tomer, 2011). Validating and processing grief in a safe and supportive setting promotes awareness, adaptability, and dignity. Therefore, engaging in and promoting grief education fosters individual and collective resilience.

1.2.2 Psychological and Emotional Benefits

Education on grief enhances coping abilities and fosters a sense of coherence, which enables individuals to better understand, manage, and make sense of life, death, and critical situations. Death and grief education reminds us to keep the "both-and" mindset, celebrating humanity while acknowledging limitations. Embracing this duality helps individuals navigate life's uncertainties with greater resilience. Whether through academic curricula, professional development, or community outreach, death and grief education equips individuals and communities with the skills and perspectives needed to confront the seemingly unbearable and draw strength during difficult times (Testoni et al., 2019).

1.2.3 Cultivating Empathy and Awareness

Death and grief education fosters empathy and connection through shared vulnerability. Confronting mortality and loss offers insight into universal struggles, deepening compassion and understanding. Education raises awareness, reduces stigma, and promotes open communication about difficult topics. This awareness deepens appreciation for life's finite nature, promoting mindfulness and presence in relationships and nurturing more authentic, compassionate interactions (Testoni et al., 2019).

1.2.4 Improving Caregiving and Professional Competence

Education on death and grief provides professionals and caregivers the skills to support those facing life-threatening illness and loss. It enhances professionals' confidence and competence in navigating difficult conversations and facing their own existential issues. Therefore, it strengthens the ability to offer compassionate, informed care while mitigating the risk of burnout and compassion fatigue (Stamm, 2013).

To summarize, death and grief education equips individuals and societies with the knowledge and compassion to navigate life's inevitable experiences with resilience and resources. By addressing these topics directly, one may develop empathy and competency to support others and themselves during difficult times. Education reduces stigma and distress, fostering open dialogue, proactive preparation, and effective care (Baier et al., 2020; Ober et al., 2012).

1.3 Personal and Professional

Thanatology is the comprehensive study of death, dying, and bereavement, encompassing psychological, social, cultural, and spiritual practices and processes related to these experiences. This multidisciplinary field draws insights from psychology, sociology, anthropology, nursing, and many other disciplines (Corr, 2024).

According to the Association for Death Education and Counseling (ADEC), **thanatologists** are "cross-disciplinary specialists who practice within the scope of dying, death, loss and bereavement. Thanatologists include front-line care providers, clinicians, practitioners, educators, researchers, administrators, and others emerging from a wide variety of educational backgrounds, professions, and occupations" (ADEC, n.d.).

The journey into the field of thanatology often emerges from a blend of personal and professional experiences, united by a shared drive to alleviate suffering. For one author, the journey began with multiple personal losses, finding healing and purpose in helping others as a "wounded healer." The other author's path grew from a lifetime commitment to addressing social problems, realizing that societal problems cannot be resolved without addressing *human* struggles. As long as a strong sense of a separated self persists, the practice of "othering" and discrimination will remain difficult to eradicate. As long as society continues to neglect individual and collective grief[3], the social justice ideal will remain elusive. These cycles of harm, left unaddressed, will perpetuate suffering at both individual and societal levels.

Breaking this cycle requires reflecting on shared humanity and creating spaces for growth and connection. Death and grief education plays pivotal roles in driving this social change. Beyond imparting knowledge, it deepens appreciation for life and fosters connection. It encourages society to examine its narratives around death and grief, embracing the full range of human experiences with greater understanding. Structured exploration of these topics invites meaningful dialog and nurtures a compassionate and resilient culture.

Professionals are also drawn to this field because of the compassionate and supportive culture it fosters. Dr. Robert A. Neimeyer, renowned grief expert and director of the Portland Institute for Loss and Transition, remarked, "Humility comes as we realize, as a species, our lives are short and history-bound. In our field, we pour our own small cup of inspiration into the common sea of practices in which we all swim" (Neimeyer, email correspondence, March 2024).

The social and cultural context shapes individual attitudes and beliefs, influencing how people interact with others. These experiences—whether joyful or painful, personal or professional—continually shape attitudes and perceptions. When engaging with the material in this book, readers are invited to reflect on their own perceptions and experiences: How do these help deepen the understanding and strengthen the ability to support oneself and others?

1.3.1 Therapeutic Alliance and the Self as an Instrument

People often come to death and grief studies for two primary reasons: personal growth and/or professional development. Some seek to understand their own grief experiences, whereas others want to be prepared to support others when the time comes. Many, including nurses, educators, counselors, and social workers, strive to enhance their competency in supporting the ability to support others during challenging times. They soon discovered that in human services, especially end-of-life and grief support, the personal and professional are deeply interconnected and mutually reinforcing.

[3] *Collective loss and grief* refer to entire communities, social groups, or societies experiencing loss and grief simultaneously. This can result from systemic injustices-structural forms of inequality embedded in institutions and social norms-such as racism, sexism, ageism, and events such as mass shootings, natural disasters, or war, which can produce feelings of powerlessness and hopelessness. Such grief transcends individual relationships, reflecting shared responses to communal, national, or global challenges. For a detailed discussion, refer to Chap. 3.

As educators, practitioners, and caregivers, individuals support and inspire others, facilitating self-exploration, growth, and healing. End-of-life and grief support fundamentally require *using the self as an instrument* to guide and accompany others through dying or grieving. The connection between personal and professional roles, along with the importance of a strong therapeutic alliance, is well-recognized in human service professions (Chan & Tin, 2012). This relational aspect is vital, as the strength of the therapeutic alliance often determines the effectiveness of care and support.

1.3.1.1 Therapeutic Alliance

Empirical research consistently highlights the pivotal role of therapeutic alliance in outcomes (Flückiger et al., 2018). It functions as an active therapy component, independent of specific techniques, and serves as a universal mediator of positive change across psychotherapeutic approaches (Baier et al., 2020).

Three elements are essential to building strong therapeutic relationships: empathy, unconditional positive regard, and congruence (Rogers, 1995). This person-centered approach creates a safe, supportive environment that fosters personal growth and self-discovery.

In end-of-life care, a strong therapeutic alliance is consistently linked to improved quality of life for patients with advanced cancer (Thomas et al., 2021). In grief counseling, experts highlight that while techniques such as eye movement desensitization and reprocessing (EMDR), journaling, and guided visualization are valuable, "nonspecific, relational, and contextual aspects" are often more crucial (Jordan & Neimeyer, 2003, p. 780). Effective bereavement support relies on compassionate, empathically attuned caregivers who provide mourners with the healing experience of being understood and supported (Harris & Winokuer, 2021).

To form a strong therapeutic alliance for those who are dying or grieving, Alan Wolfelt (2003) advocates for "companioning," focusing on presence and support rather than directing or "fixing." This is echoed in the renowned doctor Elisabeth Kübler-Ross's account: simply "sitting with" patients, listening to them, and hearing them (Kübler-Ross, 1983).

1.3.1.2 Self as an Instrument

Forming and facilitating a "therapeutic alliance" requires professionals to willingly and skillfully use *the self as an instrument*. This approach highlights the connection between the "professional" and "personal" in the following key areas:

1. **Personal integration**: Humans inevitably bring who they are into their work. Experiences with death, loss, and grief shape how professionals perceive and approach death and grief. Many educators teaching grief content reported they were motivated by their own losses (Wheat et al., 2022). Attitudes toward death

and coping mechanisms inform how they model behaviors and support those they serve. Self-reflection, addressing unresolved grief, and developing effective coping mechanisms are as important as acquiring technical knowledge. For that reason, many experts advocate for experiential learning and contemplative pedagogy to prepare professionals for effective end-of-life and grief support (Hill et al., 2018; Horn et al., 2013).

2. **Cultural sensitivity and humility**: Death and grief are deeply embedded in and impacted by cultural factors. This requires self-reflection and awareness of how one's experiences and perspectives may affect service. Being culturally sensitive involves understanding and respecting the diverse ways people experience and express grief, which enhances the support provided. Cultural humility recognizes the need for ongoing self-evaluation and learning, acknowledging that we do not have all the answers and must remain open to understanding and respecting cultural differences. Refer to Chap. 2 for detailed discussions.
3. **Self-competence as death competence:** Gamino and Ritter (2012) introduced the term "death competence" to describe the specialized skill of tolerating and managing clients' issues related to dying, death, and bereavement. This competence is crucial for helping professionals effectively support individuals while navigating the profound emotional and existential impacts of their work. Chan and Tin (2012) expanded this idea with "self-competence in death work," which involves necessary personal resources and the ability to cope with the emotions and existential issues arising from professional work. Developing self-competence not only benefits clients but also strengthens professionals' death competence. On the other hand, professional growth in death competence also fosters personal growth and resilience.
4. **Genuine relationship**: Human service professionals' relationships with those they are serving are often "genuine and reciprocal," meaning that the emotions and stories of both parties impact each other. Maintaining empathy while maintaining ethical, personal, and emotional boundaries is essential for a healthy therapeutic relationship (Harris & Winokuer, 2021).
5. **Mutual growth and compassion satisfaction**: While clients' needs are central, the therapeutic relationship offers mutual benefits. As professionals help clients harness their strengths and resources, they also learn from these experiences, fostering personal and professional growth. Engaging with clients from diverse cultures and perspectives enriches understanding and practice. Compassion satisfaction, defined by Stamm (2013) as the pleasure derived from helping others, builds resilience and a sense of fulfillment. Vicarious posttraumatic growth may also occur, where exposure to clients' transformative journeys promotes personal growth and a deeper sense of compassion and professional effectiveness (Ogińska-Bulik & Juczyński, 2024). This shared development exemplifies reciprocal growth.

In summary, personal and professional connections thrive on compassionate, congruent intrapersonal and interpersonal relationships. Although challenging, this approach is profoundly fulfilling and rewarding. Using the self as an instrument enables professionals to deliver person-centered, sustainable care while fostering personal and professional growth, reflecting the interconnectedness of humanity.

1.4 Forms of Death and Grief Education

Death and grief are universal, yet how they are learned and understood varies greatly. Views on these topics significantly influence how individuals cope with these experiences and support others. The need for structured, comprehensive death education has become increasingly evident as studies across various disciplines highlight gaps in preparedness and competency.[4] Like other educational fields, death education may occur in two primary formats: formal and informal.

Formal death and grief education occurs in structured settings such as schools, professional training programs, volunteer initiatives, and community workshops. These programs aim to deliver systematic knowledge on death, dying, and grief by integrating theories, research, and practical skills. While most formal education focuses on bereavement, most conceptual and practical approaches can also be applied to nonfinite losses, such as the end of relationships or loss of employment.

In contrast, most people first encounter ***death education informally,*** often through socialization, such as the parent's explanation about the loss of a pet or the death of a relative. Informal education typically arises through *teachable moments*—unanticipated life events that offer opportunities for learning and personal growth (Havighurst, 1953). These early experiences, deeply embedded in cultural contexts, shape initial attitudes and coping with death and grief. In addition to family socialization, informal death and grief education is influenced by other agents, including media, peers, and religious institutions. This type of education often reinforces cultural myths and norms surrounding death, grieving, and coping.

Table 1.2 provides a comparative overview of formal and informal death and grief education across key aspects.

Table 1.2 Formal vs. informal death and grief education

Aspect	Formal education	Informal education
Setting	Schools, professional training, community workshops	Family experiences, personal life events, media, peers, religion
Format	Planned, organized, structured, with learning objectives	Spontaneous and situational "teachable moments"
Content	Theoretical perspectives, empirical research, practical skills, competencies	Cultural and life-experience-based
Common myths	Minimize myths by emphasizing evidence-based understanding	Reinforces cultural myths and norms about death and grieving

[4] Refer to Sect. 2.5: Need for Integrative Training

1.5 Need for Integrative Training

Over the past few decades, there has been a widespread call across fields to enhance professional training and competency on death and grief. This includes nurses, college counselors, psychological therapists, and more (Hsiao et al., 2023; Jankauskaite et al., 2021; Ober et al., 2012). Many stress the importance of incorporating death and grief education into academic curricula and ongoing professional development. Research on training and preparedness for grief support among helping professionals highlights the following key findings and recommendations:

Curriculum gaps and educational strategies: Research emphasizes the importance of death and grief education due to its pervasive role in the human experience and the inevitability that counselors, nurses, and other professionals will work with persons facing these issues. However, many programs do not require grief coursework, leading to inadequate preparedness to provide support. For example, many counselors lack updated knowledge related to grief and apply only certain outdated models. The lack of adequate training affects their confidence and competency in delivering effective care. Moreover, repeated exposure to death and suffering can lead to emotional and existential challenges (Blueford et al., 2022; Horn et al., 2013; Ober et al., 2012).

To address these needs, there is a widespread call to incorporate grief content into counseling programs accredited by the Council for Accreditation of Counseling and Related Educational Programs (CACREP) (Wheat et al., 2022). Research indicates that training in nursing improves competence, increasing nurses' confidence and willingness to provide anticipatory grief counseling to family caregivers of terminal cancer patients (Hsiao et al., 2023). Furthermore, recommended strategies include experiential exercises and reflective assignments to enhance training (Horn et al., 2013; Hill et al., 2018).

Personal dynamics and self-awareness: Professionals' personal experiences with loss and their views on death strongly influence their preparedness and effectiveness. Self-awareness and the ability to process personal grief are crucial for effective counseling (Blueford et al., 2022; Horn et al., 2013; Ober et al., 2012).

Cultural sensitivity and competence: Understanding the cultural dimensions of death and grief is crucial for providing person-centered support. Integrating cultural competence into grief education prepares professionals to work with diverse populations (Horn et al., 2013; Hill et al., 2018).

Ongoing professional development: Continued learning and professional development are necessary to enhance competence and confidence. This includes pursuing certifications and memberships in grief-related organizations (Jankauskaite et al., 2021; Wheat et al., 2022; Ober et al., 2012).

Experiential learning and contemplative pedagogy: Many studies show that experiential learning, contemplative pedagogy, and reflective assignments enrich training and deepen learning in death and grief education (Horn et al., 2013; Hill et al., 2018).

To summarize, comprehensive education on death and grief prepares professionals to offer effective end-of-life and grief support. Given the dual nature of the human services profession, training should incorporate both professional and personal development. Effective programs should encourage professionals to examine their attitudes, beliefs, and experiences related to death and grief while providing a solid conceptual understanding and practical tools to enhance holistic well-being. This approach helps professionals incorporate "self-competence" and "death competence" into their practice.

In academic curricula, professional development, or community education programs, promoting self-reflection and fostering cultural humility is crucial to enable compassionate, culturally sensitive support.

1.6 Death Attitudes and Encounters

Death, loss, and grief are natural, transitional processes in life. Everyone will eventually face death, whether that of family members, loved ones, or themselves. How individuals experience death and grief is influenced by their attitudes and encounters with death. These attitudes are shaped by socialization and personal experiences, which in turn affect the strategies and skills used during challenging times. Therefore, each experience of death and grief is both universal and uniquely personal.

1.6.1 Death Attitudes

Death attitudes refer to the set of beliefs, feelings, and behavioral tendencies toward death, dying, and the deceased. These attitudes are shaped through socialization and influenced by various factors, such as social class, ethnicity, gender, religion, and media. For instance, gender norms and roles can affect how men and women perceive and react to death and grief, with social expectations varying significantly across cultures.

Cultural and individual attitudes toward death vary greatly, but could be roughly categorized into two perspectives (Feifel, 1977):

- **A Door**: Death is viewed as a transition, a passage from one life form to another.
- **A Wall**: Death is viewed as the absolute end, marking the cessation of life and experience.

Death attitudes influence whether death is seen as positive or negative, subsequently shaping personal experiences. One extensively studied death attitude is *death anxiety*. In *The Denial of Death* (1973), Ernest Becker argued that the fear of death is a fundamental motivator of human behavior, driving the creation of "immortality projects"—efforts to achieve symbolic or literal permanence beyond physical life.

Immortality projects manifest on both individual and collective levels. Individually, artistic, scientific, and creative endeavors—such as painting, writing, or invention—enable people to achieve symbolic immortality, leaving a legacy that outlasts their physical existence. Similarly, raising children provides a way to pass on values, beliefs, and lineage, ensuring a sense of continuity across generations.

On a collective level, religious practices and shared cultural beliefs offer spiritual continuity and a sense of eternal belonging. Actions like promoting national pride or defending communal values also contribute to collective legacies, providing a buffer against death anxiety.

While Becker highlights the motivational power of these projects, he also notes their potential downsides. The quest for legacy can fuel competitiveness, where others are seen as rivals rather than allies. This can lead to ethical compromises and strained relationships. Excessive focus on symbolic immortality risks disconnecting individuals from authentic living, aligning life around societal approval and accomplishments. The psychological burden of pursuing immortality projects can lead to burnout and intensify existential fears.

At a societal level, nationalistic or religious pursuits can justify harmful actions and create conflicts, such as exclusion or warfare, in the name of protecting collective legacies.

Becker's work reveals a profound paradox: the denial of mortality fuels both inspiring achievements and detrimental behaviors. This urges balancing the pursuit of meaningful legacies with an acceptance of life's impermanence.

Death attitudes are dynamic, evolving through personal experiences, cultural context, and psychosocial development. While some may approach death with fear or denial, others find ways to embrace it as a natural part of life. One approach to understanding this is through **meaning management theory (MMT),** which emphasizes the importance of constructing meaning in life and death (Wong, 2007). Unlike terror management theory (TMT), which focuses on defensive reactions to death fear (Greenberg et al., 1986), MMT encourages individuals to reflect upon mortality without succumbing to fear or denial. Meaning management approach can be particularly empowering for terminal-illness patients during their final stage of life (Thibault, 2002).

In summary, while death is an inevitable part of life, views toward it impact death experience and quality of life. Meaning-seeking and meaning reconstruction can transform death anxiety from a source of fear into a catalyst for self-actualization and fulfillment. This approach aligns with the broader goals of death studies: enabling individuals and society to face mortality with peace and purpose and fostering a deeper appreciation of life quality and fullness.

1.6.2 Death Encounters

Death encounters refer to the ways individuals experience and interact with death, measured through metrics such as death rates, life expectancy, causes of death, death trajectories, and places of death. In the United States, these encounters have shifted significantly over the past century. In the early 1900s, death typically occurred at home, allowing family members to be closely involved.

Modernization has significantly shifted the experience of death, moving it to institutional settings managed by medical professionals. This transition has transformed death into a clinical process, often reducing families to the role of observers. These changes prompted a growing movement in recent years to return the persons to their families in the familiar home environment, supported by hospice and outpatient services.

The causes and trajectory of death (Lunney et al., 2003) greatly affect the experiences of death and grief.[5] Sudden and traumatic deaths, such as accidents or suicides, often leave unresolved issues, disrupt stability, and challenge deeply held beliefs about the world and self. Terminal illnesses can bring anticipatory grief, compounded by financial and psychological burdens. Organ failure, marked by gradual decline and sudden acute episodes, fosters uncertainty and disrupts daily routines. Frailty, often linked to advanced age or dementia, involves a gradual loss of independence that can be emotionally and physically taxing for everyone involved. Ambiguous loss may arise as family and friends grapple with the psychological absence of a physically present loved one.

1.6.3 Impact of Death Attitudes

Death attitudes are not static; they evolve with personal experiences, life stages, and reflections (Tomoi, 2024). It may also fluctuate depending on social-psychological situations. For example, an elderly patient who once prioritized their health may shift their focus to burdening their family with high end-of-life care costs. On the other hand, a person with spiritual maturity may find their death anxiety decreasing, finding comfort in beliefs about the afterlife or the natural cycle of life and death. Death attitudes can adapt to each loss, allowing for varied reactions and coping responses.

While loss and grief are unavoidable parts of life, attitudes toward them affect people's experiences, hindering or facilitating healing and growth. Making peace with death and loss is a challenging journey that is unique for each experience. Allowing time, patience, support, and self-compassion is essential. Practicing compassion and understanding the complexities of grief not only helps individuals navigate their experiences but also empowers them to support others in meaningful ways (Cacciatore et al., 2021). Acknowledging the struggle as a natural part of healing fosters such a process.

---

[5] For a more comprehensive exploration of death trajectories and end-of-life care, see Chap. 5.

1.7 The Death Awareness Movement

Reflections on death and grief have been integral to human civilization for thousands of years, expressed through philosophy, art, music, literature, and more. In contemporary times, the aim to study these experiences scientifically has resulted in the development of death studies, a multidisciplinary field encompassing psychology, sociology, anthropology, nursing, and more (Corr, 2024). The emergence of death and grief as a field of academic study is a significant milestone of the modern death awareness movement, which gained momentum in the second half of the twentieth century.

1.7.1 Modern Death Awareness Movement

The term **death awareness movement** refers to a loosely defined but interrelated network of individuals, organizations, and groups advocating for including death and dying as part of relevant discussions of life and living (Doka, 2003). This movement emerged in response to the social environment of mid-twentieth-century Western societies, where death was often seen as a "taboo topic" and considered unsuitable for academic endeavors or public discussion. The movement aimed to bring death out of the shadows and promote open discussions about mortality, thereby transforming societal attitudes and policies surrounding death.

The movement was shaped by various historical and social factors during the mid-twentieth century. Demographic shifts increased interest in studying aging and dying, while historical events such as the advent of the nuclear age, environmental crises, and the emergence of diseases like AIDS heightened societal awareness of mortality. Sociological trends of the 1960s in the United States, which emphasized freedom, rights, and dignity, further influenced the movement. Moreover, secularization reduced the influence of traditional religious narratives, calling for more open and meaningful discussions about death (Doka, 2003).

This movement includes a diverse range of pioneering scholars and practitioners, advocates, and community networks. This led to new types of research, educational programs, and the establishment of hospice care for dying and support groups for bereaved individuals. The movement also led to the development of *thanatology*, viewed as "the study of life with death left in" (Kastenbaum, 2004). Elisabeth Kübler-Ross's work helped extend discussions from academia to healthcare practices. Accompanying academic and clinical endeavors are many grassroots efforts.

1.7.2 Early Influences and Pioneers

The Modern Death Awareness Movement has diverse origins.

Émile Durkheim, the founding father of sociology, produced pioneering work with *Suicide* (1897), which explored differing suicide rates among Protestants and

Catholics, finding that stronger social control among Catholics resulted in lower suicide rates. This work became a groundbreaking contribution to sociology and a scientific case study on death.

Sigmund Freud's influential essay, *Mourning and Melancholia* (1917/1953), was viewed as the first modern work to treat grief as a subject that could be explored in academic studies and clinical practice. Freud's psychotherapy approach inspired further academic and clinical exploration into the realm of grief. Subsequent publications built upon Freud's initial work, each contributing to the development of the movement.

The first empirical study was conducted by Erich Lindemann on the mourners of the Cocoanut Grove fire in Boston (1944). Lindemann collected data on survivors of those killed in war or the Coconut Grove fire. His work identified acute grief as a syndrome with clear symptomatology and identified various ways grief can manifest physically, mentally, and spiritually, including delayed, exaggerated, or absent grief responses. Lindermann argued that maladaptations can be transformed into normal grief.

Death attitudes and anxiety are central subjects in the field of thanatology. Geoffrey Gorer's analysis (1955) of modern society's tendency to ignore or deny death laid the groundwork for exploring how attitudes toward death are shaped and formed, laying the foundation for rich studies on this topic.

These early works laid the foundation for academic studies of death, dying, and bereavement. The second half of the twentieth century witnessed extensive development and popularization of death studies. A number of influential works have been published across various fields, from psychology, sociology, and philosophy to medicine, nursing, pastoral care, funeral service, and theology. This firmly established the multidisciplinary nature of death studies (Doka, 2003).

Elisabeth Kübler-Ross, a Swiss-American psychiatrist, extended the studies of death beyond academic boundaries into healthcare and the public sphere. Her stage theory of grief became popularly known, but more importantly, she emphasized a humanistic approach to end-of-life care, advocating for dignity and opportunities for personal growth even at life's end—a message that remains deeply relevant today. In her view, the primary concern should not be dying but living (Kübler-Ross, 1983). The key to caring for the dying is to recognize that they are living persons with their own wishes, emotions, and dignity despite the limitations imposed by impending death. Her stage theory and clinical legacy sparked significant academic debate and led to the growth of hospices and other forms of end-of-life care.

The modern hospice movement was founded by Cicely Saunders in the 1960s and focused on providing multidisciplinary care to terminally ill patients. Her holistic approach addressed not only physical needs but also emotional and spiritual well-being, ensuring a dignified and comfortable end-of-life experience. Saunders established St. Christopher's Hospice in London in 1967, which became the model for hospice care worldwide. Her work highlighted the importance of pain management and the integration of psychological and spiritual support for patients and their families. In 1978, the US Department of Health, Education, and Welfare recognized that "the hospice movement as a concept for the care of the terminally ill and their families is a viable concept and one which holds out a means of providing more humane care for Americans dying of terminal illness while possibly reducing costs. As such, it is the proper subject of federal support" (U.S. Department of Health, Education, and Welfare, 1978). Since the 1980s, hospice and palliative care have been more widely adopted in the United States.

1.7.3 Organizations, Journals, and Formal Education

The establishment of death studies as an academic discipline in the second half of the twentieth century was marked by the creation of professional organizations, journals, and educational programs.

In 1976, the Association for Death Education and Counseling (ADEC) emerged from the Forum for Death Education and became a premium broad-based professional association. Its members include a wide array of psychologists, counselors, social workers, educators, researchers, hospice personnel, clergy, and volunteers (ADEC, n.d.). Together with the International Work Group on Death, Dying, and Bereavement established in the 1970s, these professional organizations provided platforms for scholars and practitioners to collaborate and advance the field.

Journals dedicated to thanotology began to emerge over time. *Omega: Journal of Death and Dying*, which started as a newsletter, transitioned into a formal journal by 1970. *Death Education*, later renamed *Death Studies*, was founded in 1977. These specialized platforms provide central venues for scholarly discussions and the dissemination of research on the subject. Academic courses on death and dying were first offered in US colleges and universities in the late 1960s. These courses laid the groundwork for formal educational programs, including majors, certificates, and master's degrees in grief counseling. Despite advancements, death-related courses remain vulnerable and often rely on the efforts of individual professors rather than institutional support (Doka, 2003). As a result, incorporating death and grief topics into formal or professional training remains inconsistent. Over the years, there has been an increasing call for the inclusion of grief content in many professional trainings, such as accredited counselor education programs and nursing curricula, as discussed in Sect. 1.5.

1.8 Diversity and Autonomy: Contemporary Development

The death awareness movement, including death and grief studies, has entered the twenty-first century with renewed momentum, driven by both individual and collective efforts alongside significant social and historical events. A central theme of diversity and autonomy has emerged, highlighting respect for individual choices and the diverse needs of people from various social and cultural backgrounds. This shift is accompanied by initiatives for a more open, positive approach to death

(Incorvaia, 2024) and a more equitable, person-centered framework for addressing death, dying, and grief. The themes of diversity and autonomy in the contemporary era are evident across a broad spectrum of areas, including general attitudes, clinical practices, scholarship, and policy advocacy. These developments include promoting cultural diversity and sensitivity, expanding the understanding of grief beyond bereavement, advocating for greater autonomy in end-of-life decision-making, fostering community engagement and policy development, incorporating diverse therapeutic perspectives and techniques, and examining the complexities of death and grief in the digital age.

(1) **Cultural Diversity and Sensitivity**

There is increased recognition that death, dying, and grief experiences vary significantly among different groups—including social class, race, gender, sexual orientation, religious orientation, national origins, and their intersections. Social movements such as "MeToo" and "Black Lives Matter" have highlighted the varied lived realities and priorities related to death and grief encounters among different groups. These movements have heightened public awareness of the collective grief and trauma arising from systemic injustice. There is a general call for improvement at both the policy and institutional levels, alongside cultural sensitivity in care delivery, all of which are essential for just, equitable, and person-centered care.

In academia, scholarship is expanding beyond the traditional focus on American Caucasian widowed women, who constitute the major research population of most classical grief models. There has been a shift toward incorporating multiple perspectives, moving beyond a Euro-American lens to include non-Anglo-Saxon viewpoints and experiences. These diverse scholarships and perspectives pave important conceptual and research foundations for culturally responsive care. Cultural themes are elaborated in Chap. 2.

(2) **Diverse Forms of Grief**

Contemporary society faces various individual and collective losses, traumas, and grief, prompting an expansion of studies and support for nonfinite losses. This includes but is not limited to unemployment, the ending of relationships, collective grief resulting from racism and sexism, traumatic losses due to suicide and mass shootings, and ecological grief.

One developing area of research is ecological grief. Comtesse et al. (2021) described ecological grief as a response to environmental disasters and changes, demonstrating typical grief-like psychological reactions. This type of grief can lead to mental health issues or increased environmental activism. Related concepts include *solastalgia* (Albrecht et al., 2007), a form of emotional or existential distress that occurs when individuals face ecological damage to environments to which they are connected, and eco-anxiety, which is the response to anticipated future ecological loss. These ecological losses have a wide impact but particularly affect communities that rely on the environment for social, spiritual, and recreational activities. The diverse forms of loss and grief are discussed in Chap. 4.

(3) **Diversity and Agency in End-of-Life Decisions and Arrangements**

The quest for autonomy and dignity at the end of life has gained significant momentum, reflecting an effort to exert individual agency and control in what Beck (1992) terms the postmodern "risky society" and institutionalization of death. This includes the rise of end-of-life doulas providing nonmedical companionship, the expansion of medical aid in dying policies in the United States and globally, and the practice of voluntarily stopping eating and drinking as a viable end-of-life option. Additionally, interest in environmentally friendly burial options, such as water cremation (alkaline hydrolysis) and human composting (natural organic reduction), is increasing. Chapter 5 addresses key issues in end-of-life decisions and ethical considerations.

(4) **Diverse Forms of Community Involvement**

Grassroots movements and community-based initiatives have played a pivotal role in the death and grief awareness movement since its onset. Early efforts included self-help networks and support groups for individuals coping with terminal illness or bereavement. These formats have continued to evolve, growing in diversity and accessibility to address a broader range of needs.

Community education and engagement programs, such as death cafés and death-over-inner events, aim to increase awareness of death and help people make the most of their finite lives. Death cafés were initiated by Swiss sociologists and anthropologist Bernard Crettaz in 2004. These informal gatherings allow people to discuss death over refreshments, providing accessible and respectful spaces for open conversations about the "taboo" topic. Since spreading to London in 2011 and the United States in 2012, the movement has grown significantly. By July 2024, two decades after its first event, there have been over 14,000 Death Café gatherings in 84 countries (Death Café, 2024).

Organizations like Death with Dignity and Compassion & Choices advocate for end-of-life autonomy and options, including medical aid in dying. Recently, nonprofit activist groups have focused on creating equitable bereavement care systems and policies. One example is advocating for federal bereavement leave legislation in the United States, reflecting a growing recognition of grief as a societal issue that requires systemic solutions.

(5) **Diverse and Expanded Modalities and Techniques**

In response to the complex and evolving landscape of grief, various innovative modalities and techniques have emerged. The ongoing struggle to balance efforts to normalize grief and attempts to intervene in maladaptation persists. This is exemplified by the debate around the inclusion of "prolonged grief disorder" in the latest *Diagnostic and Statistical Manual of Mental Disorders*, 5th Edition (DSM-5).

Validating the normality of grief while identifying cases that need intervention provides fertile ground for counseling and intervention techniques. A variety of counseling and therapy techniques have been developed to focus specifically on grief. Equipment-based psychotherapy methods have been developing fast. AI-driven virtual reality simulations are increasingly used for both mental health and severe illness. Interactive or holistic therapies integrating Eastern spiritual practices, such as mindfulness, embodiment exercises, and guided imagery, are also gaining popularity.[6]

The digital age further broadened support and care-delivery options, providing new avenues such as Internet support groups and teletherapy, making it easier for individuals to access the help they need from anywhere in the world. The next section delves into the nuances of death and grief in the digital age.

1.9 Death and Grief in Digital Age

Technology has long influenced cultural norms and practices surrounding death, dying, and grief. In the nineteenth and twentieth centuries, industrialization and medical advancements shifted death from a personal, family-centered event to a clinical, hospital-managed experience. The rise of mass media expanded communal grief by publicizing obituaries and death-related news, which had previously been limited to private circles (Beaunoyer & Guitton, 2021).

In today's world, digital technology permeates nearly all aspects of life, including death and grief. The Internet and social media offer new ways to connect, allowing people to engage in mourning rituals across geographical boundaries. Online memorials, forums, and social media platforms have become spaces for sharing experiences, finding comfort, and building supportive communities. These digital spaces, along with teletherapies, provide essential support when traditional resources are unavailable.

The effectiveness of Internet-based interventions (IMIs) has been supported by studies indicating their potential as beneficial tools for addressing grief, depression, and posttraumatic stress following bereavement (Zuelke et al., 2021). IMIs offer advantages such as accessibility, flexibility, and privacy, making them particularly useful for individuals who may face barriers to face-to-face therapy or fear stigmatization.

However, these platforms also present challenges that need careful consideration. Overreliance on digital support can lead to superficial interactions that may not fully meet mourners' deeper emotional needs. Moreover, while IMIs can be effective, most existing studies have focused on guided interventions, emphasizing the importance of structured support to optimize outcomes (Zuelke et al., 2021).

The permanence of online memorials can also remind individuals of their loss, potentially prolonging grief. Privacy concerns and algorithm-generated reminders can disrupt the healing process, adding complexity to digital grief experiences.

---

[6] For example, see Benton and Yarbrow (2024) for a thorough exploration of the use of virtual reality in health care for symptom and pain management, anxiety control, helping patients find meaning especially near end of life.

1.9.1 Benefits of Digital Support

Digital platforms transcend barriers of time and geography, offering diverse spaces and formats for support (Beaunoyer & Guitton, 2021). They have revolutionized memory preservation and the ongoing relationship with the deceased. Social media platforms like Facebook and Instagram enable users to share tributes, photos, and memories, fostering connection and extending emotional support. Virtual grief communities such as Grieving.com and Grief in Common provide resources and peer support, while forums like Reddit and Discord create spaces for shared learning and connection.

These digital spaces nurture a sense of community, building resilience and offering comfort through shared stories and emotional expressions. Online memorials and tributes also give new meaning to the "continuing bonds" theory, helping individuals maintain ongoing connections with the deceased (Bell et al., 2015).

Instant connectivity has transformed how support is sought, making resources accessible 24/7 and overcoming geographical barrier. During the COVID-19 pandemic, when traditional mourning practices were restricted, online spaces, live streams of funerals, and more played an important role (Beaunoyer & Guitton, 2021). The global reach of digital support groups has further enriched perspectives, enabling individuals to find solace across cultural and social boundaries (Moore et al., 2019; Selman et al., 2022).

1.9.2 Challenges of Digital Grief

Despite their benefits, digital platforms present unique challenges. One significant drawback is the lack of physical presence essential for human healing. Hugs, affection, and being physically near loved ones convey empathy and understanding in ways that virtual connections cannot fully replicate (Cacciatore et al., 2021). The absence of tangible support and nonverbal cues can heighten feelings of isolation, making it harder for mourners to feel genuinely understood and connected.

Overreliance on digital connections can create a false sense of companionship. Virtual interactions often lack the richness of nonverbal communication and shared physical space, leading to relationships that may feel superficial. This superficiality can hinder mourners from fully expressing their emotions and engaging in the deep processing needed for healing. Additionally, digital inequalities, highlighted during the COVID-19 pandemic, have shown that disadvantaged populations often struggle with limited access to reliable digital connections. This disparity exacerbates feelings of isolation and highlights the unequal availability of digital grief support (Beaunoyer & Guitton, 2021).

The permanence of online memorials and tribute presents another challenge. While these platforms provide spaces for remembrance, they can also continuously remind individuals of their loss, potentially prolonging grief. The enduring nature of digital identities creates a "digital legacy" that can be both comforting and disruptive. Persistent online traces can complicate the grieving process by maintaining the deceased's presence in unexpected ways, contributing to a complex emotional experience for those left behind (Beaunoyer & Guitton, 2021). Privacy concerns add further complexity, as algorithm-generated reminders or targeted content can unexpectedly evoke memories, disrupting the healing process.

Another emerging concern is behaviors such as "grief hyper jacking," where collective grief is exploited for personal or social gain on public platforms. This behavior can dilute the sincerity of digital mourning and erode the authenticity of supportive spaces (Abidin, 2022). Additionally, some digital memorials attract "RIP trolling," a phenomenon where negative or disruptive behaviors target online spaces meant for grief, undermining the supportive nature of these communities (Beaunoyer & Guitton, 2021).

In summary, while digital platforms provide valuable avenues for connection and support, they have limitations. The absence of physical presence, reliance on virtual interactions, digital inequalities, privacy concerns, and the risk of superficial or exploitative engagement underscore the need for balance. Integrating digital and in-person support helps ensure a comprehensive approach to grief that fosters authentic connections and true emotional healing.

1.9.3 Cyberthanatology

The digital age has profoundly changed how individuals experience and process grief, offering valuable opportunities alongside challenges. Online platforms offer immediate access to support networks, enabling connections cross time and geography. These digital spaces have redefined memorial landscapes by enabling memory preservation and continuing bonds with the deceased (Beaunoyer & Guitton, 2021). However, limitations such as the absence of physical presence, the potential superficiality of online interactions, and privacy concerns highlight the need to balance digital and in-person support.

Technology has deeply influenced death-related experiences throughout human history, but today's ubiquitous digital presence has amplified its impact. Researchers have coined the term "cyberthanatology" to describe the integration of death and its related practices within the digital sphere (Beaunoyer & Guitton, 2021).

As society continues to evolve within an increasingly digital landscape, it is necessary to examine both the benefits and limitations of digital spaces in the areas of death and grief support. Technology can enhance connectivity and provide comfort, but the unique value of physical presence and authentic human interaction remains vital for healing. Integrating digital tools with traditional forms of support offers a balanced, holistic approach that embraces new advances while maintaining essential human connections during times of loss.

1.10 Concluding Reflections

Death, dying, and grief touch all aspects of society—medical, social, psychological, legal, and more. The evolution of death and grief studies illuminates the profound ways society engages with mortality. As the field progresses, it reveals not only the psychological aspects of loss but also the cultural, social, and spiritual dimensions that shape responses and experiences. The development of this discipline reflects historical movements, demographic shifts, and technological advancements.

The recent global pandemic highlighted the diverse types and forms of grief experienced by individuals and communities. Systematic reviews of grief studies during COVID-19 reveal a spectrum of grief forms, including nonfinite, disenfranchised, complicated, ambiguous, anticipatory, and delayed grief (Kumar, 2023). Post-pandemic reflections stress the importance of expanding education and research on death, dying, and grief, emphasizing the need for more inclusive and holistic support systems at the individual, institutional, and societal levels (Harrop et al., 2023).

Death and grief studies continue to respond to historical and technological shifts. While digital spaces provide new avenues for connection and memorialization, they also present challenges and ethical considerations. Navigating these changes requires a balanced approach that honors traditional practices while integrating contemporary innovations to deliver meaningful and effective support.

In conclusion, incorporating death and grief education into professional and personal spheres fosters open dialogue, reduces stigma, and enhances well-being. It encourages individuals and communities to approach mortality with awareness and compassion, enriching the experience of both living and grieving. The continued growth of this field has nurtured resilience, empathy, and a deeper appreciation for the shared human journey to navigate life, with death left in.

References

Abidin, C. (2022). Grief hypejacking: Influencers, #ThoughtsAndPrayers, and the commodification of grief on Instagram. *The Information Society, 38*(3), 174–187.

Albrecht, G., Sartore, G. M., Connor, L., Higginbotham, N., Freeman, S., Kelly, B., Stain, H., Tonna, A., & Pollard, G. (2007). Solastalgia: The distress caused by environmental change. *Australasian Psychiatry, 15*(Suppl 1), S95–S98. https://doi.org/10.1080/10398560701701288

Association for Death Education and Counseling. (n.d.). *What is thanatology and who are thanatologists?* Retrieved from https://www.adec.org/page/Earn_Certification#What%20is%20Thanatology

Baier, A. L., Kline, A. C., & Feeny, N. C. (2020). Therapeutic alliance as a mediator of change: A systematic review and evaluation of research. *Clinical Psychology Review, 82*, 101921. https://doi.org/10.1016/j.cpr.2020.101921

Beaunoyer, E., & Guitton, M. J. (2021). Cyberthanathology: Death and beyond in the digital age. *Computers in Human Behavior, 122*, 106849.

Beck, U. (1992). *Risk society: Towards a new modernity* (M. Ritter, Trans.). Sage. (Original work published 1986).
Beck, U., & Beck-Gernsheim, E. (2002). *Individualization: Institutionalized individualism and its social and political consequences*. Sage.
Becker, E. (1973). *The denial of death*. Free Press.
Bell, J., Bailey, L., & Kennedy, D. (2015). 'We do it to keep him alive': Bereaved individuals' experiences of online suicide memorials and continuing bonds. *Mortality, 20*(4), 375–389.
Benton, K. D., & Yarbrow, T. (Eds.). (2024). *Virtual reality for serious illness*. Taylor & Francis.
Blueford, J. M., Diambra, J. F., & Wheat, L. S. (2022). Counselor preparedness to counsel grieving clients: Insights and implications. *Death Studies, 46*(10), 2413–2423. https://doi.org/10.1080/07481187.2021.1956644
Bruce, E. J. (2007). Grief as a neuropsychological response to loss. *Journal of Palliative Medicine, 10*(3), 733–738.
Cacciatore, J., Thieleman, K., Fretts, R., & Jackson, L. B. (2021). What is good grief support? Exploring the actors and actions in social support after traumatic grief. *PLoS One, 16*(5), e0252324. https://doi.org/10.1371/journal.pone.0252324
Chan, W. C., & Tin, A. F. (2012). Beyond knowledge and skills: Self-competence in working with death, dying, and bereavement. *Death Studies, 36*(10), 899–913. https://doi.org/10.1080/07481187.2011.604465
Chödrön, P. (2022). *How we live is how we die*. Shambhala.
Ciupak, Y. (2025). *Spiral model of grief and healing: An integrative sociological, psychological, and cultural framework* [Unpublished manuscript]. Northern Michigan University.
Comtesse, H., Ertl, V., Hengst, S. M. C., Rosner, R., & Smid, G. E. (2021). Ecological grief as a response to environmental change: A mental health risk or functional response? *International Journal of Environmental Research and Public Health, 18*(2), 734. https://doi.org/10.3390/ijerph18020734
Corr, C. A. (2024). Some reflections on the history and current status of education in the field of death, dying, and bereavement at the college and university level in North America. *OMEGA - Journal of Death and Dying, 0*(0). https://doi.org/10.1177/00302228241248879
Death Café. (2024). *Welcome to Death Café*. Retrieved from https://deathcafe.com
Doka, K. (2003). The death awareness movement: Description, history, and analysis. In *Handbook of death & dying* (pp. 50–56). Sage. https://doi.org/10.4135/9781412914291
Durkheim, E. (1897). *Suicide, a study in sociology* (1951 ed., J. A. Spaulding & G. Simpson, Trans.).
Feifel, H. (1977). Death and dying in modern America. *Death Education, 1*(1), 5–14.
Flückiger, C., Del Re, A. C., Wampold, B. E., & Horvath, A. O. (2018). The alliance in adult psychotherapy: A meta-analytic synthesis. *Psychotherapy, 55*(4), 316–340. https://doi.org/10.1037/pst0000172
Freud, S. (1953). Mourning and melancholia. In J. Strachey (Ed. & Trans.), *The standard edition of the complete psychological works of Sigmund Freud* (Vol. 14, pp. 243–258). Hogarth Press.
Gamino, L. A., & Ritter, R. H. (2012). Death competence: An ethical imperative. *Death Studies, 36*(1), 23–40. https://doi.org/10.1080/07481187.2011.553503
Gorer, G. (1955). The pornography of death. *Encounter (London), 5*(4), 49–52.
Greenberg, J., Pyszczynski, T., & Solomon, S. (1986). The causes and consequences of the need for self-esteem: A terror management theory. In R. F. Baumeister (Ed.), *Public and private self* (pp. 189–212). Springer.
Harris, D. L., & Winokuer, H. R. (2021). *Principles and practice of grief counseling* (3rd ed.). Springer.
Harrop, E., Medeiros Mirra, R., Goss, S., Longo, M., Byrne, A., Farnell, D. J. J., Seddon, K., Penny, A., Machin, L., Sivell, S., & Selman, L. E. (2023). Prolonged grief during and beyond the pandemic: Factors associated with levels of grief in a four time-point longitudinal survey of people bereaved in the first year of the COVID-19 pandemic. *Frontiers in Public Health, 11*, 1215881. https://doi.org/10.3389/fpubh.2023.1215881

Havighurst, R. J. (1953). *Human development and education*. Longmans, Green.

Hill, J. E., Cicchetti, R. J., Jackson, S. A., & Szirony, G. M. (2018). Perceptions of grief education in accredited counseling programs: Recommendations for counselor education. *Journal of Social, Behavioral, and Health Sciences, 12*(1), 74–83. https://doi.org/10.5590/JSBHS.2018.12.1.05

Horn, E. A. D., Crews, J. A., & Harrawood, L. K. (2013). Grief and loss education: Recommendations for curricular inclusion. *Counselor Education and Supervision, 52*(1), 70–80. https://doi.org/10.1002/j.1556-6978.2013.00029.x

Hsiao, C.-C., Hsieh, S.-I., Kao, C.-Y., & Chu, T.-P. (2023). Factors affecting nurses' willingness and competency to provide anticipatory grief counseling for family caregivers of patients with terminal cancer. *Journal of Clinical Nursing, 32*(7–8), 1053–1064. https://doi.org/10.1111/jocn.16335

Incorvaia, A. D. (2024). Death positivity in America: The movement—Its history and literature. *OMEGA - Journal of Death and Dying, 89*(3), 1233–1252. https://doi.org/10.1177/00302228221085176

Jankauskaite, G., O'Brien, K. M., & Yang, N. (2021). Assessing knowledge and predicting grief counseling skills among university counseling center therapists. *The Counseling Psychologist, 49*(3), 458–484. https://doi.org/10.1177/0011000020983525

Jordan, J. R., & Neimeyer, R. A. (2003). Does grief counseling work? *Death Studies, 27*(9), 765–786. https://doi.org/10.1080/713842360

Kastenbaum, R. J. (2004). *On our way: The final passage through life and death*. University of California Press.

Kübler-Ross, E. (1983). *Speaks to a dying patient* [Video]. Nova Interview. Retrieved from https://www.youtube.com/watch?v=tIZ97OALEfE

Kumar, R. M. (2023). The many faces of grief: A systematic literature review of grief during the COVID-19 pandemic. *Illness, Crises, and Loss, 31*(1), 100–119. https://doi.org/10.1177/10541373211038084

Lindemann, E. (1944). Symptomatology and management of acute grief. *American Journal of Psychiatry, 101*(2), 141–148.

Lunney, J. R., Lynn, J., Foley, D. J., Lipson, S., & Guralnik, J. M. (2003). Patterns of functional decline at the end of life. *JAMA, 289*(18), 2387–2392. https://doi.org/10.1001/jama.289.18.2387

Moore, J., Magee, S., Gamreklidze, E., & Kowalewski, J. (2019). Social media mourning: Using grounded theory to explore how people grieve on social networking sites. *OMEGA - Journal of Death and Dying, 79*(3), 231–259. https://doi.org/10.1177/0030222817709691

Neimeyer, R. A., Prigerson, H. G., & Davies, B. (2002). Mourning and meaning. *American Behavioral Scientist, 46*(2), 235–251.

Ober, A. M., Granello, D. H., & Wheaton, J. E. (2012). Grief counseling: An investigation of counselors' training, experience, and competencies. *Journal of Counseling & Development, 90*(2), 150–159. https://doi.org/10.1111/j.1556-6676.2012.00020.x

Ogińska-Bulik, N., & Juczyński, Z. (2024). Vicarious posttraumatic growth: The benefits of indirect exposure to trauma. In *The Routledge international handbook of posttraumatic growth* (pp. 445–457). Routledge.

Ramirez, L., Monahan, C., Palacios-Espinosa, X., & Levy, S. R. (2022). Intersections of ageism toward older adults and other isms during the COVID-19 pandemic. *The Journal of social issues, 78*(4), 965–990. https://doi.org/10.1111/josi.12574

Rogers, C. R. (1995). *On becoming a person: A therapist's view of psychotherapy*. Houghton Mifflin Harcourt.

Selman, L. E., Farnell, D. J. J., Longo, M., Goss, S., Torrens-Burton, A., Seddon, K., Mayland, C. R., Machin, L., Byrne, A., & Harrop, E. J. (2022). Factors associated with higher levels of grief and support needs among people bereaved during the pandemic: Results from a national online survey. *OMEGA - Journal of Death and Dying*. https://doi.org/10.1177/00302228221144925

Stamm, B. H. (2013). Measuring compassion satisfaction as well as fatigue: Developmental history of the compassion satisfaction and fatigue test. In *Treating compassion fatigue* (pp. 107–119). Routledge.

Stylianou, P., & Zembylas, M. (2018). Dealing with the concepts of "grief" and "grieving" in the classroom: Children's perceptions, emotions, and behavior. *OMEGA - Journal of Death and Dying, 77*(3), 240–266. https://doi.org/10.1177/0030222815626717

Testoni, I., Cordioli, C., Nodari, E., Zsak, E., Marinoni, G. L., & Venturini, D. (2019). Language rediscovered: A death education intervention in the net between kindergarten, family, and territory. *Italian Journal of Sociology of Education, 11*(1), 331–346. https://doi.org/10.14658/pupj-ijse-2019-1-16

Thibault, J. M. (2002). Aging, spirituality, and religion: A handbook. In M. A. Kimble, S. H. McFadden, J. W. Ellor, & J. J. Seeber (Eds.), *Religion and spirituality in later life* (pp. 149–162). Fortress Press.

Thomas, T., Althouse, A., Sigler, L., Arnold, R., Chu, E., White, D. B., Rosenzweig, M., Smith, K., Smith, T. J., & Schenker, Y. (2021). Stronger therapeutic alliance is associated with better quality of life among patients with advanced cancer. *Psycho-Oncology, 30*(7), 1086–1094. https://doi.org/10.1002/pon.5648

Tomoi, K. (2024). Death attitudes among middle-aged and older adults in Japan: A qualitative study based on Erikson's theory of generativity. *OMEGA - Journal of Death and Dying, 90*(2), 536–553.

U.S. Department of Health, Education, and Welfare. (1978). *Hospice care: A viable concept for terminally ill patients and their families*. Government Printing Office.

Warraich, H. J. (2017). *Modern death: How medicine changed the end of life*. St. Martin's Press.

Wheat, L. S., Matthews, J. J., & Whiting, P. P. (2022). Grief content inclusion in CACREP-accredited counselor education programs. *Journal of Counselor Preparation and Supervision, 15*(2), Article 14. Retrieved from https://digitalcommons.sacredheart.edu/jcps/vol15/iss2/14

Wolfelt, A. (2003). *Companioning the bereaved: A soulful guide for counselors & caregivers*. Companion Press.

Wong, P. T. (2007). Meaning management theory and death acceptance. In *Existential and spiritual issues in death attitudes* (pp. 91–114). Psychology Press.

Wong, M., & Tomer, A. (2011). Beyond terror and denial: The positive psychology of death acceptance. *Death Studies, 35*, 99–106. https://doi.org/10.1080/07481187.2011.535377

Zuelke, A., Luppa, M., Löbner, M., Pabst, A., Schlapke, C., Stein, J., & Riedel-Heller, S. (2021). Effectiveness and feasibility of internet-based interventions for grief after bereavement: Systematic review and meta-analysis. *JMIR Mental Health, 8*(12), e29661. https://doi.org/10.2196/29661

Chapter 2
Culture in End-of-Life and Grief Support

2.1 What Is Culture

Humans are social beings who seek connections with others and prefer to live, work, and socialize together (Aronson et al., 2007). Social Psychology further posits that culture is an advanced way of being social, essentially setting humans apart from other social animals (Baumeister & Bushman, 2016). The United Nations Educational, Scientific and Cultural Organization (UNESCO) defines culture as "the set of distinctive spiritual, material, intellectual, and emotional features of society or a social group, encompassing art and literature, lifestyles, ways of living together, value systems, traditions, and beliefs." (UNESCO, 2001, as cited in UNESCO, 2013, p. 10).

Culture is an integrated and dynamic system comprising norms, symbols, values, practices, and technology shared by its members, encompassing both material achievements and nonmaterial aspects (Boyd & Richerson, 1988; Geertz, 1973; Tylor, 1871). Passed on through generations, culture is acquired and learned via socialization agents such as family, education, religion, and media.

Culture consists of multiple interconnected components, reflecting the complex and multifaceted nature of human societies (Castro, 1998). The most common elements include:

- A shared heritage and history passed down through generations
- Common values, beliefs, customs, behaviors, traditions, institutions, arts, folklore, and lifestyle
- Similar patterns of relationships and socialization
- A common style of communication or language
- Geographic location of residence (e.g., country, community, urban, suburban, or rural areas)
- Patterns of dress and diet

Y. Z. Ciupak, D. C. Smith, *Death, Dying, and Grief*,
https://doi.org/10.1007/978-3-031-88467-2_2

While these criteria may not apply universally to every cultural group, they effectively capture the key elements that distinguish cultural groups from one another (Substance Abuse and Mental Health Services Administration [SAMHSA], 2014). Many of the elements can be further broken down into more nuanced aspects. For instance, the SAMHSA of the US Department of Health and Human Services compiled a list of 22 common characteristics of culture (SAMHSA, 2014, p. 12).

Importantly, within each distinct culture, there is diversity and multiplicity. Therefore, to insiders, every group reveals itself not as homogeneous but as a nested series of progressively smaller groups that may hold distinct identities (UNESCO, 2013). This is linked to patient-centered care, which is "providing care that is respectful of, and responsive to, individual patient preferences, needs, and values, and ensuring that patient values guide all clinical decisions" (Institute of Medicine, 2001, p. 6). Essentially, the principles of patient-centered care reinforce the need to recognize that people should be treated first and foremost as individuals rather than as members of particular social groups.

Culture is collective yet personal, cumulative yet dynamic. It is deeply embedded in social environments through which people interpret experiences and generate behaviors (Boyd & Richerson, 1988). Culture influences perceptions and interactions, impacting basic human needs such as food and sex (Baumeister & Bushman, 2016). Although culture is collective, it remains profoundly personal, fluid, and constantly evolving through new experiences and societal changes. Individuals are not just passive recipients of culture; they actively participate in its production and transformation, whether intentionally or unintentionally. Culture is more than a backdrop for human actions; culture is embodied and lived through people. Whether attending a Catholic funeral in black, mourning in white cloth in rural China, decorating a Hindu fire puja with marigolds, or choosing a modern "celebrating life" theme, people are performing and shaping culture.

2.1.1 Cultural Significance of Rituals

Across history and cultures, communities have formed rich traditions and rituals surrounding death and mourning (Silverman et al., 2021). Simultaneously reflecting and shaping cultural attitudes, rituals play a vital role in private and public lives. Émile Durkheim, a foundational figure in sociology, emphasized that rituals surrounding death reinforce the collective consciousness—the shared beliefs and values that unify society. By participating in these communal practices, individuals reconnect with the social fabric, helping to mitigate the disruptive effects of death on social order. Durkheim's concept of *collective effervescence*—the shared emotional energy and harmony generated during communal rituals—captures the powerful sense of solidarity that arises in the face of loss (Olaveson, 2001).

Durkheim's sociological perspective emphasizes the critical role mourning rituals play in restoring social equilibrium. He viewed mourning not just as an individual experience but as a deeply social act shaped by the expectations and norms of the surrounding cultural context. According to Durkheim, funerary rites provide a structured space for collective emotional expression while reinforcing social cohesion and ensuring the continuity of social order.

Arnold Van Gennep (2019), another influential thinker, framed death rituals as essential rites of passage, emphasizing their role in helping individuals and communities transition from one state of existence to another. These structured rituals offer a social framework that guides mourners through the stages of grief, facilitating both personal and communal healing. The involvement of the broader community in these rites further underscores their sociological importance, as they help integrate the loss into the community's collective experience.

In modern times, research has expanded on the sociological foundations of grief rituals, examining how they have evolved in response to social changes. Studies during the COVID-19 pandemic, for example, illustrate how disruptions to traditional mourning practices impacted emotional and social coping mechanisms, underscoring the deep sociological importance of these rituals (Mazid, 2021). Even in secular societies, death rituals continue to play a critical role in maintaining social ties and collective memory, demonstrating their ongoing significance (Prickett & Timmermans, 2022).

Anthropological perspectives further deepen the understanding of the social dimensions of death rituals. These practices not only honor the deceased but also ensure the continuity of the community, reflecting collective beliefs about life, death, and the afterlife while helping the living find closure and reinforcing social structures (Abramovitch, 2015).

However, it is essential to recognize the potential shortcomings of certain rituals and promote practices that align with the values and needs of grieving people. In some cases, individuals may feel pressured to conform to cultural or social norms, participating in rituals that do not align with their personal beliefs or emotional needs. Additionally, the financial costs of traditional practices can impose significant stress on families during an already difficult time. Sociological and anthropological insights emphasize the importance of rituals in helping individuals and communities navigate grief while also inviting reflection on more equitable and compassionate approaches. Across cultures, communal rituals remain a vital source of healing, reaffirming the bonds that hold communities together.

2.1.2 Multidimensions of Cultural Diversity

Cultural identities are complex and shaped by the interplay of various elements. Individuals belong to multiple cultural groups that collectively influence their identities, perspectives, and behaviors. Several conceptual models are popularly used as frameworks for understanding culture, such as Loden and Rosener's (1991) "four layers of diversity" model. This widely recognized model, presented in their book *Workforce America: Managing Employee Diversity as a Vital Resource*, outlines four layers of diversity: personality, internal dimensions, external dimensions, and organizational dimensions. The model is aimed primarily at managing employee diversity in the workplace.

Based on the Spiral Model of Grieving and Healing (Ciupak, 2025), three dimensions of culture are identified as interacting with an individual's micro-level state (biological, affective, cognitive, behavioral, and spiritual) when navigating death, dying, and grief:

1. **Social identity and positions**: Age, gender, sexual orientation, race/ethnicity, nationality/immigration status, socioeconomic class, and able-bodiedness
2. **Institutional elements**: Family, community, workplace, policies, laws, and care system
3. **Broader macro dimensions**: Encompassing historical, geographical, economic, and political contexts

Social identities and positions form the core of self-concepts and shape the fundamental expectations of oneself and others. These identities influence behaviors, social interactions, and access to resources, creating both opportunities and barriers. For example, age, gender, race, and socioeconomic class can affect the types of support available during periods of grief and how one's expressions of mourning are perceived by society. Many of these identities and positions are fluid and evolve to a certain degree, depending on how a society allows such fluidity and mobility.

The various social markers also "intersect" to create unique systems of privilege and disadvantage. Rather than viewing these social identities and positioning in isolation, individuals often face multiple, interconnected forms of advantage or disadvantage due to complex intersectionality (Crenshaw, 1989).

For example, a woman from a minority community who works an hourly wage job and has lost her husband may face unique and compounded challenges during her grieving process. Economic insecurity from losing vital income can amplify her stress, especially if her job does not offer bereavement leave or flexibility. Being part of a marginalized racial or ethnic group may further complicate her access to adequate mental health support and resources, as systemic barriers can limit availability and inclusivity. Intersectionality helps illustrate how her grief is not only shaped by personal loss but also intensified by the intersection of her socioeconomic status, minority background, and gender.

Institutional elements, such as family structures, community connections, workplaces, and policies, play crucial roles in shaping how individuals experience death and grief. This includes healthcare providers, palliative care and hospices that deliver end-of-life care, funeral homes that manage post-death arrangements, and religious institutions that provide spiritual services. Legal frameworks govern processes such as advance directives and estate handling, whereas cemeteries and crematoria facilitate final body dispositions. These systems collectively set norms and practices that support or hinder grieving, influencing how individuals navigate loss within their cultural and social contexts.

All these dimensions are interwoven with and influenced by **macrostructures** such as historical, economic, political, and geographical contexts. For example, economic conditions can impact access to quality end-of-life care, whereas historical and cultural norms shape attitudes toward death and grief. Geographical location can dictate the availability of resources, support networks, and traditional practices, further affecting how death and grief are experienced and processed. This complex interplay of various dimensions of culture affects how individuals perceive and navigate death, dying, and grief. Figure 2.1 illustrates the self and the multi-dimensions of culture based on the Spiral Model.

The Spiral Model offers a logical and comprehensive perspective from the micro, meso, and macro dimensions, serving as both a conceptual and practical framework to understand and address how various social-cultural factors interact in complex situations. Consider the following example:

A healthcare provider is working with an immigrant patient nearing the end of life. Patient *social identity and position* include factors such as age, race, socioeconomic class, and language barriers. The *institutional* context involves the policies and support provided by the healthcare system, community resources, and family dynamics. Macro dimensions include cultural norms around death and grieving from the patient's country of origin and the historical context shaping trust in

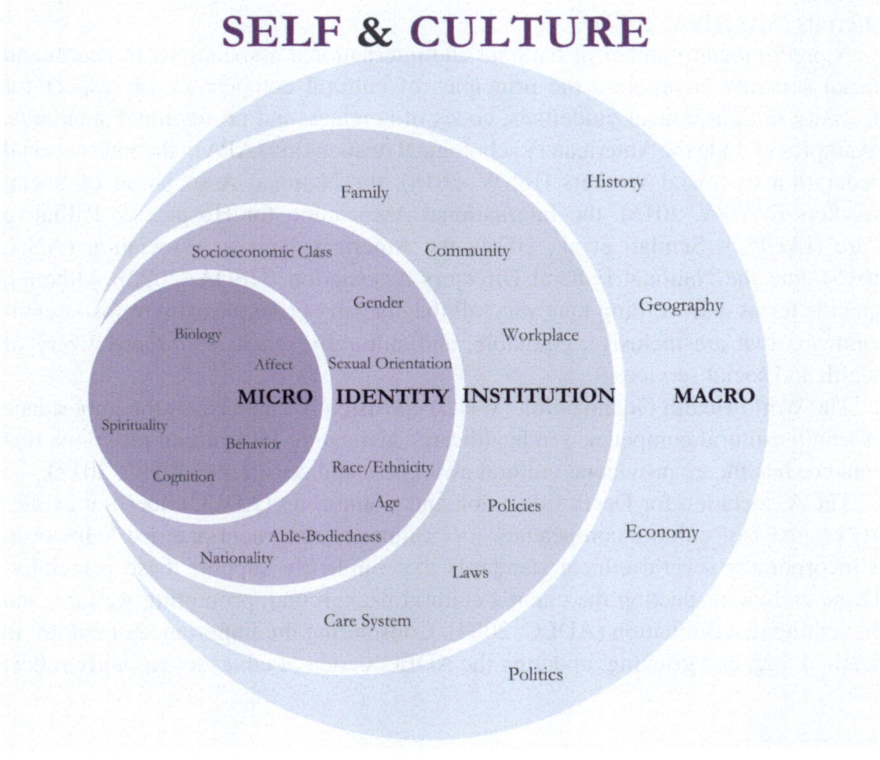

Fig. 2.1 Self and culture. Source: Based on Spiral Model of Grieving and Healing (Ciupak, 2025)

healthcare. Navigating these influences allows providers to deliver culturally sensitive and informed care.

The multidimensional nature of culture highlights the importance of diversity sensitivity and an understanding of *intersectionality*. This involves recognizing how different forms of cultural diversity and social indicators—such as age, class, race/ethnicity, gender, sexual orientation, immigration status, and religion—interact with and mutually shape identities and experiences within social structures. Understanding this complexity helps professionals ensure that effective policy and practice responses address all factors contributing to the risk of exclusion (WHO, 2020, p. 9).

2.2 Culturally Responsive Policies and Practices

Integrating culturally responsive policies and practices benefits clients, staff, organizations, and the community. It supports the sustainability of services by valuing diversity and responsiveness, meeting regulatory requirements, and enhancing risk management. Culturally competent and responsive services improve access to care, assessment, treatment planning, and communication, ultimately leading to better therapeutic outcomes and reducing the risk of misunderstandings and inappropriate referrals (SAMHSA, 2014).

A predominant number of national and international associations of health and social services incorporate the principles of cultural competency or respect for diversity in their ethical guidelines, codes of conduct, and professional standards. Examples include the American Psychological Association (APA),[1] the International Federation of Social Workers (IFSW, 2018), the National Association of Social Workers (NASW, 2015), the International Association for Hospice & Palliative Care (IAHPC) (Semlali et al., 2020), the American Nurses Association (ANA, 2015), and the National Funeral Directors Association (NFDA, 2022). Although specific terms and wording may vary, all the diversity principles aim to foster environments that are inclusive, equitable, and culturally sensitive in the delivery of health and social services.

The World Health Organization (WHO) consistently emphasizes the importance of (multi)cultural competence in healthcare, advocating for training programs that enhance healthcare providers' cultural awareness and sensitivity (WHO, 2018).

The Association for Death Education and Counseling (ADEC) does not explicitly emphasize "cultural competency" or "culturally congruent practice." However, it incorporates several ethical standards that implicitly support these principles. These include respecting the client's cultural background, promoting welfare, and preventing discrimination (ADEC, 2004). Considering the importance of culture in death, dying, and grieving, updating the ADEC's code of ethics to explicitly reflect

[1] The APA website contains a number of practice guidelines for multicultural practice serving various groups: https://www.apa.org/practice/guidelines

cultural sensitivity, competency, and humility could reinforce its commitment to these values and practices.

Prioritizing cultural responsiveness, competence, and humility enables organizations to create inclusive environments that respect and celebrate diversity. This approach contributes to better health outcomes and stronger community relationships. Understanding the importance and complexity of culture and enhancing cultural competence are essential for providing person-centered care and support. More fundamentally, cultivating cultural awareness and humility is critical to achieving cultural competency.

2.3 Culture Awareness, Competence, and Humility

Cultural awareness, humility, and competence are crucial for delivering compassionate and effective care in end-of-life and grief support. Cultural awareness involves recognizing and understanding the multidimensional nature of culture and the interactions of various social markers *(intersectionality)*. This is essential for providing care that respects and responds to the diverse ways individuals and communities experience loss, mourning, and healing. Cultural humility further enhances this competence through ongoing self-reflection, an openness to share power, and a commitment to learning. Together, these interconnected principles foster person-centered service and reduce healthcare disparities among vulnerable populations (Kleinman et al., 1978; Giger et al., 2007).

2.3.1 Cultural Awareness

Most professional training programs today include components of cultural awareness or competence. Cultural awareness involves recognizing and understanding cultural differences and similarities, allowing professionals to engage effectively with diverse groups. This concept was significantly advanced by anthropologist Edward T. Hall, who pioneered the field of intercultural communication. His influential mid-twentieth-century work, particularly the book *The Silent Language* (1959), illustrated how cultural norms shape communication and behavior.

For human service professionals, such as those involved in healthcare, social work, and education, cultural awareness is crucial for building trust and rapport. It involves being conscious of one's cultural values, biases, and assumptions and understanding how these values may impact perceptions and interactions with others. It requires a willingness to learn about and respect different cultural practices, beliefs, and traditions and to adapt one's approach to meet the unique needs of each individual. Fostering cultural awareness enhances the overall quality and equality of care and services, contributing to a more just and compassionate culture.

A lack of cultural awareness can lead to misunderstanding, miscommunication, and adverse outcomes. One well-documented case is detailed in *The Spirit Catches You and You Fall Down* by Anne Fadiman (1999). The book recounts the tragic story of Lia Lee, a young Hmong girl with severe epilepsy. Her family's cultural beliefs, rooted in a spiritual understanding of her condition known as "quag dab peg," conflict with the American medical system's approach. While her parents turned to traditional healing, her doctors prescribed a complex regimen of medications. Miscommunication and cultural misunderstandings resulted in inconsistent treatment, worsening Lia's condition and leading to severe seizures that left her in a persistent vegetative state.

Kleinman, Eisenberg, and Good's classical work on clinical lessons related to multicultural cases (1978) used sociological and anthropological concepts to inform clinical strategies, looking at the varied cultural views of sickness and care. They highlighted that a lack of cultural awareness among healthcare providers often results in ineffective clinical treatment and poor health outcomes.

One example involved a 33-year-old Cantonese-speaking man treated at Massachusetts General Hospital. He presented with fatigue, dizziness, and insomnia and attributed his symptoms to "wind" and "not enough blood," rooted in traditional Chinese medicine. He initially resisted Western psychiatric care and continued traditional remedies, including herbal treatments and consultations with community "experts." This case demonstrated how divergent cultural explanatory models could lead to patient resistance and gaps in treatment if healthcare providers do not engage with patients' beliefs.

Another case described a 26-year-old Guatemalan woman who was receiving treatment for severe regional enteritis. She believed her condition was caused by witchcraft and was influenced by traditional health beliefs related to the balance between heat and cold. These beliefs led to withdrawal and noncooperation with her treatment. It was only when a psychiatric consultant acknowledged her cultural framework and listened without judgment that her cooperation improved, underscoring the importance of cultural sensitivity in patient care.

Cultural incompetence often leads to significant healthcare disparities. For example, a case study detailed a Latino patient with limited English proficiency who experienced complications during childbirth due to the healthcare team's inability to communicate effectively and address her cultural needs (Betancourt et al., 2003). These examples highlight the pressing need for cultural awareness and competence. Racial and ethnic disparities in healthcare further emphasize the importance of culturally responsive practices to improve outcomes and promote equity (Nelson, 2002).

These clinical lessons demonstrate the vital role that cultural awareness plays in professional practice, especially in supporting people in vulnerable moments. Understanding and respecting cultural diversity helps professionals avoid miscommunication and build stronger, more effective relationships. This has propelled the rise of cross-cultural psychology (Berry, 2002) and enriched scholarship and training in cultural competency and intercultural sensitivity (Bennett, 1993).

2.3.2 *Cultural Competence: Definition and Dimensions*

Countless scholars and organizations have explored and developed the concept of cultural competence. The Office of Minority Health (U.S. Department of Health and Human Services, Office of Minority Health, 2013) synthesizes several definitions to conclude that:

> Cultural and linguistic competence is a set of congruent behaviors, attitudes, and policies that come together in a system, agency, or among professionals that enables effective work in cross-cultural situations. 'Culture' refers to integrated patterns of human behavior that include the language, thoughts, communications, actions, customs, beliefs, values, and institutions of racial, ethnic, religious, or social groups. 'Competence' implies having the capacity to function effectively as an individual and an organization within the context of the cultural beliefs, behaviors, and needs presented by consumers and their communities. (p. 28)

Cultural competence requires coordinated efforts at the individual, programmatic/clinical, organizational, and national or international levels. At the institutional level, healthcare organizations should adopt policies and practices that promote cultural competence. This can include ongoing training, the development of culturally appropriate health materials, and fostering an environment that supports interprofessional collaboration, respect, and the accommodation of diverse cultural needs. Institutional commitment may also involve partnerships with community organizations and intercultural mediators to bridge communication gaps and reduce cultural barriers.

On a national or international scale, initiatives to promote cultural competence might include creating frameworks and standards to guide healthcare practices across regions and countries. This can involve developing national registries for intercultural mediators, establishing international guidelines for culturally competent care, and sharing best practices across borders to improve healthcare quality for diverse populations. These comprehensive strategies help ensure that cultural competence is integrated at every level of the healthcare system, creating more equitable and effective care for all.

Case Study: Successful Intercultural Mediation Programs in Healthcare: Lessons from Belgium, Catalonia, and Rome

A World Health Organization publication highlighted three cases exemplifying the successful implementation and impact of intercultural mediation programs in healthcare settings.

Belgium initiated an intercultural mediation project in 1991 and integrated it into the healthcare system by 2000. Subsequent training was provided to ensure its ongoing relevance and updates. Numerous general and psychiatric hospitals employ onsite intercultural mediators who facilitate communication, provide multicultural education, and offer advocacy. In 2013 alone,

(continued)

(continued)

mediators handled over 110,000 interventions. Evaluations demonstrated increased care quality, and the project has expanded to include online mediation and plans to cover nonresidential care. It is recognized as a model of good practice in the WHO European Region.

The Migrant-Friendly Health Centers project in Catalonia, Spain, was launched between 2003 and 2006 by the Asociación Salud y Familia (ASF) and the public health system (PHC), which aimed to improve healthcare for immigrants. Objectives included increasing culturally adapted services, breaking down language and cultural barriers, reducing intercultural conflict, and enhancing patient satisfaction. Twenty-five intercultural mediators worked in five hospitals and 19 primary healthcare centers, supporting over 38,000 immigrant patients. The public health system adapted materials and procedures with an intercultural focus and increased intercultural training for staff. The project led to immediate care improvements and significantly enhanced staff intercultural competencies, making intercultural organizational development a part of the public health agenda.

In Rome, Italy, the Public Registry of Intercultural Mediators was established in 2006 by the Rome Municipality for Rome and the Lazio Region. Enrollment is required for mediators to work in public offices, including social services, hospitals, and schools, with strict criteria for language skills and competence. The registry is updated annually to verify qualifications and provide relevant training courses. Within a decade, the registry included 520 mediators from 80 different countries, highlighting the program's diversity and extensive reach.

These cases illustrate the important role of intercultural mediation or liaison and demonstrate that cultural competency is beyond individual professional practice. Structured programs and systematic endeavors can enhance communication, reduce cultural barriers, and improve overall care quality for diverse populations. Belgium's long-term integration, Catalonia's collaborative model, and Rome's formal registry system have each offered valuable lessons and inspirations for implementing effective culturally competent strategies at the broader level to meet diverse needs.

Source: World Health Organization. Regional Office for Europe. (2020). Migration and health: enhancing intercultural competence and diversity sensitivity. World Health Organization. Regional Office for Europe. https://iris.who.int/handle/10665/332186.

2.3.2.1 Components of Cultural Competence

A useful framework for understanding cultural competence in practice is the tripartite model, which encompasses three core components: cultural awareness/attitudes, cultural knowledge, and cultural skill development (SAMHSA, 2014; Sue et al.,

1992). Synthesizing the guidelines from the American Psychological Association (APA, 2017) and SAMHSA (2014), providing culturally competent services requires counselors, clinical staff, and organizations to:

1. Become aware and reflective of their own cultural background and understand how it influences their attitudes, beliefs, and assumptions about others. Professionals must acknowledge their cultural perspectives and strive to mitigate biases (**i.e., Awareness/attitudes**).
2. Develop an understanding and cultural knowledge of the individuals they serve, recognizing that identity is dynamic and shaped by intersecting social and contextual factors (**i.e., Knowledge**).
3. Develop competence in clinical skills to ensure the delivery of culturally appropriate treatment interventions. This includes promoting culturally adaptive and strength-based approaches that build resilience and reduce trauma within diverse sociocultural contexts (**i.e., Skills**).

The classical tripartite model continues to guide the research, practice, and training of medical and mental health care workers. The Standards and Indicators for Cultural Competence in Social Work Practice (NASW, 2015) expanded the tripartite model to ten standards. These standards include ethics and values, self-awareness, cross-cultural knowledge and skills, service delivery, empowerment and advocacy, a diverse workforce, professional education, language and communication, and leadership to advance cultural competence.

Cultural groups are diverse and continuously evolving, making it impossible to rely on a static set of knowledge about specific populations. Therefore, cultural competence is a dynamic, ongoing developmental process that requires long-term commitment. It requires professionals to continuously strive to learn, understand, and work within their clients' cultural contexts. This process involves humility, ongoing self-reflection, education, and a commitment to embracing and respecting cultural diversity.

2.3.2.2 Culturally Competent Practices

What do culturally competent practices look like? According to the *Treatment Improvement Protocol: Improving Cultural Competence* (SAMHSA, 2014), culturally competent counselors:

- Frame issues in culturally relevant ways
- Allow for the complexity of issues based on cultural context
- Make allowances for variations in the use of personal space
- Are respectful of culturally specific meanings of touch (e.g., hugging)
- Explore culturally based experiences of power and powerlessness
- Adjust communication styles to the client's culture
- Interpret emotional expressions in light of the client's culture
- Expand roles and practices as needed

Cultural competence is essential for providing effective and equitable care, particularly for professionals working with individuals who are dying or grieving. Researchers emphasize that cultural beliefs and practices significantly impact decision-making processes, pain management, and perspectives on death and dying (Kagawa-Singer & Blackhall, 2001). Incorporating these beliefs into care plans leads to higher patient satisfaction and better treatment adherence (Betancourt et al., 2003). Care providers who understand and accommodate their patients' diverse cultural backgrounds are better equipped to navigate differences in communication styles, family dynamics, and spiritual beliefs. Building cultural competence applies not only to individual staff members but also to the care team, institutions, and, at times, national or international frameworks.

2.3.2.3 Moving Forward with Cultural Competence

Despite its recognized importance, achieving cultural competence remains challenging, and the effects of cultural competence training are controversial. Professionals often struggle with integrating it into practice because of a lack of clear definitions and operational guidelines. Additionally, there is a risk of superficial understanding, where professionals may display cultural competence only to meet social desirability rather than genuinely integrating it into their practice (Henderson et al., 2018). Cultural competency training that emphasizes knowledge and skills could risk stereotyping and othering people and overlook intersectionality, which may undermine the recognition of patients' multiple social statuses, shaping their beliefs and behaviors (Lekas et al., 2020). Therefore, some scholars and practitioners propose reconceptualizing or even abandoning the term in favor of cultural humility or other frameworks (Hook et al., 2017; Lekas et al., 2020; Tervalon & Murray-García, 1998).

The concept of "cultural competence" or "multicultural competence" remains valuable for achieving culturally responsive care. However, it should be expanded to include multidimensional aspects, intersectionality, cultural humility, and an understanding that it is an ongoing process rather than an end goal. Integrating these broader perspectives allows rich resources and discussions around cultural competence to be used effectively. This approach ensures a more comprehensive and nuanced method of care. The expanded framework addresses the limitations of traditional models and fosters a deeper understanding of and responsiveness to patients' diverse cultural contexts.

A notable example is the 2015 update by the National Association of Social Workers to its *Standards and Indicators for Cultural Competence in Social Work Practice*. This revision broadened the concept of culture beyond race and ethnicity to include aspects such as sexual orientation, gender identity or expression, and religious identity or spirituality. The updates also highlighted the importance of cultural humility, emphasizing a lifelong commitment to self-evaluation and self-critique. Additionally, they incorporated intersectionality, acknowledging the complexity of individuals' experiences shaped by multiple intersecting identities.

The *Treatment Improvement Protocol: Improving Cultural Competence* (SAMHSA, 2014) provides invaluable resources and practical guides for culturally competent and responsive services applicable to individuals and organizations in healthcare and other sectors. Similarly, the *Enhanced National Standards for Culturally and Linguistically Appropriate Services in Health and Health Care* (OMH, 2013) aim to reduce disparities, enhance the quality of care, and promote health equity through a comprehensive framework for healthcare delivery.

Cultural competence training that emphasizes cultural humility helps professionals develop higher levels of moral reasoning and genuine respect for cultural differences. Cultural humility recognizes that one can never fully understand another's cultural background or master the knowledge of their culture. Therefore, it is acknowledge our limitations and be open to learning, allowing clients to lead and guide us in understanding what different issues mean to them. This approach fosters a deeper and more authentic application of cultural competence in professional practice.

Case Study: Cultural Competence Leading to Stereotype

A program for Somali Bantu refugees at a community health center near Boston faced significant challenges. Cultural variations and subethnic conflicts emerged alongside individual differences. For instance, a patient identified as Bantu by the clinic rejected this label, preferring to associate with the higher-status Madibaan group and struggling to fit in with the Bantu community at the clinic. Additionally, the Somali staff, comprising both Bantu and non-Bantu members, frequently argued about patient assignments based on ethnic identities. Detailed cultural information about the Bantu group was provided and communicated to medical personnel beforehand to strengthen their cultural competence. However, the standardized cultural information and rigid grouping led to stereotyping and othering and was not deemed to improve the quality of care.

Source: Migrant Integration Policy Index (2015). (MIPEX). (2015). How countries promote the integration of immigrants. Barcelona/Brussels: CIDOB and MPG. Retrieved from http://www.mipex.eu/

2.3.3 Cultural Humility

Cultural humility involves an ongoing commitment to self-reflexivity, appreciating cultural complexity, addressing power imbalances, and developing mutually respectful partnerships for more equitable care and an inclusive society. It encompasses competence, attitudes, quality, and embodied practices that value diversity and empowers individuals and communities. The concept was first proposed by Tervalon and Murray-García (1998) and was subsequently developed by scholars and practitioners in various fields to address the limitations of the cultural competence framework (Hook et al., 2017; Chávez, 2022). Tervalon and Murray-García famously noted that "cultural competency is a process rather than an end product. From this perspective, competency involves more than gaining factual knowledge; it also includes our ongoing attitudes toward both our clients and ourselves" (p. 122).

Unlike cultural competence, which traditionally focuses on building knowledge of cultural content areas or mastery of cultural differences, cultural humility invites professionals to engage in self-reflection as an ongoing, life-long commitment to personal and institutional growth in understanding and respecting cultural diversity. It focuses on maintaining an interpersonal stance that is open to the cultural identity aspects most important to a particular individual. It involves recognizing and challenging power imbalances and developing partnerships on the basis of mutual respect and learning.

Renowned psychological counselors such as Hook et al. (2017) advocate that mental health professionals focus on what they do not know about the client sitting across from them rather than relying solely on prior clinical or educational experiences. Their book, *Cultural Humility: Engaging Diverse Identities in Therapy*, proposes shifting from multicultural competence to a multicultural orientation, with cultural humility as its foundation. They suggest multicultural orientation as "how a therapist thinks about and values diversity, which necessarily affects the therapist's work with diverse clients" (p. 9). While multicultural competence focuses on "ways of doing" therapy, including the effective implementation of cultural knowledge and skills, multicultural orientation emphasizes "ways of being" with clients, incorporating cultural humility, cultural comfort, and seizing cultural opportunities (Owen, 2013, as cited in Hook et al., 2017).

The key components of cultural humility, as identified by various scholars and practitioners (Chávez, 2022; Gottlieb, 2020; Hook et al., 2017; Tervalon & Murray-García, 1998), include the following:

1. **Cultural self-awareness**: Being aware of one's own cultural influences and how these influences affect interactions with others. This self-awareness helps professionals understand the impact of their cultural identity on their perceptions and behaviors.
2. **Life-long self-reflection and self-critique**: Continuously engaging in self-reflection and self-assessment to understand and address personal biases and assumptions.
3. **Openness and willingness to learn**: Maintaining an open attitude toward learning from individuals from different cultural backgrounds, recognizing that this learning process is never complete.
4. **Other-oriented stance**: Prioritizing the perspectives and experiences of the individuals being served rather than assuming that one's own cultural knowledge is sufficient or superior.
5. **Development of mutually respectful relationships and partnerships.**
6. **Recognition of power dynamics**: Identifying and addressing power imbalances in relationships, striving to develop equitable partnerships with individuals and groups advocating for others.

7. **Institutional accountability**: Ensuring that organizations and institutions hold themselves accountable for promoting cultural humility and addressing systemic inequities.

The HUMBLE model, commonly used in cultural humility training, provides a clear and practical framework for cultural humility practices (School of Social Work, 2021):

- **H**: Be humble about the assumptions you make.
- **U**: Understand your own background and culture.
- **M**: Motivate yourself to learn more about the other person's background.
- **B**: Begin to incorporate this knowledge into your work.
- **L**: Commit to lifelong learning.
- **E**: Emphasize respect and negotiate service plans

2.3.4 Integrating Cultural Awareness, Humility, and Competence

Integrating cultural awareness, humility, and competence is critical to compassionate and person-centered service. Cultural awareness lays the foundation for cultural competence, and cultural humility further facilitates it. These principles work synergistically to ensure that care is sensitive, inclusive, and responsive to diverse cultural contexts.

Cultural awareness serves as the foundation for competence by fostering an understanding of how cultural aspects shape attitudes and experiences surrounding death, dying, and mourning. It begins with recognizing one's own cultural biases, which can influence interactions with those receiving service and care. Professionals need to actively educate themselves about the cultural traditions and values of the communities they serve, moving beyond factual knowledge to appreciate the emotional and symbolic meanings embedded in cultural practices.

Cultural humility is crucial in end-of-life and grief support because it encourages caregivers to approach each individual openly and respectfully. Cultural humility recognizes and respects that each person has unique cultural identities, experiences, and perspectives. This practice involves active listening, validating experiences, and sometimes authentically admitting a lack of knowledge, demonstrating a willingness to learn from those they serve. It requires acknowledging the limits of one's cultural knowledge and being prepared to seek guidance from cultural informants or the persons themselves. For example, some cultures may view death as a transition rather than an end, with specific rituals and ceremonies to honor the deceased and support the grieving process. Understanding and respecting these practices can help strengthen relationships, build rapport, and provide more effective support for healing.

Cultural competence in end-of-life and grief support requires a multifaceted and expanded approach beyond the classical dimensions of cultural awareness, knowledge, and skills. Professionals must continuously engage in learning and self-reflection to understand and appreciate the cultural lenses of those they support because culture is fluid and dynamic and also because of heterogeneity within the same cultural categories. This involves not only acquiring knowledge about different cultural practices and beliefs but also developing the skills to apply this knowledge sensitively and respectfully. Practices helpful for delivering culturally competent end-of-life care and grief support include exploring culturally relevant language, addressing the complexity of issues within specific cultural contexts, and adapting to variations in personal space and touch preferences. Other strategies include adjusting communication styles to align with cultural norms, interpreting emotional expressions within cultural frameworks, and adapting roles and practices as needed. These practices ensure that caregivers are not only aware of cultural differences but also capable of addressing them effectively in their interactions.

Embracing cultural awareness, humility, and competence in end-of-life and grief support is essential for providing compassionate and effective care. These principles help professionals navigate the diverse ways in which individuals and communities experience death, dying, loss, and grief. By fostering a deeper understanding of cultural diversity and maintaining openness to learning, caregivers can offer more meaningful and sensitive support, ultimately contributing to a more inclusive and equitable approach to end-of-life care and grief support. This comprehensive approach ensures that care is respectful, individualized, and responsive to the unique cultural context, enhancing the overall quality and effectiveness of services.

2.4 Practical Guidelines for Culturally Responsive Care

With the ever-changing and complex demographic landscape, embracing cultural diversity is one thing; embodying it in day-to-day, case-to-case situations is another. Various professional organizations have issued guidelines for clinical practices. For example, the National Coalition for Hospice and Palliative Care (2018) issued detailed clinical practice guidelines for quality palliative care. It covers communication and language, screening and assessment, and treatment. The following outlines practical guides for professionals to improve their cultural awareness and competence. This way, culture becomes a strong resource instead of a barrier to support and services. These guides aim to provide actionable steps for integrating cultural sensitivity into practice.

1. **Ascertain cultural preferences:** Identify an individual's cultural preferences upon admission and continue to refine understanding during care plan development and implementation. This should include attention to language needs, non-verbal communication preferences, and cultural customs related to end-of-life care. For example, incorporating interpreters or bilingual staff can bridge lin-

guistic gaps, and understanding how different cultures view autonomy and decision-making helps ensure respect for cultural norms. Beliefs and practices related to death, dying, and grief vary significantly across cultures. For example, many cultures have taboos against discussing death openly, which can influence end-of-life care approaches. Other cultures have specific mourning periods and practices essential for grieving, and ignoring these can lead to disenfranchised grief and emotional distress for the bereaved.

2. **Practice person-centered care:** Engage with clients and their families to honor their cultural identities and needs. Interactions should be guided by openness and cultural humility. It is crucial to remember that culture is dynamic, and individuals may not fit into predefined cultural categories. Asking open-ended questions about cultural backgrounds and preferences builds trust and aligns care with clients' values.
3. **Providing culturally sensitive spiritual care:** Respectfully meeting patients' spiritual needs and meaning-making efforts. Initial and regular spiritual screening and assessments should be integrated to explore spiritual language, beliefs, existential concerns, and sources of strengths. Addressing spiritual distress and involving chaplains or spiritual care specialists ensures a comprehensive response to patient and family needs (NCP, 2018).
4. **Empower the client and address power imbalances:** Empower clients by balancing power dynamics in interactions to foster mutual respect and collaboration. Respect the client's autonomy and involve family members in care decisions to mitigate feelings of powerlessness (Tervalon & Murray-García, 1998). Collaborate with culturally relevant support systems, such as family and faith community leaders, when requested to ensure culturally congruent care (Simpson, 2022).
5. **Communicate sensitively and maintain a compassionate presence:** Facilitate communication by respecting family dynamics, culturally appropriate language, and nonverbal cues. Using symbols and language reflective of cultural and spiritual practices enhances understanding (NCP, 2018). Employing interpreters and community spiritual leaders supports nuanced communication that respects patient and family preferences (NCP, 2018). Linguistic or cultural barriers can be challenging, but they should not deter human communication, as communication is fundamentally about forming understandings and connections. Cultivating a compassionate presence and being open to listening and learning helps with such a connection. The renowned doctor Elisabeth Kubler-Ross noted, "I've not done anything except sit with people and listen to them and hear them" (Kubler-Ross, 1983).
6. **Ensuring institutional accountability and support:** Foster environments that support cultural humility and competence. Ongoing staff training focused on the cultural and spiritual beliefs of diverse populations should be provided to cultivate cultural humility, empathy, and skills in recognizing spiritual distress, as well as an open approach to care. Implement policies that promote diversity and equity and ensure that services are both linguistically and culturally appropriate (NASW, 2015; NCP, 2018).

7. **Interprofessional allies and collectivity:** Recognize that death, dying, grieving, and healing are collective human experiences best supported through interprofessional collaboration. This involves teamwork with social workers, chaplains, translators, and other professionals who ensure integrated care. Partnerships with community spiritual care providers enhance well-rounded care (NCP, 2018).

Case Study: Culturally Responsive End-of-Life Care and Grief Support

1. **A Latino Family Confronts End-of-Life Decisions:** An elderly Puerto Rican immigrant with diabetes faced end-of-life decisions. The family prioritized collective decision-making, requiring the healthcare team to navigate cultural nuances and involve the family in all critical discussions. This approach ensures that the patient's and family's values are respected, leading to more culturally sensitive care (Markkula Center for Applied Ethics, 2021).
2. **Orthodox Jewish Family During Sabbath:** An Orthodox Jewish couple faced challenges during childbirth on the Sabbath, which restricted their ability to drive, use the phone, or handle money. The healthcare team arranged for the husband to stay with his wife and accommodate their dietary needs, demonstrating cultural competence and sensitivity to religious practices.
3. **Supporting a South Asian Family in Grief:** A South Asian family faced challenges in accepting pain management for a terminally ill family member due to cultural and religious beliefs. The healthcare team engaged a cultural liaison to facilitate discussions, respecting the family's values while ensuring the patient's comfort. This approach helped bridge cultural gaps and provided more effective and compassionate care.
4. **Navigating Grief with an African American Family:** A young African American boy with uncontrolled asthma returned to the clinic owing to his family's mistrust of the healthcare system. Healthcare providers work to build trust through consistent, empathetic communication and the involvement of community leaders. This approach helped the family feel respected and supported, improving the child's health outcomes and overall well-being.

2.5 Concluding Reflection

Culture shapes the human psyche and behaviors, making cultural awareness, competence, and humility essential for human service professionals, particularly in end-of-life and grief support. Cultural awareness is a prerequisite, and humility serves as the foundation for enabling cultural competence. Humility ensures professionals remain open, adaptable, and free from assumptions, allowing for genuine and compassionate care.

While cultural competency training and shared group membership may enhance skills and knowledge, yet without humility, these can easily lead to stereotypes. Approaching individuals first and foremost as unique, holistic beings helps foster trust and uncovers strengths. Cultural diversity could pose challenges, but it is also an important strength and resource. Tapping into these resources transforms care into an opportunity for connection, growth, and enriched understanding.

When cultural humility leads, competence becomes a powerful tool, much like the bow of a sailboat cutting through waters, guided by cultural awareness as the sail. The multicultural perspectives explored in this chapter—and throughout this book—highlight how diverse culture enriches human experiences, presenting invaluable resources for healing and growth.

References

Abramovitch, H. (2015). Death, anthropology of. In *International Encyclopedia of the social & behavioral sciences* (Vol. 5, pp. 870–873). Elsevier.

American Nurses Association (ANA). (2015). *Nursing: Scope and standards of practice* (3rd ed.). American Nurses Association.

American Psychological Association. (2017). *Multicultural guidelines: An ecological approach to context, identity, and intersectionality*. Retrieved from http://www.apa.org/about/policy/multicultural-guidelines.pdf

Aronson, E., Wilson, T. D., & Akert, R. M. (2007). *Social psychology* (6th ed.). Pearson.

Association for Death Education and Counseling (ADEC). (2004). *ADEC code of ethics*. Retrieved from https://www.adec.org/page/code_of_ethics

Baumeister, R. F., & Bushman, B. J. (2016). *Social psychology and human nature* (4th ed.). Cengage Learning.

Bennett, M. J. (1993). Toward ethnorelativism: A developmental model of intercultural sensitivity. In R. M. Paige (Ed.), *Education for the intercultural experience*. Intercultural Press.

Berry, J. W. (2002). *Cross-cultural psychology: Research and applications*. Cambridge University Press.

Betancourt, J. R., Green, A. R., Carrillo, J. E., & Ananeh-Firempong, O. (2003). Defining cultural competence: A practical framework for addressing racial/ethnic disparities in health and health care. *Public Health Reports, 118*(4), 293–302. https://doi.org/10.1093/phr/118.4.293

Boyd, R., & Richerson, P. J. (1988). *Culture and the evolutionary process*. University of Chicago Press.

Castro, F. G. (1998). Cultural competence training in clinical psychology: Assessment, clinical intervention, and research. In A. S. Bellack & M. Hersen (Eds.), *Comprehensive clinical psychology: Sociocultural and individual differences* (Vol. 10, pp. 127–140). Pergamon.

Chávez, V. (2022). Cultural humility and social inclusion. In P. Liamputtong (Ed.), *Handbook of social inclusion*. Springer. https://doi.org/10.1007/978-3-030-89594-5_7

Ciupak, Y. (2025). *Spiral model of grief and healing: An integrative sociological, psychological, and cultural framework* [Unpublished manuscript]. Northern Michigan University.

Crenshaw, K. (1989). Demarginalizing the intersection of race and sex: A black feminist critique of antidiscrimination doctrine, feminist theory and antiracist politics. *University of Chicago Legal Forum, 1989*(1), 139–167.

Fadiman, A. (1999). The spirit catches you and you fall down: A Hmong child, her American doctors, and the collision of two cultures. *Journal of Public Health Policy, 20*(4), 504–507.

Geertz, C. (1973). *The interpretation of cultures: Selected essays*. Basic Books.

Giger, J. N., Davidhizar, R., Purnell, L., Harden, J. T., Phillips, J., & Strickland, O. (2007). American Academy of Nursing expert panel report: Developing cultural competence to eliminate health disparities in ethnic minorities and other vulnerable populations. *Journal of Transcultural Nursing, 18*(2), 95–102.

Gottlieb, M. (2020). The case for a cultural humility framework in social work practice. *Journal of Ethnic & Cultural Diversity in Social Work, 30*(6), 463–481. https://doi.org/10.1080/15313204.2020.1753615

Hall, E. T. (1959). *The silent language*. Anchor Books.

Henderson, S., Horne, M., Hills, R., & Kendall, E. (2018). Cultural competence in healthcare in the community: A concept analysis. *Health & Social Care in the Community, 26*(5), 590–603. https://doi.org/10.1111/hsc.12556

Hook, J. N., Davis, D., Owen, J., & DeBlaere, C. (2017). *Cultural humility: Engaging diverse identities in therapy*. American Psychological Association.

Institute of Medicine (US) Committee on Quality of Health Care in America. (2001). Crossing the quality chasm: A new health system for the 21st century. *National Academies Press (US).*

International Federation of Social Workers (IFSW). (2018). *Global social work statement of ethical principles*. Retrieved from https://www.ifsw.org/global-social-work-statement-of-ethical-principles

Kagawa-Singer, M., & Blackhall, L. J. (2001). Negotiating cross-cultural issues at the end of life: "You got to go where he lives". *JAMA, 286*(23), 2993–3001. https://doi.org/10.1001/jama.286.23.2993

Kleinman, A., Eisenberg, L., & Good, B. (1978). Culture, illness, and care: Clinical lessons from anthropologic and cross-cultural research. *Annals of Internal Medicine, 88*(2), 251–258. https://doi.org/10.7326/0003-4819-88-2-251

Kubler-Ross, E. (1983). *Elisabeth Kubler-Ross speaks to a dying patient*. Nova Interview. YouTube. Retrieved from https://www.youtube.com/watch?v=tIZ97OALEfE

Lekas, H. M., Pahl, K., & Fuller Lewis, C. (2020). Rethinking cultural competence: Shifting to cultural humility. *Health Services Insights, 13*, 1178632920970580.

Loden, M., & Rosener, J. B. (1991). *Workforce America!: Managing employee diversity as a vital resource*. Business One.

Markkula Center for Applied Ethics. (2021). *Cases on culturally competent care*. Retrieved from https://www.scu.edu

Mazid, S. (2021). Grieving the dead: A sociological analysis of mourning in a pandemic. *The JMC Review: An Interdisciplinary Social Science Journal of Criticism, Practice, and Theory, 5*, 98–114.

Migrant Integration Policy Index (MIPEX). (2015). *How countries are promoting integration of immigrants* [website]. CIDOB and MPG. Retrieved from https://www.mipex.eu

National Association of Social Workers (NASW). (2015). *Standards and indicators for cultural competence in social work practice*. Retrieved from https://www.socialworkers.org/LinkClick.aspx?fileticket=PonPTDEBrn4%3D&portalid=0

National Consensus Project for Quality Palliative Care (NCP). (2018). *Clinical practice guidelines for quality palliative care* (4th ed.). National Coalition for Hospice and Palliative Care. Retrieved from https://www.nationalcoalitionhpc.org/ncp

National Funeral Directors Association (NFDA). (2022). *Code of professional conduct*. Funeral Home Directors Code of Professional Conduct.

Nelson, A. (2002). Unequal treatment: Confronting racial and ethnic disparities in health care. *Journal of the National Medical Association, 94*(8), 666.

Office of Minority Health (OMH). (2013). *Enhanced national standards for culturally and linguistically appropriate services in health and health care*. U.S. Department of Health and Human Services. Retrieved from http://www.thinkculturalhealth.hhs.gov

Olaveson, T. (2001). Collective effervescence and communitas: Processual models of ritual and society in Emile Durkheim and Victor Turner. *Dialectical Anthropology, 26*, 89–124.

Owen, J. (2013). Early career perspectives on psychotherapy research and practice: Psychotherapist effects, multicultural orientation, and couple interventions. *Psychotherapy, 50*(4), 496.

Prickett, P. J., & Timmermans, S. (2022). "If no one grieves, no one will remember": Cultural palimpsests and the creation of social ties through rituals. *The British Journal of Sociology, 73*(2), 244–258.

School of Social Work. (2021). *Master learner workbook: Cultural humility*. University of Illinois at Urbana-Champaign. Retrieved from https://socialwork.illinois.edu/app/uploads/2021/09/Master-Learner-Workbook-Cultural-Humility-1.pdf

Semlali, I., Tamches, E., Singy, P., & Weber, O. (2020). Introducing cross-cultural education in palliative care: Focus groups with experts on practical strategies. *BMC Palliative Care, 19*(1), 171. https://doi.org/10.1186/s12904-020-00678-y

Silverman, G. S., Baroiller, A., & Hemer, S. R. (2021). Culture and grief: Ethnographic perspectives on ritual, relationships, and remembering. *Death Studies, 45*(1), 1–8. https://doi.org/10.1080/07481187.2019.1661133

Simpson, J. (2022). Culturally competent end of life care in district nursing. *Primary Health Care, 33*, 36. https://doi.org/10.7748/phc.2022.e1783

Substance Abuse and Mental Health Services Administration (SAMHSA). (2014). *Improving cultural competence*. Treatment Improvement Protocol (TIP) Series No. 59. Retrieved from https://www.ncbi.nlm.nih.gov/books/NBK248431/

Sue, D. W., Arredondo, P., & McDavis, R. J. (1992). Multicultural counseling competencies and standards: A call to the profession. *Journal of Counseling and Development, 70*(4), 477–486. https://doi.org/10.1002/j.1556-6676.1992.tb01642.x

Tervalon, M., & Murray-García, J. (1998). Cultural humility versus cultural competence: A critical distinction in defining physician training outcomes in multicultural education. *Journal of Health Care for the Poor and Underserved, 9*(2), 117–125. https://doi.org/10.1353/hpu.2010.0233

Tylor, E. B. (1871). *Primitive culture*. Harvard University Press.

UNESCO. (2001). *UNESCO Universal Declaration on Cultural Diversity*. UNESCO.

UNESCO. (2013). *Intercultural competences: Conceptual and operational framework* (W. Leeds-Hurwitz, Ed.). UNESCO. Retrieved from https://unesdoc.unesco.org/ark:/48223/pf0000219768

Van Gennep, A. (2019). *The rites of passage*. University of Chicago press.

World Health Organization (WHO). (2018). *WHO global competency model*. World Health Organization.

World Health Organization (WHO). (2020). *Migration and health: Enhancing intercultural competence and diversity sensitivity*. World Health Organization. Retrieved from https://iris.who.int/handle/10665/332186

Part II
Theories and Concepts in Loss, Grief, and Dying

Chapter 3
Loss and Grief: Concepts and Types

3.1 Introduction

Loss and grief are integral to the human experience, touching everyone at various points in their lives. The way individuals experience and express grief varies significantly across different cultures and developmental stages. Loss and grief can significantly alter one's social role, emotional state, and even physical and economic conditions. Losses can be tangible and finite, such as the death of a loved one, or symbolic and nonfinite, such as a career setback or the end of a relationship. Regardless of the type, loss signifies an absence of something or someone important to us. Physical losses are concrete and irreversible, exemplified by death, which results in the permanent absence of a loved one. Symbolic losses reshape social and psychological landscapes, often altering one's sense of identity. Grief is the natural, albeit painful, response to these losses. Grief is rooted in the human survival needs of attachment and love. A popular quote circulated online poetically captures this paradox between grief and love and vividly captures the various ways grief may manifest:

> *Grief, I've learned, is truly just love. It's all the love you want to give, but cannot. All of that unspent love gathers in the corners of your eyes, the lump in your throat, and in the hollow part of your chest. Grief is just love with no place to go.*[1]

Love, particularly attachment, developed as a human survival mechanism through evolution. As human infants are born immature, human attachment ensures the necessary tending and care. The flip side of the coin is grief when such an attachment is broken or when the attached objects become absent. Therefore, grief is a natural and normal response to a loss. It is a "dis-ease," not a disease, something not

[1] This quote has been shared in personal blogs, social media posts, or grief support communities without clear and verifiable source.

Y. Z. Ciupak, D. C. Smith, *Death, Dying, and Grief*,
https://doi.org/10.1007/978-3-031-88467-2_3

to be cured but rather a process to be navigated. These basic principles of grief are rooted in the depth of human connections and resilience.

Major losses like the death of a close family member or traumatic losses like sexual assault can have lasting impacts on our lives. They challenge our sense of control, shatter the "assumptive world" (Janoff-Bulman, 1992), and often leave a lasting imprint on the consciousness, influencing future interactions and relationships. The intensity and duration of grief vary among individuals and are shaped by many factors: the death encounter, death attitude, personal history, cultural background, the nature of the lost relationship, and more.

Grief extends beyond individuals and families to communities and even the entire society. The global grief experienced during the COVID-19 pandemic is a stark example. The widespread loss of life, disruptions to daily routines, and breakdown of social connections have created a collective wave of grief that continues to ripple through societies.

Historical events, such as the terrorist attack of September 11, and more recent tragedies, such as wars and mass shootings, leave deep scars on communities, becoming significant sources of collective grief and anxiety. Systematic issues such as racism, sexism, and ageism (often embedded in institutional and cultural practices) also contribute to pervasive grief within affected communities. Systemic racism, for example, results in chronic stress and trauma, with high-profile incidents of racial violence and discrimination resonating deeply, leading to widespread grief and demands for social justice. Similarly, sexism and ageism lead to significant collective grief, which impacts mental health and social cohesion.

Grief and loss weave through every stage of life (Hooyman & Kramer, 2006). Everyday losses, such as unmet expectations and life changes, add to the ongoing experience of grief. Childhood experiences, such as the death of a pet, a change in family structure, or relocation, can create an early sense of loss. Adolescents may encounter grief through the end of friendships or romantic breakups that challenge their self-concept. When these losses are not adequately processed, they accumulate, creating a burden of unresolved grief that can significantly impact mental well-being and social behavioral patterns.

Young adulthood brings its own losses, such as career challenges or setbacks, which can evoke feelings of failure and uncertainty, or the loss of social networks when moving for a job or education, which disrupts established support systems. Middle adulthood often involves significant losses like the death of parents, which can evoke deep grief and force an individual to confront their own mortality. Experiences such as divorce or job loss can lead to major life disruptions and identity distress. For older adults, grief can stem from the death of a spouse, which leaves behind profound loneliness, or the loss of independence due to declining health or mobility. During this stage, individuals may experience a loss of social roles, such as transitioning from being a provider or caregiver to retirement. This shift can lead to a feeling of reduced purpose, especially in cultures that place a high value on performance and productivity.

Any grief that is insufficiently validated and processed becomes cumulative. This cumulative grief can manifest as chronic stress, depression, physical illness, or a reduced ability to cope with new losses.

Recognizing and addressing unprocessed grief, especially disenfranchised grief, is crucial for maintaining overall well-being and resilience. Major losses often trigger memories of previous losses, especially during significant life changes such as the death of a partner in older adulthood or the realization of lost opportunities in middle age. These experiences lead to additional secondary losses, reflecting the interconnected nature of life and ever-evolving biography. Acknowledging and processing grief as it occurs helps prevent the accumulation of unresolved grief. The following sections discuss the various types of losses and grief, and Tables 3.1 and 3.2 provide a summary.

Table 3.1 Types of losses

Type of loss	Description	Example	Coping
Primary loss	Direct loss impacting core attachments	Death of a loved one	Seek support Rituals Allow processing grief
Secondary loss	Consequences of the primary loss	Loss of routines, roles, financial stability, or shared dreams	Identify tasks Adapt to new roles Validation Seek resources
Death-related loss (finite loss)	Irreversible and tangible, involving existential reflections	Death of a family member, a friend	Meaning-making Belief reflection Supportive rituals
Nonfinite loss (symbolic loss)	Persistent psychological/social disruptions	Divorce, unemployment, infertility	Acknowledge and validate the loss Explore "lossography" Address unresolved grief
Ambiguous loss (physical absence)	The person is physically missing but remains psychologically present	Missing persons, incarceration	Name the ambiguity Practice both-and thinking Use relational interventions such as family and community-based
Ambiguous loss (psychological absence)	The person is physically present but psychologically unavailable	Dementia, traumatic brain injury	
Traumatic loss	Sudden and violent loss	Accidents, homicides, suicides, sexual abuse, wars	Meaning reconstruction Mindfulness-based practices "Healing relationships" with professionals

Table 3.2 Types of grief

Type of grief	Description	Example
Traumatic grief	Grief resulting from sudden or violent circumstances	War, abuse, homicide, suicide, accident
Anticipatory grief	Grief experienced before an expected loss	Terminal illness
Disenfranchised grief	Grief not socially recognized or validated	Loss of a pet, miscarriage, breakup
Vicarious grief	Grief experienced in response to another's loss	Empathy-driven; grief amplified by personal experiences
Collective grief	Shared grief across communities or societies due to large-scale events	Racism, sexism, mass shootings, natural disasters
Cumulative grief	Multiple, unprocessed losses compounding over time	Series of personal losses across the lifespan
Prolonged grief disorder (PGD)/complicated grief	Persistent and pervasive grief response disrupting daily functioning significantly exceed cultural norms	Pervasive and persistent beyond 6 months (ICD) or 12 months (DSM)

3.2 Primary and Secondary Loss

A primary loss, such as the death of a loved one or the end of a marriage, occurs when a close attachment or relationship is terminated. These losses affect the core of an individual's life and necessitate substantial adaptation. The immediate impact of a primary loss often disrupts an individual's social roles and emotional equilibrium, resulting in a profound grieving process.

A secondary loss follows a primary loss, emerging from the consequences and changing circumstances of the initial loss. For example, after the death of a spouse, an individual may experience the loss of social connections with in-laws, the end of shared activities and routines, and potential financial instability. These losses extend the impact of the primary loss, adding layers of grief that need to be addressed. Taking the death of a spouse, for example, secondary losses may entail any combination of the following:

- Decreased **emotional and physical health:** The stress and emotional toll of grief can lead to increased anxiety, depression, or other mental health challenges. It can also affect physical health, causing fatigue, sleep disturbances, or a weakened immune system.
- **Altered belief system or cognitive framework:** A significant loss poses a challenge to one's meaning system. Individuals may experience profound questioning or alteration of their religious beliefs or assumptions about the world or themselves.
- **Loss of activities and routines**: Shared hobbies and daily routines that involve the loved one may end, leading to a significant void and need for adaptation in daily life.

- **Changes in identity and role:** The bereaved person may struggle with changes in their social role within the family or community, such as transitioning from being a spouse to being single. These changes impact the internalized identity related to social roles.
- **Loss of future dreams and plans:** The bereaved person might grieve the loss of plans and aspirations that involved the deceased, leading to feelings of uncertainty and disorientation.
- **Decreased financial security or quality of life:** The death of a spouse can result in a loss of income and financial instability, affecting the overall quality of life.
- **Loss of social network or support system**: Relationships with friends and family connected to the deceased may weaken or dissolve, and the bereaved person might feel a loss of support from those who do not understand their grief or who distance themselves.

Loss and grief are complex and multifaceted experiences. Understanding primary and secondary losses helps identify the major coping tasks and provides effective support.[2] Addressing the various layers of loss and grief assists in navigating the complex grieving process and facilitates adaptation.

3.3 Death-Related Loss and Nonfinite Loss

Death-related losses (finite losses) are permanent and cannot be recovered or reverted. This type of loss brings human mortality to the forefront of consciousness, provoking existential reflections and biopsychological responses to a broken attachment. Even for those who believe in an afterlife or some form of continuation beyond death, the absence of a physical presence necessitates profound adjustments. The tangible loss of touch, voice, and daily interactions creates a void that fundamentally alters one's daily life and requires significant adaptation.

Death-related losses can be sudden or anticipated, and the circumstances can significantly influence the grieving process in addition to the relationship. For example, witnessing a mass shooting at an elementary school or surviving a car accident that claims a loved one's life can have a more traumatic impact.

Child loss is one of the most intense stressors and is often considered the most difficult type of grief. Bereaved family members are at an elevated risk of prolonged depression and anxiety, with these effects potentially lasting for up to a decade. Additionally, parents facing this loss are more susceptible to a range of physical health issues (Hooyman & Kramer, 2006).

Nonfinite losses (symbolic losses) are those not directly related to death but can still significantly affect an individual. These losses encompass events such as divorce, unemployment, disability, infertility, and loss of social reputation. Nonfinite

[2] Refer to Chap. 4 for discussions of grieving tasks and support strategies.

losses can involve ongoing and unresolved elements that create a persistent sense of grief and loss.

Nonfinite losses are not necessarily less stressful or impactful than death-related losses. For example, the end of a significant relationship can trigger a profound grief response, which is sometimes more intense than the grief experienced after the death of a distant relative. Additionally, the potential for reconciliation in nonfinite losses, such as the hope for a relationship to mend, can challenge acceptance and complicate the grieving process.

Nonfinite losses could also induce disenfranchised grief-grief that is not socially recognized or validated as significant. A couple of years ago, a local high school student took his life after experiencing sextortion. The threat of the perceived loss of his public image was so overwhelming that it led to a tragic outcome. This incident illustrates how deeply nonfinite losses can affect individuals, leading to extreme emotional distress and life-altering consequences. This tragedy indicates the importance of building resilience at both the community and individual levels, fostering a compassionate culture and social buffer against the stigmas attached to victims of sex crimes.

For both death-related and nonfinite losses, each person's response is highly individual, shaped by unique personal history, cultural background, and available support systems. The significance and impact of the loss can only be subjectively evaluated by the person grieving it, not by any standardized stress scale. Acknowledging and validating different types of losses and grief important to the grieving individual is a fundamental principle of grief support. Exploring one's "lossography"—the various types of losses throughout one's lifetime—helps understand the development of coping styles and grief responses.

3.4 Ambiguous Loss

In the mid-1970s, Dr. Pauline Boss coined the term "ambiguous loss" to describe a situation of unclear loss that remains unverified and thus without resolution (Boss, 2018). There are two classifications of ambiguous loss: physical and psychological.

Physical absence with respect to psychological presence occurs when families do not know where their loved ones are or even whether they are dead or alive. This type of loss happens when there is a physical absence of a loved one, but a psychological presence lingers. Examples include missing persons, war, incarceration, and divorce.

Psychological absence with physical presence involves a physical presence but a psychological absence, which is not associated with death. This type of loss can result from cognitive impairment, traumatic brain injury, Alzheimer's disease, or other forms of dementia. There is a distinct emotional or cognitive disconnection correlated with psychologically ambiguous loss.

In recent years, ambiguous losses have gained global recognition, particularly following the COVID-19 pandemic. During lockdown periods and social distancing procedures, individuals across the globe experienced various forms of ambiguous loss and uncertainty. The death of loved ones during this time was especially difficult, as many people died in hospitals or institutions with restricted or no access to family or loved ones (Boss, 2022). Other forms of loss, such as global climate change, also contribute to ambiguous losses through the collective loss of clean water resources, fertile lands, and loss of life.

According to Dr. Pauline Boss, ambiguous losses within the United States may be rooted in generational trauma stemming from the slavery era. The legally enforced separation of families and cultural communities resulted in trauma and ambiguous loss across generations, even in modern society. Similarly, ambiguous losses are also found among indigenous peoples around the world due to colonization and assimilation efforts legally enforced by the government. Both slavery and colonization resulted in oppressed, traumatized generations of people who rarely received recognition or amends for what they lost and endured along the way.

Coping with and Supporting Ambiguous Loss

Dr. Pauline Boss emphasized the importance of meaning reconstruction for both types of ambiguous loss through a paradox of absence and presence (Boss, 2018). She noted that human beings seek certainty over closure after experiencing a loss, meaning that people search for assurance that the loss is real and valid. Individuals experiencing ambiguous loss try to remember the bond or connection and find meaning and certainty in such loss. To manage the complex emotions and reactions associated with ambiguous loss, several coping strategies can be particularly effective:

- **Naming the Ambiguity**: Identifying the ambiguous element of the loss may help bereaved individuals express and process their emotions attached to the loss. Naming the ambiguous factor may aid in effective, productive grief work.
- **Dialectical Thinking**: This enables bereaved people to hold opposing thoughts, emotions, and actions around the loss. Allowing oneself to engage in nonrigid or nonbinary thinking permits us to confront the multitude of emotions and reactions we may experience with grief and loss.

Practicing *both/and thinking* provides an avenue for coping with and supporting ambiguous loss. This method empowers bereaved people to articulate the array of emotions that come with grief and loss. For example, people may feel mournful for the loss and grateful for the memories and experiences shared with the deceased. Utilizing both/and thinking accounts for the complicated and often conflicting emotions that follow loss and grief. Pauline Boss captures this complexity, stating, "I intentionally hold the opposing ideas of absence and presence because I have learned that most relationships are indeed both" (Boss, 2018, p. 210).

It is essential for care providers to recognize the complexity of grief and to validate oftentimes conflicting feelings. Providing a safe and supportive environment for people to express their emotions without judgment is crucial. This could include educating them about ambiguous loss, helping them find languages for their emotions and experiences, and facilitating a contextualizing of their experience.

Additionally, collaboratively exploring coping strategies and care plans can empower individuals to address uncertainties and resolve unresolved issues. This may include finding ways to maintain connections with the absent loved one, engaging in exercises like the "empty chair exercise," guiding visualization techniques, and creating meaningful rituals. Part IV "Addressing Psychosocial Needs" and Part V "Addressing Spiritual Needs in End-of-Life and Grieving" contain many such tools.

Dr. Pauline Boss stated that relational interventions, such as family- or community-based approaches, are more effective than an individualized approach (Boss, 2018). Facilitating connections with support groups or mental health professionals experienced in working with ambiguous loss can also offer valuable resources and validation. Ultimately, the core of supporting ambiguous grief is to encourage a compassionate holding of uncertainties.

3.5 Traumatic Loss and Death

Traumatic loss occurs when an event happens under sudden and violent circumstances, resulting in intense emotional and psychological distress. Such circumstances may result from human-induced acts or natural disasters. Examples of traumatic losses include war, physical/sexual/emotional abuse, car accidents, homicides, and suicides. Grieving individuals often perceive traumatic losses as avoidable or preventable, typically associated with intense emotions.

Traumatic losses can present a multitude of difficulties, including shock effects for bereaved individuals. Shock effects often overwhelm a bereaved person's ability to cope, inducing feelings of terror, fear, and anxiety alongside a sense of victimization, vulnerability, and powerlessness. Another challenge is the difficulty in making sense of the event due to the traumatic circumstances. Attempting to process and comprehend a traumatic death can be demanding because bereaved people may feel that they do not have time to address unfinished businesses or say their goodbyes. The assumption of preventability also affects a griever's ability to make sense of the loss, shattering one's *assumptive worlds* and perception of life (Janoff-Bulman, 1992; Tedeschi & Calhoun, 2004).

3.5.1 Traumatic Loss & Assumptive Worlds

Traumatic loss can shatter *assumptive worlds*, the deeply held set of beliefs about the world and the self. This set of beliefs is developed, maintained, and used to guide cognition, planning, and actions. These assumptions form the foundations of core beliefs and values essential for both psychological well-being and social interactions. Three primary assumed worlds are generally considered beneficial for mental well-being (Janoff-Bulman, 1992; Beder, 2005):

1. **The world is benevolent**: This assumption signifies that the world is generally a benevolent place where people have good intentions. Righteous and unethical actions each have corresponding consequences.
2. **The world is meaningful**: This assumption indicates that things make sense and that there is a cause-effect relationship between events and their outcomes. Events are perceived as coherent and predictable.
3. **The self is worthy**: This assumption allows us to view ourselves as decent and capable beings who, though not perfect, deserve good things.

According to Beder (2005), these *assumptive worlds* are developed and reinforced through one's life experiences. These belief systems help individuals trust that people are fundamentally good and that they live in a benevolent world where things generally make sense. However, when a traumatic death or loss occurs, these beliefs are fundamentally shattered, altering one's perspectives and creating what Durkheim refers to as "anomie" (/ˈæn.ə.miː/)—the breakdown of social or personal norms. This disruption of perceived order and meaning triggers cognitive challenges, intense emotions, and a profound sense of hopelessness (Janoff-Bulman, 1992).

3.5.2 Supporting Traumatic Loss: From Victims to Survivors

Individuals experiencing traumatic loss may face a multitude of hardships on the journey to healing. Supporting someone through a traumatic loss can be simultaneously rewarding and demanding. Research and clinical practices related to trauma have grown substantially, establishing it as a vital specialty area with abundant scholarship beyond the scope of this chapter. The posttraumatic growth literature identifies two key points that are useful for considering posttraumatic growth and productive coping strategies:

1. **Differentiating between traumatic events/deaths and traumatic bereavement**: A traumatic event may or may not cause complicated bereavement, which aligns with resilience studies. **Traumatic bereavement** refers to an intense and complicated grieving process in which the loss itself is traumatic. In traumatic bereavement, grief and trauma are intertwined, impacting a person's entire experience and processing of grief (UK Trauma Council, 2023).
2. **Possibility of posttraumatic growth**: Traumatic experiences may entail the possibility of posttraumatic growth, especially when assisted by an "expert companion," such as a grief or trauma counselor. Seeking help from a professional can assist in reconstructing meaning, addressing various dissociations, and shifting the perspective on the context of the loss and how to move forward (Tedeschi & Calhoun, 2004).

3.5.3 Mechanisms for Supporting and Coping with Traumatic Loss

Meaning Reconstruction

The way individuals experience loss and the meaning they assign to it can determine whether that loss is felt as traumatic. Reconstructing the meaning of the loss and the connection to the deceased is a healthy and effective way to cope. Meaning Reconstruction Therapy, developed by Dr. Robert Neimeyer (2001), adopts a constructionist approach that shifts the focus from achieving closure to fostering meaning. It integrates narrative therapy, storytelling, and metaphors, helping individuals reconstruct their narratives regarding their relationship with themselves, the lost person, and their life story. The aim is to rebuild a sense of coherence and purpose in life.

Frameworks for Recovery

The neurobiological connection between trauma and the body has been thoroughly researched, particularly in Bessel van der Kolk's classic *The Body Keeps the Score.* This research points to somatic therapy as an important approach for releasing trauma. Somatic therapy focuses on increasing awareness of bodily sensations and reactions to stress and trauma, intentionally releasing these sensations (Van der Kolk, 2014).

Mindfulness-based approaches, such as the "five-step unblending" method discussed by Fisher (2017), distance the internal reactions of fragmented parts and reconnect them to the present. This approach recommends the following five steps:

Step 1: Pause and notice: Notice the overwhelming thoughts and emotions without judgment. View them as messages from various inner parts. Describe them as "their" reactions (e.g., "They are upset," "They are overwhelmed") to create emotional distance.

Step 2: Create separation: Foster a slight separation from these feelings by adjusting posture (e.g., lengthen your spine, sit back) and affirming, "They are feeling ______." This helps reduce intensity and allows you to maintain self-awareness.

Step 3: Engage with compassion: Use a calm, supportive mindset to reassure the parts. Acknowledge their fear, sadness, or shame as you would for a friend or colleague. Respond with kindness and ask what they need to feel safer or less distressed.

Step 4: Check feedback: Check if your responses help. Ask what they need right now to feel more supported or less alone. Reassure them with promises of continued care and attention.

Informed by internal family systems, the "five-step unblending" approach draws from techniques of mindfulness. This method aims to help create a separation between their adult self and reactive, fragmented parts that have developed as a result of trauma.

Stages of Trauma Recovery

According to Herman (2022), the stages of trauma recovery include establishing safety, remembering and mourning, and reconnecting with ordinary life. This journey of recovery can be facilitated by a "healing relationship" with a professional. Creating a safe and non-judgmental space and empowering the survivor is essential in facilitating recovery (Herman, 2022, p. 191).

3.5.4 Transitioning from Grief to Growth

Traumatic losses are often associated with more challenges for bereaved individuals. The nature of the traumatic loss (e.g., violent or unexpected death) may lead individuals to ruminate more about their loss than if the loss was expected. Posttraumatic growth is not a linear or immediate process; it requires time, effort, and, most importantly, self-compassion in the grieving process.

The transition from victim to survivor involves reconstructing a sense of safety and meaning in life after a traumatic loss. The journey involves acknowledging and integrating the trauma and reconstructing the shattered assumptive world, which assists in finding new ways to engage with life and relationships. This rebuilding of the assumptive world is not about returning to a state of naive optimism but rather achieving a balanced and resilient perspective that acknowledges both the potential for disaster and the capacity for healing. Janoff-Bulman (1992) beautifully elaborates on this transformation:

> These survivors recognize the possibility of tragedy but do not allow it to pervade their self- and worldviews. For such survivors, the world is benevolent, but not absolutely; events that happen make sense, but not always; the self can be counted on to be decent and competent, but helplessness is at times a reality… There is disillusionment, yet it is generally not the disillusionment of despair. Rather, it is disillusionment tempered by hope… [In the end, this view] involves an acknowledgement of real possibilities, both bad and good—of disaster in spite of human efforts, or triumph in spite of human limitations. (Janoff-Bulman, 1992, pp. 174–175)

3.6 Anticipatory Grief

Anticipatory grief refers to grieving experiences that occur prior to and in connection with a significant, expected loss. It is increasingly recognized as a significant stressor for both terminally ill patients and their social networks (National Cancer Institute, 2024). Anticipatory grief may encompass the total set of cognitive, affective, cultural, and social reactions to the expected death. The signs of anticipatory grief often resemble those experienced after a loss. The National Cancer Institute (2024) identified the most common signs of anticipatory grief as follows:

- Depression
- Heightened concern for the ill
- Rehearsal of the loved one's end-of-life
- Attempts to adjust to the consequences of the loved one's end of life
- Anxiety and worry
- Increased irritability
- Mourning changes in the loved one's personality or physical appearance

While often associated with aging and end-of-life processes, anticipatory grief can also stem from circumstances such as a progressive illness, the decline of a loved one with dementia, or preparing for life-altering changes like separation or relocation. These experiences affect both the individual and their support network.

Coping Mechanisms and Social Support

Anticipatory grief and loss can cast a shadow of doubt, sadness, existential concerns, and other challenges. Effective coping mechanisms and social support are crucial in mitigating these challenges. Social support, interpersonal bonds, stress management, and spiritual exploration can enhance the journey of coping with the continuous journey from anticipatory to post-death grief (Prati & Pietrantoni, 2009; Tedeschi & Calhoun, 2004). These factors foster a positive relationship, helping to manage grief and strengthen bonds. The key aspects of coping and support may include the following:

1. **Proactive care and coping strategies:** Proactive coping strategies prepare individuals and families for mental and emotional challenges during grief. These strategies include learning what to expect and making practical arrangements, such as organizing finances, end-of-life care, and medical planning. Such preparation provides reassurance and control during anticipatory grief.
2. **Social support:** The role of social support in personal growth is vital to fostering resilience while preparing for loss. Mental health professionals, clients, and others involved in end-of-life care often face anticipatory grief. Asking for help or relying on a support network can strengthen bonds with other loved ones. Proactive coping and social support can significantly aid growth during this challenging time (Rogalla, 2020).
3. **Meaning construction and focus on life:** Even in the context of end-of-life care, hope can be nurtured through immediate, achievable goals. Families and caregivers can find purpose in daily moments of connection, seeking "good" days marked by comfort and holistic well-being. This shift brings fulfillment and supports meaning-making during anticipatory grief. Reflecting on shared experiences, creating rituals, and cherishing present moments help build healing, empowering narratives.

While anticipatory grief can be painful, it can also act as a powerful motivator to address unresolved issues and create a supportive environment where positive experiences and memories can be formed. Research shows that anticipatory grief can lead to positive, proactive preparation for loss, stronger relationships, and personal growth (Rogalla, 2020). Chapter 5, which focuses on dying and end-of-life care, features in-depth discussions on this topic. Additionally, Part III and Part IV of this book, Addressing Psychosocial Needs and Spiritual Needs in End-of-Life and Grieving, offer a variety of practical tools to help individuals and their families navigate the challenges of dying and anticipatory grief.

In conclusion, adopting a compassionate and mindful approach to anticipatory grief can effectively manage emotional strain while improving the quality of time spent together. It also addresses practical matters associated with end-of-life planning. By enriching daily life and tackling unfinished business, dying persons and their families can find comfort during this difficult period, which ultimately promotes healthier grieving and coping processes after a loved one's passing.

3.7 Disenfranchised Grief

Disenfranchised grief is grief that is not or cannot be openly acknowledged, publicly mourned, or socially supported. Since Dr. Kenneth J. Doka introduced this concept in his 1989 book *Disenfranchised Grief: Recognizing Hidden Sorrow,* this valuable concept has expanded and applied widely.[3] This type of grief occurs when the loss experienced by an individual is not recognized or is dismissed by societal norms and expectations. This lack of recognition can leave individuals without the necessary social support to process their grief effectively.

Grief can be disenfranchised in terms of the structural elements of bereavement or functional elements. The structural elements of bereavement may be as follows:

- **Relationship**: When the relationship is not granted social approval, such as secret relationships, extramarital affairs, or same-sex relationships in nonaccepting communities.
- **Loss**: When the significance of the loss is not recognized by society. This can include losses such as miscarriage, the death of a pet, or the loss of a job.
- **The griever**: When the individual is not viewed by society as entitled to the experience of grief or the processes of mourning. This often happens with sibling grief, ex-spouses, individuals with intellectual disabilities, or those perceived to be emotionally strong.

Grief can also be disenfranchised in terms of the dynamic or functional elements of bereavement:

- **The grief reactions**: When the individual's experience and expressions of grief are viewed by society as inappropriate. This can include the absence, intensity, or length of mourning that does not conform to societal expectations of how one should grieve for their social roles or relationships with the deceased.

[3] See Doka's (2020) article that discusses the evolution of the concept and integrate literature exploring the phenomenon.

- **Mourning responses**: When the individual's ways of coping with grief and loss are rejected by society. This can include nontraditional mourning practices or personal rituals that are not understood or accepted by others.

Two Examples of Disenfranchised Grief
Romantic breakups frequently go unrecognized as "real" grief despite the significant psychosocial distress they can cause. These breakups can lead to various emotional and behavioral problems. Young adults, in particular, often experience negative self-concepts following a romantic heartbreak. This experience can mirror prolonged grief typically associated with the death of a loved one (Hooyman & Kramer, 2006). Society's lack of validation and support for grief from romantic breakups indicates how these losses exemplify disenfranchised grief.

Another example of common disenfranchised grief is pet loss. Numerous studies and cross-cultural explorations have highlighted the importance of the human–animal bond, which can manifest as an emotional attachment similar to that of human relationships. The grief from losing a pet can be as profound as losing a human loved one (Lavorgna & Hutton, 2019). However, grief following the loss of a beloved pet is frequently minimized and goes unnoticed. This can result in depression, regret, intrusive thoughts, and loneliness (Packman et al., 2014). The lack of social support and the tendency to suppress grief further contribute to disenfranchised grief (Cesur-Soysal & Ari, 2024).

Challenges of the Disenfranchised Grief
Individuals experiencing disenfranchised grief face significant psychological and social challenges in mourning their losses. They may experience isolation and shame, question the legitimacy of their feelings, and struggle to seek support from others who may not understand or acknowledge their pain. This lack of validation can hinder the grieving process, as individuals find expressing and processing their emotions difficult.

A lack of social approval and support may intensify reactions, such as heightened anger, guilt, or loneliness. They might also internalize the lack of recognition, leading to internal conflict and minimizing their feelings. This can result in unresolved grief, where individuals are unable to fully process their loss, potentially leading to long-term issues in mental health and social interactions.

Coping Strategies
To cope with disenfranchised grief, individuals can consider several strategies:

1. **Social support**: Finding or creating a support system with people who understand or are willing to listen can be validating. This might include friends, family, support groups, counselling, or online communities.
2. **Engaging in personal rituals**: Personal rituals, such as writing a letter, holding a small ceremony, or engaging in cultural or religious practices, can help one express and process grief.
3. **Communication needs**: Clear communication of one's needs and feelings may help one receive the necessary support. This might involve explaining the nature of the loss and its emotional impact.

4. **Professional help**: Seeking therapy or counseling can provide a safe and non-judgmental space to process grief and develop coping mechanisms.

Supporting and Working with the Disenfranchised Grief
When supporting individuals experiencing disenfranchised grief, it is important to do the following:

- **Be sensitive to the complexity and range of losses**: Recognizing that loss is individually perceived and evaluated and that each person's grief experience is unique.
- **Validate grief**: Acknowledge the significance of their loss, even if society does not recognize it. Validating their grief can help them feel understood and supported.
- **Develop therapeutic rituals**: Encouraging the use of rituals, which can provide a structured way to express grief and help individuals feel connected to their loss and others who understand their pain. This may range from traditional practices such as fire pujas to personalized rituals, including personal altars and memorials that honor and process the loss. Part III of this book is particularly valuable for guidance on this topic, with Chaps. 10 and 13 offering a diverse array of ritual practices that can aid in the healing process.

Disenfranchised grief signifies the social aspect of grief, highlighting how the social construction of mourning, as well as support, impacts the grieving process. By acknowledging the unique challenges of disenfranchised grief and providing validation and acceptance, we can help individuals navigate their emotional journeys and find paths to healing and resilience.

3.8 Vicarious Grief

Vicarious grief (VG) refers to the grief experienced in response to someone else's loss. It was first introduced by Robert Kastenbaum in the late 1970s, who observed elderly women expressing sorrow for the death of individuals whom they did not personally know. Manifestations of VGs are similar but not identical to those of direct loss, including reactions such as weeping, feelings of emptiness and heaviness, sleep and appetite disturbances, and preoccupation with the incident.

Rando (1991) expanded on Kastenbaum's work and identified two types of VGs. In Type 1, the vicarious griever empathizes with what the bereaved must be feeling. Type 2 VGs, however, involve both vicarious and personal losses, where the vicarious mourner experiences their own grief while empathizing with the bereaved. Sometimes, these losses are indistinguishable, as another person's grief can remind one of unfinished grief. Intense reactions in Type 2 VGs can range from extreme shock to temporary impairment and may also involve a violation or destabilization of the mourner's assumptions about reality or themselves. These disruptions can trigger a crisis of meaning and a re-examination of beliefs (Sullender, 2010). The factors that determine the likelihood and potency of VGs include the following:

- **Physical distance**: The closer the second griever is to the primary griever, the more intense the vicarious grief can be. Compared with mass shootings in other states, mass shootings in a neighboring county induce more intense VGs.
- **Psychological distance**: Greater psychological closeness or identification with the primary griever increases the intensity of vicarious grief.
- **Social relationship distance**: Social connections and the degree to which relationships impact the severity of VGs.
- **Specific features of the death situation**: Factors such as unpredictability can heighten VG. Examples are traumatic death due to suicide, mass shootings, and natural or social disasters.
- **One's own unprocessed grief**: Unresolved personal grief can amplify the experience of VGs when triggered by another's loss.

The above factors align with some of the key mediators of mourning in the renowned Task Models elaborated by Worden (2008). This includes who the person died was, the nature of the attachment, and how the person died.

The phenomenon of vicarious grief is amplified by modern media, which makes distant tragedies feel immediate and personal through vivid imagery and personal accounts. Constant coverage of death and grief events encourages viewers to engage emotionally, broadening the circle of mourners beyond immediate family and friends. For example, the death of a celebrity can extend mourning to a global audience through widespread media coverage, deepening experiences of vicarious grief (Sullender, 2010).

Vicarious traumatization shares similarities with vicarious grief but, with its intensified effects, can lead to heightened stress and secondary trauma symptoms. The accessibility of social media further amplifies these effects, serving as a catalyst for both vicarious grief and traumatization. For example, the Halloween stampede in Korea in October 2022, which claimed the lives of many young people, left lasting emotional impacts on viewers worldwide. Some college students, despite being far from the event, reported experiencing distressing emotions after witnessing the tragedy through social media. This distress interrupted their daily routines, revealing the deep impact of vicarious trauma in the digital age.

Coping and Supporting Strategies for Vicarious Grief

Vicarious grief (VG) is related to compassion fatigue; both can impact professionals in care and crisis-response roles, such as healthcare workers, first responders, and social workers. Preventing and coping with vicarious grief involves identifying red flag stress signs and formulating holistic self-care plans (Harrison & Westwood, 2009). The following are some tips to cope with and support vicarious grief:

1. **Practice self-awareness and reflection:** Recognize and understand emotional responses. Notice the bodily sensations that are associated with the emotion. Reflect on triggers and develop strategies to manage them, such as through

breathing techniques. Journaling the experiences helps process and release stored emotions, gaining clarity on the impact of vicarious grief.
2. **Use mindfulness and relaxation techniques**: Incorporate mindfulness techniques such as meditation, deep breathing exercises, and yoga. These practices can reduce stress and enhance emotional regulation (Shapiro et al., 2005).
3. **Seek social and professional support**: Consult a counselor for tailored coping strategies. Join professional-facilitated or peer support groups to share experiences and learn from others.
4. **Prioritize self-care**: Examine aspects of self-care across all areas and formulate goals and plans—physical, psychological, social, spiritual, and professional.

Organizational Support Strategies
Organizations are crucial in addressing and supporting vicarious grief and resilience among care professionals. By fostering a culture of well-being and providing resources for coping with grief and trauma, organizations can create a healthier and more resilient workforce (Grauerholz et al., 2020). This may involve:

1. **Psychoeducation and professional development**: Organizations should provide comprehensive education on grief dynamics, vicarious trauma, and self-care strategies. This includes offering continuous professional development opportunities and providing resources such as training programs, workshops, and literature. Understanding these concepts and having access to professional growth tools can help professionals navigate their emotional experiences more effectively.
2. **Structured debriefing sessions**: Conduct regular debriefing sessions where professionals can discuss challenging experiences in a supportive environment. These sessions, led by experienced facilitators, help in processing emotions and developing coping strategies.
3. **Creating a supportive work culture**: Foster an environment that prioritizes holistic well-being. Encourage open communication about emotional challenges and provide access to employee assistance programs (EAPs) for additional support.
4. **Encouraging work–life balance**: Promotion of healthy work–life balance by encouraging employees to engage in nonwork-related activities and hobbies. Ensuring time to relax and recharge is crucial for mental health.
5. **Providing supportive peer networks:** Establishing peer support networks or mentorship programs where professionals can connect and share their experiences with colleagues who understand their unique challenges. These networks can offer emotional support, practical advice, and a sense of community.

In addition to the above general guidelines, Chap. 6 offers additional strategies and self-care tips to prevent compassion fatigue and address vicarious grief.

3.9 Cumulative and Collective Loss and Grief

Cumulative or compounded loss and grief describe experiencing multiple losses that occur consecutively without being adequately addressed. Various losses occur throughout one's life, as aptly captured by the title of Hooyman and Kramer's (2006) book *Living through Loss*. From childhood to adolescence, young adulthood to middle age, and into older adulthood, losses and grief accompany the entire life journey.

These losses can range from the loss of family structure, friendships, or romantic relationships to loss of identity, the death of loved ones, unemployment, and loss of mental or physical health. While adapting to these changes can strengthen resilience, unacknowledged or unprocessed grief can accumulate, leading to delayed or intensified grieving reactions. This can affect one's self-concept and "assumptive world (Janoff-Bulman, 1992)," potentially leading to mental and behavioral issues. Grief or bereavement overload occurs when multiple significant losses happen within a short period, creating an intensified magnitude of stressors. This compounded experience can make the grieving and adaptation process especially challenging, as individuals may struggle to process and cope with the cumulative burden.

Collective loss and grief refer to the shared experience of entire communities, groups, or societies feeling loss and grief simultaneously. This phenomenon can arise from systemic injustices-patterns of inequality embedded in institutional practices and social norms, including what some scholars term laissez-faire, which sustains inequality through inaction and subtle biases. These collectively-experienced injustices, such as racism, sexism, and ageism, reflect structural forces that shape life chances and access to care. Additionally, collective loss can result from significant events, including natural disasters, wars, mass shootings, and environmental crises, which often lead to feelings of powerlessness and hopelessness.

The COVID-19 pandemic created collective and cumulative grief that impacted people around the world. For many younger generations, this has been their first experience of widespread loss and grief. Every society has felt the effects, from the loss of loved ones due to the virus to the disruption of everyday normalcy and social interactions.

Collective loss and grief do not depend solely on an individual's relationship with the deceased; rather, they reflect the interconnection of humanity. Those who are grieving may find comfort in community-based and relational coping to express and process their losses. This may include community rituals, ceremonies, and workshops involving interactive activities that can effectively support collective grief. Equally important is to identify allies and consider ways to promote change and healing on the system and societal level.

In conclusion, loss and grief are intrinsically personal yet also collective and dynamic. The cumulative impact of various losses has a profound effect on a grieving person's life and concept of self and the world. The combined effects of multiple losses can amplify stress, increasing the demand for adaptation to changes. Therefore, it is crucial to understand the unique aspects of each loss and the totality of their effects to assess our grief properly. Grief mapping and other tools discussed in Chap. 10

provide methods to explore one's loss and coping experiences. The shared experience of collective grief fosters empathy, allowing people to navigate challenges and bond over common struggles. Shared grief can create a sense of solidarity and strength, enabling individuals to face adversities while promoting positive social change.

3.10 Prolonged Grief Disorder/Complicated Grief

Prolonged grief disorder (PGD) used to be termed and studied as "complicated grief" is a mental health condition characterized by intense and persistent grief that disrupts daily functioning. While most individuals adapt to grief over time, approximately 7–10% depict prevalent and persistent intense grief trajectories that are considered to warrant professional intervention (Szuhany et al., 2021).

The *International Classification of Diseases*, 11th Edition (ICD-11; World Health Organization [WHO], 2019) is a globally recognized system for classifying and coding health conditions. The *Diagnostic and Statistical Manual of Mental Disorders*, Fifth Edition, Text Revision (DSM-5-TR; American Psychiatric Association [APA], 2022) is a key resource for diagnosing mental disorders in clinical and research settings. Both manuals have recently established criteria for diagnosing PGD. However, they differ in specific symptom items and requirements.

Historically, DSM had been hesitant to recognize complicated grief as a psychiatric diagnosis because it was not clearly distinguished from uncomplicated grief or other psychiatric disorders that can be triggered by bereavement, such as clinical depression. However, the American Psychiatric Association (APA) eventually concluded that there was sufficient research-based evidence to establish that prolonged grief is a disorder distinct from the normal grieving process. As APA President Vivian B. Pender, M.D., stated, "Grief is normal, but not at certain levels and not most of the day, nearly every day for months" (American Psychiatric Association, 2021). The APA CEO and medical director Saul Levin, M.D., M.P.A., added, "Including prolonged grief disorder in the DSM-5-TR will mean that mental health clinicians, patients, and families alike share an understanding of what normal grief looks like and what might indicate a long-term problem" (2021). Table 3.3 compares PGD with common grief.

3.10.1 Definition and Diagnostic Criteria: Overview

Prolonged grief disorder is generally defined as "a disturbance in which, following the death of a partner, parent, child, or another person close to the bereaved, there is a persistent and pervasive grief response with specific characteristics" (ICD-11). Prolonged grief disorder (PGD) was recognized in both the *International Classification of Diseases*, 11th Edition (ICD-11) in 2018 and the *Diagnostic and Statistical Manual of Mental Disorders*, Fifth Edition Text Revision (DSM-5-TR) released in 2022. Both diagnostic frameworks address the persistent and impairing

Table 3.3 Prolonged Grief Disorder (PGD) vs. common grief

Aspect	Common grief	Prolonged Grief Disorder (PGD)
Duration	Response decreases over time, typically within 6–12 months	Intense response persists beyond 6 months (ICD) or 12 months (DSM) and is significantly prolonged compared to cultural norms
Emotional response	Sadness, longing, and sorrow gradually diminish	*Intense, pervasive* emotional pain, sadness, and yearning
Functionality	Daily life slowly resumes; occasional sadness may return	*Significant impairment* in personal, family, social, educational, occupational, or other important areas of functioning
Focus of grief	Grief gradually integrates into life, allowing other activities	Constant preoccupation with the deceased, difficult to allow restorative activities or breaks
Behavioral response	Grieving behaviors (e.g., avoiding reminders) diminish over time	Persistent avoidance of reminders or inability to reconnect socially.
Cultural norms	Grief reactions fall within cultural or societal context	Grief reactions and duration *exceed standard cultural or religious norms*
Co-occurring conditions	Grief usually occurs without major psychological conditions	May co-occur with PTSD, depression, or anxiety disorders

Sources: Based on *International Classification of Diseases, 11th Edition* (World Health Organization, 2019) and the *Diagnostic and Statistical Manual of Mental Disorders, Fifth Edition, Text Revision* (American Psychiatric Association, 2022)

nature of prolonged grief but differ in their criteria, timelines, and diagnostic specifics. Table 3.4 compares the major diagnostic criteria of the two systems.

Both the ICD-11 and the DSM-5-TR include core symptoms centered around intense yearning or longing for the deceased and preoccupation with the deceased. These core symptoms form the foundation for diagnosing PGD in both diagnostic systems.

3.10.2 ICD-11 Criteria for PGD

The ICD-11 criteria adopt a typological approach, emphasizing a simplified and flexible diagnostic structure accommodating cultural differences.

Core Symptoms:

- Persistent and pervasive longing or yearning for the deceased
- Persistent and pervasive cognitive preoccupation with the deceased

Additional Symptoms (at least one of the following indicators of intense emotional pain):

- Difficulty accepting death
- Feelings of disbelief or emotional numbness over the loss

Table 3.4 Comparison of PGD criteria by ICD-11 (2018) vs. DSM-5-TR (2022)

Criteria	ICD-11 (prolonged grief disorder)	DSM-5-TR (prolonged grief disorder)
Event criterion	Bereavement following the death of a partner, parent, child, or another person close to the bereaved	Death of someone close, with the death occurring at least 12 months ago (6 months for children/adolescents)
Separation distress	Persistent and pervasive grief response, characterized by either: (1) intense longing for the deceased or (2) preoccupation with the deceased	Persistent grief response characterized by either: (1) intense yearning/longing for the deceased, or (2) preoccupation with thoughts or memories of the deceased, present most days for at least the past month
Accompanying symptoms	The grief response is accompanied by intense emotional pain, such as sadness, guilt, anger, denial, or blame, and may also involve difficulty accepting the death, a sense that a part of oneself has died, an inability to experience positive emotions, emotional numbness, or difficulty engaging in social or other activities	The grief is accompanied by at least three of the following symptoms: (1) identity disruption (feeling that part of oneself has died), (2) disbelief about the death, (3) avoidance of reminders of the loss, (4) intense emotional pain (such as anger, bitterness, or sorrow), (5) difficulty reintegrating into life, (6) emotional numbness, (7) feeling life is meaningless, or (8) intense loneliness. These symptoms must be present most days for at least the past month
Functional impairment	The disturbance causes significant impairment in personal, family, social, educational, occupational, or other important areas of functioning. If functioning is maintained, it requires additional effort	The disturbance causes clinically significant distress or impairment in social, occupational, or other important areas of functioning

(continued)

Table 3.4 (continued)

Criteria	ICD-11 (prolonged grief disorder)	DSM-5-TR (prolonged grief disorder)
Cultural and time context	The grief persists for an atypically long period following the loss, markedly exceeding expected social, cultural, or religious norms for the bereaved's culture and context (generally persisting for more than 6 months)	The grief reaction persists for at least 12 months for adults (6 months for children/ adolescents), significantly exceeding expected social, cultural, or religious norms for the individual's cultural context
Exclusion of other conditions	The symptoms are not better explained by another mental disorder, such as major depressive disorder or posttraumatic stress disorder (PTSD), and are not attributable to the physiological effects of a substance or another medical condition	The disturbance is not better explained by major depressive disorder, PTSD, another mental disorder, or attributable to the effects of a substance or another medical condition

Sources: Based on *International Classification of Diseases, 11th Edition* (World Health Organization, 2019) and the *Diagnostic and Statistical Manual of Mental Disorders, Fifth Edition, Text Revision* (American Psychiatric Association, 2022)

- Difficulty engaging in social or other activities
- Identity disruption (feeling lost or incomplete without the deceased)
- Intense emotional pain (such as sadness, guilt, anger, denial, and blame)
- Difficulty moving on with life (e.g., problems making plans for the future, engaging in new activities, or maintaining relationships)

Duration:

- Symptoms must persist for at least 6 months after bereavement.

3.10.3 DSM-5-TR Criteria for PGD

The DSM-5-TR criteria provide a more detailed and symptom-specific framework for diagnosing PGD.

Core Symptoms:

- Persistent longing for the deceased
- Intense sorrow and emotional pain

Additional Symptoms (at least three of the following):

- Preoccupation with thoughts of the deceased
- Preoccupation with the circumstances of death
- Marked difficulty accepting the death
- Avoiding reminders of the loss
- Inability to move on with life, such as difficulties in engaging with friends, pursuing interests, or planning for the future

- Feeling that life is meaningless or empty without the deceased
- Intense loneliness (feeling alone or detached from others)
- Disbelief or emotional numbness can occur during loss
- Feeling that a part of oneself has died along with the deceased
- Difficulty in trusting others since death
- Experiencing identity disruption (e.g., feeling that a part of oneself has died)

Duration:

- Symptoms must persist for at least 12 months after bereavement.

3.10.4 Summary on ICD-11 and DSM-5-TR Criteria for PGD

In summary, both major diagnostic systems recognize PGD as a mental health issue and have reached a consensus on the term previously referred to as "pathological grief" or "complicated grief" in research and practice. The ICD-11 requires symptoms to persist for at least 6 months, whereas the DSM-5-TR stipulates a duration of 12 months (for children and adolescents, it should persist for at least 6 months). With respect to symptom quantity, the ICD-11 requires only one additional symptom, whereas the DSM-5-TR requires three. The DSM-5-TR places more emphasis on cognitive and behavioral symptoms, such as preoccupation with thoughts of the deceased and avoidance of reminders, whereas the ICD-11 focuses more on emotional pain and difficulty moving on with life. Furthermore, the DSM-5-TR criteria are more detailed, with more specific additional symptoms than the ICD-11 criteria do.

Despite these differences, both sets of criteria recognize intense emotional pain and maladaptation as core aspects of PGD. They both acknowledge the significant impact on social functioning and identity disruption as key components of the disorder. Moreover, both cultural and developmental considerations are emphasized in the context of diagnosis. These nuances reflect the evolving attempts in mental and social services to provide necessary interventions to ensure appropriate care while avoiding pathologizing normal human experiences.

3.10.5 Boundary with Posttraumatic Stress Disorder and Depressive Episodes (ICD-11)

According to ICD-11, prolonged grief disorder could occur in individuals who experience bereavement as a result of the death of a loved one occurring in traumatic circumstances. In PGD, the person may be preoccupied with memories of the circumstances surrounding the death. However, unlike those with PTSD, they do not re-experience these memories as occurring again both here and now.

Some common symptoms of prolonged grief disorder are similar to those observed in a depressive episode, such as sadness, loss of interest in activities, social withdrawal, feelings of guilt, and suicidal ideation. However, PGD is differentiated from a Depressive Episode because its symptoms are specifically focused on the loss of the loved one, whereas depressive thoughts and emotional reactions typically encompass multiple areas of life. Additionally, other common symptoms of PGD, such as difficulty accepting the loss, feeling angry about the loss, and feeling as though a part of the individual has died, are not characteristic of a depressive episode. The timing of the onset of symptoms in relation to the loss is also crucial in making this distinction. Despite these differences, PGD and mood disorders can co-occur, and both should be diagnosed if the full diagnostic requirements for each are met.

Research indicates a significant comorbidity between major depressive disorder (MDD) and complicated/prolonged grief disorder. Moreira et al. (2022) reported that individuals with MDD presented significantly higher rates of CG than did those without a history of depression. Moreover, bereavement can precipitate depressive symptoms, especially when grief becomes prolonged or complicated. Factors influencing the risk of comorbid depression and prolonged grief include pre-existing mental health conditions, social support availability, and the nature of the loss. In addition, unexpected or traumatic losses increase the likelihood of both complicated grief and depression, as these types of losses disrupt an individual's ability to find meaning and adapt. This aligns with findings from other studies indicating that prolonged or complicated grief often coexists with depressive disorders, particularly when vulnerabilities such as poor social support or prior mental health challenges are present.

3.10.6 Cultural and Developmental Considerations

An individual experiencing a grief reaction that is within a normative period, given their cultural and religious context, should not be assigned a diagnosis of prolonged grief disorder. ICD-11 suggests considering whether other people who share the bereaved person's cultural or religious perspective (e.g., family, friends, community) regard the response to the loss or duration of the reaction as abnormal.

Children and adolescents may respond to the loss of a primary attachment figure (e.g., a parent or caregiver) with an intense and sustained grief response, which may be greater in intensity, symptomatology, and duration because of the role these individuals play in the child's life. Aspects of the grief response may be retriggered at various points during the individual's development, for example, as new needs arise that would normally be supplied by the parent or caregiver. ICD-11 recommends that these reactions be regarded as normal, and the diagnosis of prolonged grief disorder should be assigned with caution to children and adolescents in this situation.

3.10.7 *Concerns and Challenges*

Even before the inclusion of prolonged grief disorder (PGD) in diagnostic manuals such as the DSM-5-TR, there had been two decades of debate surrounding its classification. Proponents argue that the classification enhances practitioner knowledge, increases access to resources, raises public awareness, and establishes a benchmark for research (Shear, 2022). However, many researchers and practitioners have continued to express concerns about the implications of formal inclusion and challenges in the diagnosis of PGD (Eisma, 2023). These concerns revolve around the medicalization of normal grief responses, the risk of pathologizing natural emotional reactions, and the broader societal and clinical impacts of such a diagnosis.

Potential Pathologization Critics caution that classifying complicated grief as a disorder might pathologize typical grief reactions, which are often intense and persistent yet still within the range of normal responses to a significant loss. This could result in normal grief being inappropriately treated as a mental illness, potentially leading to stigmatization and unnecessary treatment (Bergsmark & Ramsing, 2023; Weir, 2018).

Inappropriate Medication and Training There is a risk that antidepressants, which have not been proven effective for grief-related issues, may be prescribed more frequently to bereaved individuals. Antidepressants are typically prescribed for depression, and their use in treating grief could lead to inadequate and potentially harmful treatment. Most prescriptions for antidepressants are written by primary care physicians rather than psychiatrists, who may lack specialized training in addressing grief (Attig et al., 2013).

Criteria and Timing Differentiating between normal and pathological grief is challenging, with debates over appropriate time frames and symptom criteria for accurately diagnosing PGD without pathologizing normal grief processes (Weir, 2018).

Stigmatization The establishment of PGD as a diagnosis may lead to stigmatization. Individuals diagnosed with PGD might face negative societal reactions, including labelling, stereotyping, and discrimination. Stigma can lead to increased depression, social isolation, and reduced help-seeking behavior (Bergsmark & Ramsing, 2023).

Pharmacotherapy Risks The inclusion of PGD might promote pharmacotherapy for grief despite its equivocal efficacy and potential adverse side effects. Pharmacological treatment risks include blunting emotional processing, which is essential for adapting to loss and reducing social connectedness by dampening emotional engagement (Shear, 2022). The effectiveness of antidepressants, such as SSRIs, in directly addressing grief-specific symptoms remains limited, with side effects like nausea, fatigue, and weight gain adding to the concerns.

Overmedicalization and reliance on medication may shift focus away from psychotherapeutic and holistic interventions that support natural recovery (Eisma, 2023).

Cultural issues Cultural differences play a significant role in shaping the expression, recognition, and response to grief, including prolonged grief disorder (PGD). However, current diagnostic criteria for PGD are largely derived from studies conducted within Western populations, offering limited cultural relevance for diverse groups. Researchers increasingly advocate for cross-cultural studies to enhance the development and validation of screening tools and culturally attuned interventions, ensuring they address the unique needs of various communities (Hilberdink et al., 2023).

While the inclusion of PGD in the ICD-11 and DSM-5-TR introduces standardized criteria for diagnosing pathological grief, it also raises concerns and challenges in application. Addressing these issues requires continued research and careful consideration of cultural contexts to avoid the pitfalls of medicalizing normal grief and to mitigate potential negative societal impacts.

3.10.8 Practical Tips for Professionals and Practitioners

The recent inclusion of PGD in diagnostic manuals poses various opportunities and challenges for caregivers and professionals. Numerous books and articles published on grief therapies directly or indirectly address PGD.[4] The Center for Prolonged Grief at Columbia University provides valuable resources and training designed to support those dealing with PGD. In addition to the general principles and guidelines, such as forming "therapeutic allies" and cultural sensitivity, some general practical tips and considerations are as follows:

1. **Focus on healing milestones**: Structure therapy around the key healing milestones/tasks, which may include accepting the reality of the loss, processing grief, adjusting to a world without the deceased, facilitating continuing bonds while integrating the loss into life, and more (Worden, 2008).
2. **Person-centered interventions**: Employ specific, structured interventions such as cognitive-behavioral strategies and exposure-based techniques such as imaginal revisiting and memory-building exercises. These methods and many other complicated grief-focused intervention modalities can help clients process grief and build a renewed sense of identity.

[4] For a recent comprehensive discussion on the diagnosis, assessment, and treatment of PDG, refer to Szuhany et al. (2021). Dr. Neimeyer also edited a series of books published by Routledge on grief therapy assessments, intervention, and treatment techniques that could serve as valuable resources. The Center for Prolonged Grief at Columbia University offers resources and workshops for both professionals and grievers.

3. **Address roadblocks**: Preparing for managing common therapy obstacles. Maladaptive cognitions and avoidance behaviors often contribute to resistance and complex grief reactions. Practitioners should be equipped with strategies to adapt treatment plans and use case examples for learning.
4. **Regular monitoring and assessment**: Continuously assess progress through structured interviews and questionnaires designed for PGD. This ensures that the therapy remains effective and that any necessary adjustments are made promptly. Be vigilant in assessing comorbid conditions such as depression, anxiety, and PTSD.
5. **Avoid over-diagnosing**: Be cautious not to pathologize normal grief responses. Apply diagnostic criteria thoughtfully. Consider the cultural context and developmental conditions.
6. **Appropriate referrals**: Refer clients to mental health professionals with expertise in prolonged grief disorder or bereavement. Overreliance on pharmacotherapy for grief-related issues should be avoided.
7. **Professional development**: Engage in ongoing training and professional development through workshops, webinars, and self-study courses offered by reputable institutions such as the Center for Prolonged Grief at Columbia University. Such training ensures that professionals are equipped with the most current and evidence-based practices.

Life is complex, as is grief. Cultural, developmental, and social variations further complicate distinguishing between typical responses and maladaptive patterns. As research and guidelines on PGD continue to evolve, these strategies aim to provide practical guidance for professionals navigating this multifaceted landscape. It is important to maintain balance—avoiding the pathologization and overdiagnosis of grief while ensuring that individuals whose daily functioning is genuinely impaired receive accurate diagnoses and appropriate treatment.

3.11 Concluding Reflection

The chapter has explored the diverse types of loss and grief, presenting strategies for coping and support. From primary and secondary losses to finite and nonfinite losses, the breadth of loss and grief extends beyond death-related contexts. Ambiguous loss, disenfranchised grief, and anticipatory grief emphasize the need for contextual considerations and relational approaches instead of approaches narrowly focused on individuals.

The inclusion of prolonged grief disorder (PGD) in diagnostic manuals represents a significant development in grief studies, offering both opportunities and challenges for research and clinical practice. The potential benefits of standardizing PGD diagnosis are balanced by concerns about pathologizing normal grief responses. Cultural considerations are emphasized by the World Health Organization, which again highlights the importance of culturally sensitive practices in grief support.

Grief is not limited to isolated events. The concept of collective grief emphasizes the effects on entire communities or societies, whereas cumulative grief refers to unresolved grief from multiple losses compounding over time. Recognizing these dimensions underscores the need to take a historical and comprehensive view beyond the present loss and grief, respecting the diverse experiences of those who grieve.

The diversity and breadth of losses and grief require validation and compassion. The grieving and healing journey is like a tornado-shaped spiral, characterized by periods of progress interwoven with moments of regression (Ciupak, 2025). This perspective fosters compassion, patience, and hope, emphasizing that healing is not a linear path but remains within reach. Setbacks are a natural part of the process, and small victories should be celebrated as meaningful steps forward.

References

American Psychiatric Association. (2021, September 22). *APA offers tips for understanding prolonged grief disorder.* [News Release]. Retrieved from https://www.psychiatry.org/newsroom/news-releases/apa-offers-tips-for-understanding-prolonged-grief-disorder

American Psychiatric Association. (2022). *Diagnostic and statistical manual of mental disorders* (5th ed., text rev.). American Psychiatric Publishing.

Attig, T., Nilsson, M., Kissane, D. W., Breitbart, W., Kacel, E., Jones, E. C., & Prigerson, H. G. (2013). Underutilization of mental health services among bereaved caregivers with prolonged grief disorder. *Psychiatric Services, 62*(10), 1225–1229. https://doi.org/10.1176/ps.62.10.pss6210_1225

Beder, J. (2005). Loss of the assumptive world--How we deal with death and loss. *Omega: Journal of Death and Dying, 50*(4), 255–265. https://doi.org/10.2190/GXH6-8VY6-BQ0R-GC04

Bergsmark, L. P. S., & Ramsing, F. (2023). Which considerations are lost when debating the prolonged grief disorder diagnosis? *Theory & Psychology, 33*(6), 856–872.

Boss, P. (2018). *Loss, trauma, and resilience: Therapeutic work with ambiguous loss.* W. W. Norton & Company.

Boss, P. (2022). *The myth of closure: Ambiguous loss in a time of pandemic and change.* W.W. Norton & Company.

Cesur-Soysal, G., & Arı, E. (2024). How we disenfranchise grief for self and other: An empirical study. *OMEGA - Journal of Death and Dying, 89*(2), 530–549.

Ciupak, Y. (2025). *Spiral model of grief and healing: An integrative sociological, psychological, and cultural framework* [Unpublished manuscript]. Northern Michigan University.

Doka, K. J. (2020). Disenfranchised grief: An exposition and update. In *Readings in thanatology* (pp. 275–283). Routledge.

Eisma, M. C. (2023). Prolonged grief disorder in ICD-11 and DSM-5-TR: Challenges and controversies. *Australian & New Zealand Journal of Psychiatry, 57*(7), 944–951.

Fisher, J. (2017). *Healing the fragmented selves of trauma survivors: Overcoming internal self-alienation.* Routledge/Taylor & Francis Group.

Grauerholz, K. R., Fredenburg, M., Jones, P. T., & others. (2020). Fostering vicarious resilience for perinatal palliative care professionals. Frontiers in Pediatrics, 8, 572933. doi:https://doi.org/10.3389/fped.2020.572933.

Harrison, R. L., & Westwood, M. J. (2009). Preventing vicarious traumatization of mental health therapists: Identifying protective practices. *Psychotherapy: Theory, Research, Practice, Training, 46*(2), 203–219.

Herman, J. L. (2022). *Trauma and recovery: The aftermath of violence*. Basic Books.

Hilberdink, C. E., Ghainder, K., Dubanchet, A., Hinton, D., Djelantik, A. M. J., Hall, B. J., & Bui, E. (2023). Bereavement issues and prolonged grief disorder: A global perspective. *Cambridge Prisms: Global Mental Health, 10*, e32.

Hooyman, N. R., & Kramer, B. J. (2006). *Living through loss: Interventions across the life span*. Columbia University Press.

Janoff-Bulman, R. (1992). *Shattered assumptions: Toward a new psychology of trauma*. Free Press.

Lavorgna, B. F., & Hutton, V. E. (2019). Grief severity: A comparison between human and companion animal death. *Death Studies, 43*(8), 521–526.

Moreira, D., Azeredo, A., Moreira, D., Favero, M., & Sousa-Gomes, V. (2022). Why does grief hurt?: A systematic review of grief and depression in adults. *European Psychologist, 28*, e490. https://doi.org/10.1027/1016-9040/a000490

National Cancer Institute. (2024). *Grief, Bereavement, and Coping with Loss (PDQ®)–Health Professional Version.* Retrieved from https://www.cancer.gov/about-cancer/advanced-cancer/caregivers/planning/bereavement-hp-pdq

Neimeyer, R. A. (Ed.). (2001). *Meaning reconstruction & the experience of loss*. American Psychological Association. https://doi.org/10.1037/10397-000

Packman, W., Carmack, B. J., Katz, R., Carlos, F., Field, N. P., & Landers, C. (2014). Online survey as empathic bridging for the disenfranchised grief of pet loss. *OMEGA - Journal of Death and Dying, 69*(4), 333–356.

Prati, G., & Pietrantoni, L. (2009). Optimism, social support, and coping strategies as factors contributing to posttraumatic growth: A meta-analysis. *Journal of Loss and Trauma, 14*(5), 364–388. https://doi.org/10.1080/15325020902724271

Rando, T. A. (1991). *How to go on living when someone you love dies*. Bantam Books.

Rogalla, K. B. (2020). Anticipatory grief, proactive coping, social support, and growth: Exploring positive experiences of preparing for loss. *OMEGA - Journal of Death and Dying, 81*(1), 107–129.

Shapiro, S. L., Astin, J. A., Bishop, S. R., & Cordova, M. (2005). Mindfulness-based stress reduction for health care professionals: Results from a randomized trial. *International Journal of Stress Management, 12*(2), 164–176.

Shear, K. (2022). Benefits of PGD inclusion. *American Journal of Psychiatry, 179*(4), 399–406. Retrieved from https://www.example.com

Sullender, R. S. (2010). Vicarious grieving and the media. *Pastoral Psychology, 59*, 191–200.

Szuhany, K. L., Malgaroli, M., Miron, C. D., & Simon, N. M. (2021). Prolonged grief disorder: Course, diagnosis, assessment, and treatment. *Focus, 19*(2), 161–172.

Tedeschi, R. G., & Calhoun, L. G. (2004). Posttraumatic growth: Conceptual foundations and empirical evidence. *Psychological Inquiry, 15*(1), 1–18.

UK Trauma Council. (2023). *What is traumatic bereavement?* Retrieved from https://uktrauma-council.org/resource/what-is-traumatic-bereavement-2?cn-reloaded=1

Van der Kolk, B. A. (2014). *The body keeps the score: Brain, mind, and body in the healing of trauma*. Viking.

Weir, K. (2018, November). *New paths for people with prolonged grief disorder*. Monitor on Psychology. Retrieved from https://www.apa.org/monitor/2018/11/ce-corner

Worden, J. W. (2008). *Grief counselling and grief therapy: A handbook for the mental health practitioner* (4th ed.). Springer.

World Health Organization. (2019). *International classification of diseases for mortality and morbidity statistics* (11th ed.). Retrieved from https://icd.who.int/

Chapter 4
Grieving Process Models and Theories

4.1 Introduction

The American Psychological Association defines grief as "the anguish experienced after significant loss, usually the death of a beloved person" (APA, 2018). Although the definition of grief has remained relatively stable across history and culture, the understanding of how people grieve and how we support bereaved people has evolved significantly. Scholars, practitioners, and cultural perspectives have all contributed to a more nuanced, multidimensional comprehension of grief over time.

Several key developments have emerged in the evolution of grief theories. First, there has been a shift from stage-based, linear models, such as Freud (1917)'s "grief work" and Kübler-Ross's Five Stages of Grief (1969), toward more individualized, dynamic, and nonlinear approaches. Models such as Worden's task model (2008) emphasize active coping and tasks that the bereaved can revisit. The Dual Process Model (Stroebe & Schut, 1999) illustrates the oscillation between loss-oriented and restoration-oriented coping. The Spiral Model of Grieving and Healing synthesizes and advances existing understanding, presenting a spiral trajectory of grieving as a nonlinear, dynamic, and socioculturally embedded process (Ciupak, 2025).

Second, the understanding of emotional ties to the deceased has evolved. Freud's early theory suggested that grieving individuals must detach and sever their emotional bonds to heal. In contrast, contemporary models now emphasize the concept of continuing bonds, where maintaining a connection with the deceased is seen as a healthy and integral part of the healing process. These bonds, which may manifest through memory, rituals, or ongoing emotional connections, allow individuals to integrate the loss while moving forward.

Third, contemporary models increasingly consider cultural and religious variations in grief. Scholars critique the ethnocentric focus of many early Western models and highlight the importance of diverse worldviews in shaping the grieving

Y. Z. Ciupak, D. C. Smith, *Death, Dying, and Grief*,
https://doi.org/10.1007/978-3-031-88467-2_4

process (Hooyman et al., 2021). Today, grief models are more inclusive of cultural and spiritual differences, recognizing that grief is a deeply personal experience influenced by various social, religious, and philosophical contexts.

Fourth, there is a growing recognition of the potential for personal growth through grief. Rather than viewing loss solely as a stressor that requires adaptation, this perspective emphasizes meaning-finding, meaning-making, and reconstructing personal narratives. "Meaning reconstruction (Neimeyer, 2020)" suggests that grief can foster transformative growth as individuals work to find new meaning in life and reshape their identities in the aftermath of loss.

Additionally, there has been a decades-long, ongoing struggle to identify the boundaries between normal grief and pathological grief (maladaptation). This has led to considerable debate regarding how long is "too long" and how intense is "too intense." These discussions culminated in the eventual inclusion of prolonged grief disorder in diagnostic manuals. This struggle underscores the tension between validating the natural and deeply personal experience of grief and recognizing when professional intervention is necessary to support those whose grief becomes prolonged or severely disruptive to daily life.

The breadth of grief theories and scholarship is so vast that it defies an exhaustive review. Therefore, this chapter offers a focused and comprehensive introduction to the key frameworks that have shaped our understanding of grief in modern times. By examining the evolution from classical models to more contemporary approaches, this chapter guides the reader through historical development and the most up-to-date understanding of grieving.

4.2 Classical Perspectives and Models

From ancient philosophical contemplations to modern psychological frameworks, scholars and practitioners have long sought to understand the multifaceted nature of suffering and grief. Freud's psychoanalysis theory and the essay *Mourning and Melancholia* (1917) were revolutionary works on modern grief intake. His work profoundly inspired many other researchers and shaped clinical practices. Legendary physician Kübler-Ross's stage model, which was developed based on her keen observation of terminally ill patients whom she was tending, became widely known and popular.

4.2.1 Freud's "Grief Work"

Freud published his influential essay *Mourning and Melancholia* in 1917. Even though it was not a direct response to World War I, against the historical backdrop of widespread loss, trauma, and upheaval, Freud's conceptualization of *"grief work"* and psychoanalytic approach provided a groundbreaking way to understand

and support grieving and mental health. According to psychoanalytic theory, when a loved one dies, the bereaved person faces the challenge of severing ties and releasing the energy invested in the deceased person. This essay proposed that when an individual encounters the loss of a loved one, they embark on a journey of "*decathexis*," wherein they gradually withdraw libido/emotional energy from the departure to facilitate emotional reattachment to the external world. This concept depicts mourning as a gradual disinvestment of emotional energy from the lost object, fostering the internalization of the object's absence and the eventual redirection of emotional focus toward new connections. The psychological function of grief is to free the person from ties to the deceased, achieving gradual detachment through a process of "grief work": the psychological labor necessary to disengage from emotional ties with the deceased and realign oneself with new relationships and experiences. According to Freud, mourning entails a series of psychological efforts, including processing painful emotions intertwined with grief and integrating the memory of the lost individual into the internal world through symbolic representation.

Importantly, Freud (1917) never aimed to pathologize grief. In contrast, in his renowned essay, he explicitly stated:

> Although mourning involves grave departures from the normal attitude to life, it never occurs to us to regard it as a pathological condition and to refer it to medical treatment. We rely on it being overcome after a certain lapse of time, and we look upon any interference with it as useless or even harmful (p. 243).

Although Freud's work paved the way for including grief in psychiatry and advocated that the grieving person detach their emotional energy from the deceased and sublimate it in other areas of living, he neither viewed grief as pathological nor considered that grief work could/should ever be completely resolved.

Freud's work has profoundly shaped the landscape of grief psychology, influencing subsequent theorists such as Abraham (1927) and John Bowlby (1979). Freud emphasized the sublimation of cathartic energy, whereas Abraham focused on internalizing the lost object during mourning. According to Abraham, the grieving individual's "grief work" entailed incorporating the deceased person into oneself as a means of healing from the loss. He expressed this idea by stating, "The process of mourning thus brings with it the consolation; 'My loved object is not gone, for now, I carry it within myself and can never lose it'" (Abraham, 1927, pp. 436–437).

Bowlby was a British psychologist and pioneer in studies on attachment. Drawing upon evolutionary biology and observations of the separation of children and their parents, Bowlby argues that attachment forms a protective biological mechanism that serves to ensure the survival of an individual species and derives from the basic need for security. In the classical book *Attachment and Loss* (1969), Bowlby depicts grief as a normal adaptive response to a broken affective bond/system, and responses are based on the social environment and psychological makeup of the griever. Later, with his colleague Colin Parkes, he broke down this natural adaptive grief response into four phases of grief: Phase 1: Shock and numbness; Phase 2: Yearning and searching; Phase 3: Despair and Disorganization; and Phase 4: Reorganization and Recovery.

Like Freud and Bowlby, many others view the process of grieving as involving a certain amount of "grief work" that involves a period of intense emotional distress and pain that must be expressed, fully experienced, and "worked through.[1]" This dominant perspective has not been without question about its adequacy, as the "grief work" perspective focuses on emotions and assumes a universal human affective experience of mourning.[2] However, in the field, there remains an overall emphasis on grieving as an active and ongoing effort to process the cognitive and emotional difficulties associated with the loss of a relationship. Through this grief work, individuals are believed to come to terms with their loss and reduce their grief over time.

4.2.2 *Kübler-Ross's Stage Theory*

The classical perspectives and assumption of a universal human response to loss led to various phase- or stage-based models. Many prominent theorists have developed various phase-based models over the past few decades.[3] Among these, the psychiatrist Elisabeth Kübler-Ross's stage model has gained widespread recognition. The five stages of her theory are (1) shock and denial, (2) anger, resentment, and guilt, (3) bargaining, (4) depression, and (5) acceptance (Kübler-Ross, 1969). Her model implies that the failure to complete any of these stages could result in incomplete healing and unfinished business.

According to the stage model, the first stage, shock, and denial, is characterized by the feeling of numbness and moving on as if nothing happened. The anger stage is characterized by negative emotions aimed at either the one who died, the person, or the situation as a whole. Bargaining is known as the stage of "what ifs." Those facing grief look at the past and think of times when things could have gone differently, and they often look toward their religious figures for answers. The depression stage begins with intense feelings of sadness and grief. Kübler-Ross stated that this stage can last from many months to many years. The final stage in the model is acceptance. This stage does not mean that people "get over" a loss but rather that they learn how to live with the loss.

Kübler-Ross developed the stage model based on her extensive clinical work with terminally ill patients, not bereaved persons. She also made it clear that there are individual variations. Despite that, the stage model is often misinterpreted and misused. An essential issue is the indication of a universal linear framework for

[1] The concept of "grief work" as a necessary process for overcoming loss has been detailed in foundational works, emphasizing the need for the bereaved to engage with their emotions fully and often suggest active professional interventions (Rando, 1993; Sanders, 1999; Hooyman et al., 2021)

[2] The adequacy of "grief work" has been debated, with some scholars questioning its assumption of a universal emotional response and risks of overintervention. Contemporary scholarship suggests that cultural and social variations may challenge the traditional view of grief work. For example, Harris et al. (2021).

[3] A couple examples are: Jacobs, S. (1993) and Sanders, C. M. (1999).

grieving. This perspective has led to discussions, research, and diagnostic manuals that try to define what is considered a "normal" duration for mourning, which types of grieving experiences are acceptable, and the expectation that individuals will smoothly transition through different "stages" of grief. Corr et al. (2019) summarized the critiques of stage- and phase-based models as follows:

1. The existence of these stages has not consistently been demonstrated.
2. Sufficient empirical evidence has not been presented that people actually do move from stage 1 through stage 5.
3. Limitations of the methods, especially the narrow study population.
4. The line is blurred between description and prescription.
5. The totality of the person's life is neglected.
6. The resources, pressures, and characteristics of the immediate environment are not considered.
7. The model suggests that how all human persons respond to the stress of dying is independent of any social or cultural influence.

Due to the above limitations, many scholars and clinicians have cautioned healthcare professionals about applying stage/phase models to individuals experiencing grief and mourning (Stroebe et al., 2017). Nevertheless, Kübler-Ross's stage theory continues to play a prevalent role in the public's understanding of and ability to cope with grief and continues to be widely accepted and promoted with limited caution. A recent article conducted a systematic analysis of the Stages of Grief portrayed on the internet (Avis et al., 2021). The authors reported that 61% of the 72 eligible websites presented the Stage Model without any evaluative commentary or mention of limitations or cautions. The article concludes that a definitive and uncritical portrayal of the model is highly misleading, implying that navigating these stages represents the exclusive and normal journey of grieving. This may cause harmful consequences for bereaved persons and alienate and invalidate those experiences that the model does not apply. The authors recommend that the presentation of the model should be limited to acknowledging its historical importance with critical appraisal and present more updated models that more accurately and comprehensively represent the process of grieving.

A counselor in a training program mentioned that her client insisted on the stage model because she felt that it provided a roadmap to avoid unbearable pain. This aligns with what Holland and Neimeyer (2010, p. 116) suggest: "Human beings are inveterate seekers of patterns to organize the flux of experience in a fashion that enhances their sense of prediction and control." Therefore, holding onto a rigid and leaner roadmap with a seemingly predictable process, no matter how misleading it might be, may provide a sense of control in times of chaos and despair. However, this effort may undermine one's unique grieving styles and experiences and eventually lead to self-doubt for failure to reach the next stage.

Recognizing the historical significance and limitations of classical grief models, contemporary theories emphasize active coping and individualized, nonlinear grieving processes.

4.3 Worden's Task Model of Mourning

In 1982, psychologist J. William Worden introduced a ground-breaking concept by proposing an approach to mourning tasks rather than stages or phases. Worden began his research on grief in 1968 at Massachusetts General Hospital, aiming to create training for human service professionals to support grieving individuals and families. Drawing inspiration from developmental psychology, Worden proposed that mourners work through specific tasks to process their loss, which could be revisited as needed based on the individual's unique circumstances. This flexible approach acknowledges the different challenges that different mourners may face depending on their grieving process and loss experience.

The Tasks
Worden identified four key tasks of mourning:

1. Accept the reality of the loss.
2. Process the pain of grief.
3. Adjust to a world without the deceased.
4. Find an enduring connection with the deceased while continuing with life.

Unlike stage-based models, Worden's tasks offer a nonlinear approach, acknowledging that grief does not follow a direct path. Mourners may move between these tasks at their own pace, revisiting them as necessary depending on the complexity of the loss.

The 6 Mediators
Integral to the task model, Worden identified six mediators that significantly influence the grieving process and affect how individuals navigate the four tasks of mourning. These mediators, which shape the unique experience of grief for each survivor, include the following:

1. **The nature of the survivor's relationship with the deceased** (kinship or familial connection).
2. **The strength and type of attachment** between the survivor and the deceased.
3. **The circumstances surrounding the death**, such as whether it was sudden, expected, or traumatic.
4. **The survivor's history with previous losses** and how they have processed grief in the past.
5. **Personality factors and social variables**, including lingering grief from cumulative losses or preexisting mental health conditions such as mood or personality disorders.
6. **The level of emotional and social support available**, as well as any additional stresses the survivor may face, such as economic hardships or substance abuse.

The task model has been applied to a wide range of settings. Khosravi (2021) applied these mediators to examine the grief experienced by survivors during the COVID-19 pandemic. During this period, many of the mediators were heightened, particularly the circumstances of death, which were often sudden and unexpected due to the pandemic. Preexisting mental health conditions are exacerbated by prolonged quarantine and social isolation, depriving survivors of time with loved ones and intensifying their grief. Additionally, the economic instability caused by the pandemic, including job losses, added further stress to the already overwhelming experience of bereavement.

Clinical Applications

Worden's task model closely aligns with Freud's concept of grief work and provides a practical framework for clinical application. For example, caregivers and counselors can identify the specific tasks through which their clients work and offer targeted support. For clients working on **Task I** (accepting the reality of the loss), emotional or cognitive turmoil may arise, especially for those whose grieving style is either expressive (emotionally focused) or instrumental (focused on problem solving). In this task, the role of the counselor is to guide the client in confronting and accepting the loss.

When supporting **Task II** (processing the pain of grief), counselors can adopt an empathetic-abiding presence, providing companionship and understanding as clients navigate the emotional pain associated with loss. For **Task III** (adjusting to a world without the deceased), the counselor helps the client integrate the loss into their life by assessing the client's situation and creating strength-based care and action plans to assist in their adjustment.

In **Task IV** (finding an enduring connection with the deceased while moving forward), grief support facilitates the mourner's process of emotionally relocating the deceased. This includes enabling the individual to maintain continuing bonds with the deceased while encouraging healthy adaptation to life after loss.

Table 4.1 provides a detailed overview of the four tasks of the Mourning and support strategies:

4.4 Dual Process Model

To address the limitations of stage- and phase-based models, psychologists Stroebe and Schut (1999) developed the dual process model of coping with grief. This model emphasizes an oscillation or alternation between two dynamic and complementary grief-coping processes: *loss-oriented* and *restoration-oriented* coping. The dual process model proposes that individuals move back and forth between focusing on their grief and addressing the secondary losses and new challenges brought on by death. This back-and-forth movement is seen as essential to healthy coping, as it allows the griever to balance the emotional processing of the loss with the necessity of adapting to life changes. This oscillation represents a balance between the emotional impact of the loss and the potential for positive growth and change (Fiore, 2021). Additionally, the dual process model recognizes that grief coping can vary widely among individuals depending on personal and cultural backgrounds and may shift from moment to moment.

Table 4.1 Overview of Worden's tasks of mourning and support strategies

Task number	Name of task	Brief description	Support strategies
Task I	Accept the reality of the loss	Acknowledge and come to terms with the fact that the loss has occurred. This involves overcoming denial and accepting the permanence of the loss	– Encourage open discussions about the deceased and the circumstances of the death. – Participate in rituals such as funerals or memorial services to reinforce the reality of the loss. – Provide a supportive environment where the mourner feels safe to express feelings and thoughts about the deceased
Task II	Process the pain of grief	Experience and work through the emotional pain associated with the loss, rather than avoiding or suppressing it	– Offer empathetic listening to allow the mourner to express feelings of sadness, anger, guilt, or anxiety. – Encourage the use of creative outlets like journaling, art, or music to process emotions. – Be patient and understanding, recognizing that the intensity and duration of grief can vary among individuals
Task III	Adjust to a world without the deceased	Adapt to the environment in which the deceased is missing, which may involve internal, external, and spiritual adjustments	– Assist in developing new routines and roles that the deceased once fulfilled. – Encourage the mourner to build new relationships or strengthen existing ones to fill social voids. – Support the exploration of new interests or activities that provide a sense of purpose and fulfillment
Task IV	Find an enduring connection with the deceased while moving on	Develop a way to maintain a connection with the deceased while continuing to live a fulfilling life. This involves keeping memories alive without hindering personal growth	– Encourage the creation of lasting tributes, such as photo albums, memory boxes, or charitable donations in the deceased's name. – Support the mourner in finding personal rituals or traditions that honor the deceased's memory.– Help the mourner understand that moving forward does not mean forgetting the deceased but integrating the loss into their ongoing life

Source: Based on Worden, J. W. (2008)

Dual Processes

The **loss-oriented process** involves confronting the immediate emotional impact of the loss, including the effects on daily life, reworking bonds with the deceased, and often avoiding restoration tasks. This type of coping is common in the early stages

Table 4.2 Key activities of dual-process

Loss oriented	Restoration-oriented
• Grief work • Intrusion of grief • Relinquishing-continuing-relocating bonds • Denial/avoidance of restoration changes	• Attending to life changes • Doing new things • Distraction from grief • Denial/avoidance of grief • New roles/identities/relationships
Everyday life experience is an oscillation between the two orientations.	

Source: Based on Stroebe, M., & Schut, H. (1999)

of bereavement and can encompass both expected and unexpected emotions.[4] While this process is crucial for emotional processing, experts caution that prolonged reliance on it may hinder healing, potentially leading to behavioral avoidance and difficulty acknowledging the loss. Excessive focus on loss-oriented coping has been linked to complicated grief, depression, loneliness, and prolonged grief disorder.[5]

The **restoration-oriented process** shifts focus to adapting to life after the loss, addressing new challenges, and engaging in new activities. This approach helps bereaved persons rebuild their identity and relationships, promoting well-being, personal growth, and self-care. Active engagement with life enables individuals to navigate their new reality effectively. Striking a balance between loss-oriented and restoration-oriented coping is crucial for healthy outcomes, as both processes complement each other to support the mourner's adaptation over time.[6]

Table 4.2 summarizes the key activities and aspects associated with the loss-oriented and restoration-oriented processes within the dual process model of grief.

Discussions on the Dual Process Model

The dual process model has been instrumental in shaping contemporary understandings of grief as nonlinear. It is not without limitations. For example, the model has been criticized for its limited consideration of grief overload, where individuals face the combined demands of loss- and restoration-oriented tasks, leading to internal conflict. Critics also challenge its assumption that these processes cannot occur simultaneously, noting they are often interwoven, especially in cases of traumatic bereavement. Additionally, the concept of oscillation disregards moments of respite, where individuals temporarily disengage from both grief and restoration stressors. These limitations suggest a need for further refinement to address the nuanced experiences of grief (Fasse & Zech, 2016; Fiore, 2021; Worden, 2008).

[4] See Fasse and Zech (2016), Fiore (2021) on descriptions of loss-oriented coping processes and early bereavement stages.

[5] Prolonged reliance on loss-oriented coping and associated risks have been discussed by Stroebe and Schut (2016), Tang and Chow (2017), and Fiore (2021).

[6] Numerous studies have discussed the restoration-oriented process, its benefits, and the importance of balancing coping processes. For example, Fasse and Zech (2016), Tang and Chow (2017). Fiore (2021) provides a systematic comprehensive review of studies using the dual process model.

4.5 Grieving Styles

Doka and Martin (2011) identify four types of grievers that exist along a continuum. At one end are **intuitive grievers**, who express their grief outwardly through visible emotional displays such as crying, screaming, sadness, anger, and guilt. In contrast, **instrumental grievers** process their emotions more privately through problem-solving and cognitive processing rather than overt expressions. Instrumental grievers may engage in storytelling, creating art, or performing rituals to cope with their grief.

Among these two extremes are **blended grievers**, who show characteristics of both intuitive and instrumental grieving styles. Blended grievers may express emotions outwardly while also processing grief through behaviors and actions. Most individuals who experience grief are thought to fall into this blended category. Finally, there are **dissonant grievers** who exist outside the continuum. Dissonant grievers tend to repress their emotions, leading to a disconnect between how they feel internally and how they express their grief outwardly (Harrington & Neimeyer, 2020).

Traditionally, it has been believed that men and women grieve differently, with women being more likely to express grief outwardly (e.g., through crying) and men being more likely to withdraw socially because of societal expectations about masculinity. However, research in Western contexts has shown no straightforward correlation between gender and grieving style (Harris et al., 2021). Doka and Martin's (2011) research shows that both men and women can exhibit either intuitive or instrumental grieving styles, and many individuals fall somewhere in between. They emphasize that gender is just one of many factors that shape an individual's grieving style.

Further research is needed to explore how societal and cultural factors influence grieving styles and the manifestation of grief, both at the individual and collective levels. Figure 4.1 illustrates the various styles of grieving.

4.6 Meaning Reconstruction

Meaning reconstruction highlights the human need to impose order on life's chaos, particularly during times of loss. Meaning, as Viktor Frankl (1985) famously articulated, is fundamental to how people make sense of daily events and drives their motivations and actions. In the face of disorder or traumatic events like bereavement, reconstructing meaning helps individuals integrate the loss into their life story and move forward. This process allows the bereaved to reestablish a sense of coherence and purpose, which has been deeply disrupted by the death of a loved one.

Frankl's existential perspective emphasizes that people can find meaning even in suffering, providing a pathway to healing after loss. Neimeyer (2020) extends this

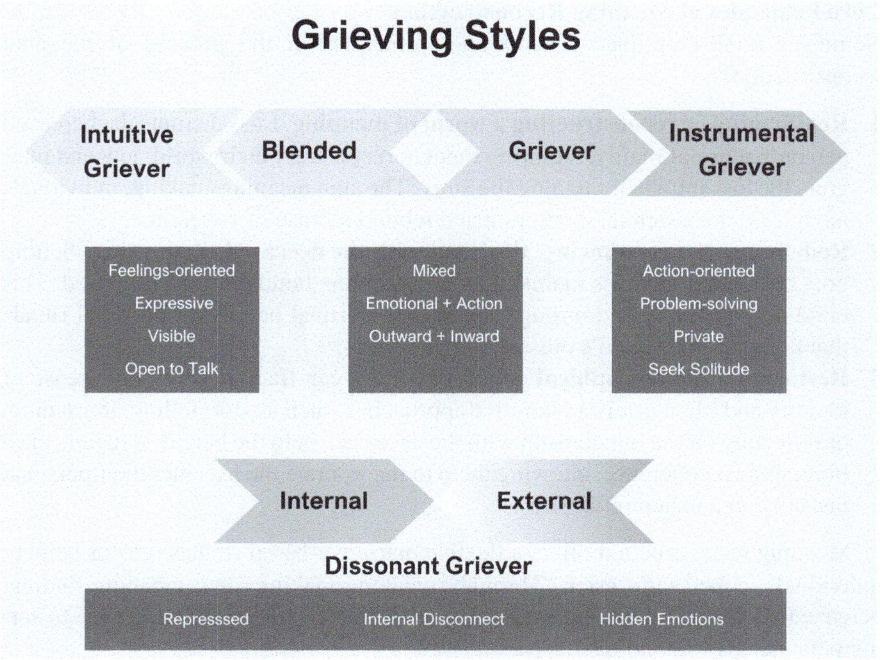

Fig. 4.1 Grieving styles

concept through his constructivist approach to grief, which focuses on how individuals actively rebuild their narrative in response to loss rather than passively progressing through emotional stages. Neimeyer identifies two integral processes in meaning reconstruction: meaning-making and meaning-finding.

- **Meaning-making** involves the creation of new interpretations of the loss, helping individuals process why the loss occurred and how it fits into their broader worldview. This cognitive process is essential in helping the bereaved restore a sense of coherence.
- **Meaning-finding** entails discovering inherent value or personal growth in life after loss. It helps bereaved people recognize the ways in which the experience of loss might transform their perspective, contributing to emotional adaptation and resilience.

These processes are not about achieving "closure" but about reauthoring one's life narrative to honor both the reality of the loss and the ongoing presence of the deceased in their memories and experiences. Meaning-making and meaning-finding are fundamental to adapting to loss by helping the bereaved reconcile the disruption caused by death and moving forward with a new understanding of their world (Milman et al., 2019).

Core Principles of Meaning Reconstruction

Neimeyer (2020) outlined several core principles in the process of meaning reconstruction:

1. **Reaffirming or reconstructing a world of meaning**: Loss disrupts the bereaved person's sense of reality, requiring them to reconstruct their worldview and integrate the loss into their ongoing life story. Through meaning-making, individuals navigate this existential disruption and rebuild a sense of coherence.
2. **Redefining, not renouncing, the bond with the deceased**: Rather than "letting go," grief often involves maintaining a continuing bond with the deceased. This bond may be expressed through memories, spiritual beliefs, or personal rituals that honor the deceased's presence in new ways.
3. **Restoring autobiographical coherence**: Loss can fracture a person's sense of identity and life narrative. Narrative approaches, such as storytelling, journaling, or reflecting on the relationship with the deceased, help the bereaved regain autobiographical coherence, allowing them to incorporate the loss into their personal narrative in a meaningful way.

Meaning reconstruction offers a flexible, narrative-based framework for helping individuals cope with grief. Through meaning-making and meaning-finding, bereaved people are able to integrate the loss into their life story, ultimately fostering personal growth and resilience.

Support Meaning Reconstruction Challenges

Traumatic or sudden losses present unique challenges in the process of meaning reconstruction. When a loss is unexpected, such as in the case of an accident or violent death, it can shatter the bereaved person's *assumptive world*—the core beliefs about safety, order, and predictability that guide their understanding of life (Janoff-Bulman, 1992). This disruption makes it significantly harder for individuals to make sense of the loss and integrate it into their life narrative. In these instances, the search for meaning can feel overwhelming, as the event challenges fundamental beliefs and creates a void that is difficult to fill. *Sense-making*—an essential aspect of meaning reconstruction—often becomes a long and complex process in the aftermath of traumatic loss.

Moreover, *social support* plays a crucial role in facilitating meaning reconstruction, particularly following traumatic events. Support from family, friends, or communities helps validate the grief experience, offering a framework within which individuals can process their loss. This validation is crucial for fostering posttraumatic growth, where individuals are able to not only adapt to the loss but also find personal growth in its wake (Neimeyer, 2020). However, when social support is absent or inadequate or when grief is *disenfranchised*, meaning-making can become significantly more difficult, increasing the risk of *complicated grief* (Milman et al., 2019).

For those experiencing *disenfranchised grief*, where their loss is not acknowledged or supported by societal norms, the challenge of meaning reconstruction intensifies. Without recognition or the ability to mourn openly, individuals may struggle to reframe their relationship with the deceased or redefine their personal narrative, leading to prolonged suffering (Neimeyer, 2020).

Attachment styles[7] also affect one's ability to engage in meaning-making. Individuals with *anxious or avoidant attachment* may have a more challenging time coping with loss, as they either avoid confronting their grief or become overwhelmed by it, further complicating their ability to reconstruct meaning (Milman et al., 2019). This can hinder their ability to find coherence in their life story after loss, delaying emotional recovery and adaptation.

In the face of these challenges, narrative techniques such as storytelling, journaling, or reflection can be powerful tools for helping bereaved people integrate traumatic or disenfranchised losses into their life narrative. These practices offer structured ways to process both the *event story* (what happened) and the *back story* (the ongoing relationship with the deceased), promoting healing and the reconstruction of meaning. In addition, Milman et al. (2019) reported that meaning reconstruction mediates the negative effects of anxious coping, spousal loss, neuroticism, and low social support. Structuring the disordered emotions surrounding grief and transforming them into an organized understanding allows grievers to release emotional tension and find peace. Additionally, the Grief and Meaning Reconstruction Inventory (GMRI) has been developed as a tool to assess levels of meaning-making in bereaved individuals, providing practitioners with valuable insights for supporting the grieving process.

4.7 Continuing Bonds

Continuing bonds refer to the enduring connections individuals maintain with deceased loved ones, challenging the views of detachment as a marker of "successful" grieving. This perspective recognizes that relationships with the deceased can evolve over time, providing comfort, meaning, and a sense of continuity in the lives of those who grieve (Klass, 2006). Research on grieving children, for instance, reveals that feeling a parent's presence—such as believing they are "watching over them"—can provide comfort even years after the loss (Mallon, 2018).

Cultural Influences

In many cultures, continuing bonds are preserved through rituals and practices that keep memories alive. Whether through memorial ceremonies, altars, or religious rites, these traditions reflect humanity's deep desire to maintain a connection with those who have passed. Practices such as celebrating death anniversaries and honoring the deceased through prayer or ritual are ways in which people around the world ensure that their loved ones remain present in their lives.

However, cultural attitudes and norms around death significantly affect the view toward continuing bonds. While some cultures actively encourage maintaining

[7] Attachment styles include **secure**, where individuals express emotions openly and seek support, showing resilience in grief; **anxious**, characterized by intense distress and fear of abandonment, many experiencing increased psychosocial challenges during loss; **avoidant**, where individuals may suppress emotions and avoid confronting grief; and **disorganized**, marked by inconsistent behaviors and may experience difficulty processing grief due to trust and emotional regulation issues. Refer to Sect. 4.8 of this chapter for more detailed discussions.

these connections, such as the Mexican tradition of honoring loved ones through Día de los Muertos (Day of the Dead), others may view them with hesitation. A meaningful understanding of continuing bonds, therefore, must include the cultural, community, and social contexts that influence how individuals construct their views and experiences.

Coping and Growth

Continuing bonds provide more than temporary emotional comfort; they may offer resilience and meaning. By bridging the past and present, these connections allow the bereaved persons to maintain a sense of coherence as they carry on life (Leichtentritt et al., 2015). Such bonds help anchor individuals in their personal history and community, fostering stability during times of upheaval. People sustain these connections in various ways, including tangible actions such as creating keepsakes and tattoos or symbolic practices such as rituals or storytelling (Leichtentritt et al., 2015; Maddrell, 2013).

Existential anthropologist Albert Piette (2015) explores how time, continuity, and finiteness influence the understanding of relationships and presence. He emphasized that bonds with the deceased are not static but evolve over time, shaped by the bereaved person's ongoing reflections and experiences. Piette's work helps to understand how these connections address fundamental existential questions, such as how love and memory endure and transform. His insights highlight the dynamic nature of human connections. Reflection on and experiences with continuing bonds, therefore, may prompt spiritual and personal growth, fostering transcendence and connection.

Meanwhile, continuing bonds are not about dwelling on the past. A constructive and meaningful continuing bond involves successfully relocating the deceased within one's life and creating a narrative around the relationship that supports adaptation to a changed world. It is not about "moving on" or remaining stagnant but about reshaping the relationship while carrying on forward (Worden, 2008).

Real Life Story: Continuing Bond

A friend is a beautiful example of living fully. She has a successful career she is passionate about, dedicates time to charity work, and makes self-care a priority through yoga, running, and other activities. Her home and garden are always filled with blooming flowers, a reflection of the life and energy she embodies.

In a conversation, she shared that her younger brother died at a young age, a loss that took her years to process. She said she felt her brother was cheated out of life, and because of that, she made the decision to live fully—for both of them. She carries this continuing bond with her brother in everything she does. Through her thriving career, her acts of kindness, her vibrant garden, and her mindful approach to life, she honors him.

Her brother continues his life through hers, in the way she embraces the world so completely. This continuing bond doesn't hold her back—it propels her forward.

4.8 Five Critical Variables that Influence the Grieving Experience

Researchers have identified five key variables that significantly shape how individuals experience and navigate grief. These variables are crucial in identifying risk factors for complicated or prolonged grief. These include (a) the circumstances of the loss, (b) the prior attachment/prior relationship, (c) the background of the bereaved person, such as gender and developmental stage, (d) coping styles and strategies, and (e) the broader social and institutional systems (Neimeyer & Burke, 2017).

(1) **Circumstances of the Loss**

The circumstances surrounding a loss play a crucial role in shaping the grieving process, as both the nature of the loss and external factors serve as significant stressors. These stressors can vary in intensity depending on whether the loss was sudden or expected, traumatic or peaceful, or complicated by external challenges such as financial or social instability. The way an individual experiences and navigates grief is directly influenced by these factors.

In cases of anticipated losses, such as the natural death of an aging loved one, the bereaved may engage in *anticipatory grief,* which allows time for emotional and practical preparation. This can sometimes soften the impact of eventual death, although the grief that follows is still significant. On the other hand, *traumatic losses*, such as those resulting from war, traffic accidents, sexual assault, robbery, or suicide, tend to amplify emotional responses such as shock, guilt, and anger. These events often occur without warning, leaving little time for emotional or psychological preparation and making the grieving process more complex.

Beyond the cause of death or the nature of the loss itself, the peri-event variables at the time of loss—such as viewing the body following a violent death, physical or mental health, or other existing stressors—can exacerbate the grief experience. *Grief overload* occurs when multiple stressors, including the loss itself, compound an already heavy emotional burden.

Consider an older adult who has been managing a chronic illness and relying on their spouse for caregiving. When the spouse dies unexpectedly, the individual not only faces the emotional weight of the loss but also must navigate the practical and physical challenges of losing their primary support. Without their spouse's care, they may struggle to manage daily tasks, access medical care, and maintain their independence.

This loss extends beyond the emotional pain of bereavement to include secondary losses, such as diminished quality of life, social isolation, and increased dependency on others. These layered stressors can intensify feelings of grief and overwhelm, leaving the individual emotionally and physically vulnerable. This example illustrates how grief overload can arise when a single loss triggers a cascade of additional challenges, emphasizing the need for holistic, multifaceted support.

In traumatic losses, survivors often struggle to make sense of the event, experiencing guilt over perceived preventability or frustration due to unresolved issues or the inability to say goodbye. Moreover, certain losses—such as those involving suicide—may carry a social stigma, further reducing the bereaved person's access to support systems, which are crucial for healing. Traumatic losses can also shatter an individual's basic beliefs about safety, predictability, and meaning in life. The bereaved are not only mourning the loss of a loved one but also grappling with a fundamental disruption to their worldview, which adds another layer of complexity to their grief. Refer to Chap. 3: Types and Concepts of Loss and Grief for more discussion on traumatic loss.

(2) **Relationship and Prior Attachments**

The relationship with the deceased significantly influences grief intensity. Immediate family members, such as spouses and children, typically experience the most severe grief. Dependency and caregiving burdens, especially in cases of long-term illness, can lead to anticipatory grief and profound post-loss distress. The bereaved person's attachment style—whether secure or insecure—also plays a crucial role, affecting their resilience and emotional response to the loss.

Psychologists such as John Bowlby and Mary Ainsworth have extensively studied the role of attachment in human development and its impact on well-being (Shear & Shair, 2005). Healthy attachments can foster resilience, improve self-esteem, and alleviate stress (Simpson & Rholes, 2017). Conversely, ambivalent or conflict-laden relationships can complicate the grieving process, as unresolved issues may surface posthumously, affecting the bereaved person's emotional well-being (Bowlby, 1969).

Phyllis Kosminsky extended these insights into the realm of grief therapy, developing "*attachment-informed grief therapy*" (Kosminsky & Jordan, 2016).

In Worden's task model, attachment is one of the key mediators and can be further broken down into five aspects that influence grief (Worden, 2008):

1. **The strength of the attachment**: Stronger bonds typically result in more intense grief.
2. **The security of the attachment**: When the deceased provides a sense of belonging, security, or self-worth, their absence may intensify feelings of insecurity, loneliness, and diminished self-esteem.
3. **Ambivalence in the relationship**: While ambivalence is common in close relationships, high levels of negative emotions or unresolved conflict can complicate the grieving process.
4. **Conflicts with the deceased**: Unresolved conflicts at the time of death or a history of tension, including abuse, can complicate grief.
5. **Functional dependency**: Individuals who rely on the deceased for daily tasks may face additional challenges as they adjust to their new circumstances.

(3) **Coping Style and Strategies**

Coping involves ongoing efforts to manage the cognitive and emotional demands that arise in stressful situations.[8] Research suggests that individuals often draw on familiar coping mechanisms when confronted with loss (Folkman, 2001). Moos and Schaefer (1986) identified three primary coping strategies:

1. **Appraisal-focused coping** involves making sense of the loss through mental preparedness and logical analysis.
2. **Problem-focused coping**: This includes taking active steps to address the loss, such as seeking support, gathering information, and finding ways to adapt.
3. **Emotion-focused coping**: Entails managing emotional responses to grief, which might include processing emotions, finding comfort, or reaching acceptance.

While some people actively cope with grief by confronting the loss, others may avoid it through *avoidant coping* strategies, such as ignoring the pain or engaging in distractions (Herman-Stahl et al., 1995).

(4) **Background of the Bereaved Person**

Demographic factors, such as gender, socioeconomic status, and developmental stage, significantly shape how individuals experience grief. Women, along with those with fewer financial resources or lower levels of education, are often more vulnerable to intense and complicated grief. These factors can limit access to essential support networks, exacerbating feelings of isolation and emotional distress. The book *Living Through Loss: Interventions Across the Life Span* (Hooyman et al., 2021) takes a much-needed life-course perspective in understanding the varying types of loss and the most effective interventions at different stages of life.

Understanding grief from a developmental perspective is crucial, especially in children and adolescents, as their cognitive and emotional capacities evolve. Children, for instance, begin to grasp the concept of death as their cognitive abilities grow. Even very young children may exhibit grief-like behaviors when they lose an attachment figure, though their understanding of death develops progressively.

Adolescents, on the other hand, are more cognitively aware of the permanence of death, but their emotional responses can be more complex. They may wrest with existential questions, search for meaning, and question how death impacts their identity. Adolescents often display grief through behaviors such as confusion, crying, and disturbances in sleep or eating. Their unique developmental task of individuation, combined with their egocentrism, can make them feel as though their grief is incomprehensible to others. This isolation can lead to expressions of grief in

[8] This definition is based on Lazarus and Folkman's transactional theory of stress and coping, which continues to be the most influential theory in psychological stress and coping. Biggs et al. (2017)'s article discusses Lazarus and Folkman's theory and two other coping taxonomies.

short outbursts or attempts to suppress it. Complicated grief may arise if there are unresolved conflicts with the deceased or if the adolescent's grief is disenfranchised—when society does not acknowledge the relationship or the grief itself. However, navigating grief during adolescence can also foster resilience and growth, resulting in emotional maturity and enhanced interpersonal skills (Hooyman et al., 2021).

(5) **Nature of the Support**

The nature and quality of support play a fundamental role in shaping the grieving experience. Social support, whether from family, friends, or professional caregivers, provides not only crucial emotional outlets but also practical assistance, which is essential for navigating the often tumultuous process of grief. Having a support network—people who truly listen and offer meaningful help—helps ease feelings of isolation and emotional distress, making the grieving process more bearable.

However, effective support must go beyond the immediate aftermath of a loss. Grief does not end with the funeral, and continued support is vital as individuals face recurring waves of grief, especially during significant dates such as birthdays, holidays, or anniversaries. Emotional support from therapy, support groups, or loved ones provides a safe space for bereaved people to explore their feelings, and the consistency of this support is key. Grief often does not follow a linear timeline, and it is important for the bereaved to have access to ongoing care long after the initial shock of the loss.

Economic factors can also significantly impact the grieving process. Financial strain following the death of a loved one—particularly when the deceased is a key provider—can compound emotional stress with practical worries. In such cases, access to financial resources, whether through aid, community support, or family, is critical to helping bereaved people focus on healing rather than survival.

An often overlooked factor is perceived social support. It is not just about whether support is available but also about whether the grieving individual feels truly supported. Lower perceived support from family or friends can lead to greater distress, with issues such as poor communication or perceived criticism further complicating the grieving process.

Finally, institutional factors also shape the bereavement journey. Compassionate care, clear communication during the end-of-life process, and emotional and informational support from healthcare settings play crucial roles in the mourner's ability to adjust post-loss. A lack of support or poor communication from institutions can create additional layers of complexity in the grieving process, leaving the bereaved feeling abandoned or ill-equipped to cope.

Ultimately, the nature of support—social, economic, emotional, or institutional—provides the foundation for a healthier grieving process. Ensuring that support is accessible, compassionate, and ongoing is essential to helping individuals navigate their grief and move toward healing.

4.9 Spiral Model of Grieving and Healing[9]

The Spiral Model of Grieving and Healing proposed by Yan Ciupak (2025) synthesizes and advances the existing understanding of grieving. It takes a holistic, interdisciplinary approach to present grief as a nonlinear, dynamic, spiral-shaped allostatic process deeply embedded in sociocultural dimensions. Unlike stage-based theories that imply a predictable, linear progression, the spiral model embraces the complexity of grief, recognizing it as an adaptive, multifaceted experience that invites growth and compassion (Refer to Fig. 1.1 in Chap. 1). This model integrates loss-oriented and restoration-oriented tasks, striking a balance between acknowledging the pain of the loss and rebuilding life.

Central to the Spiral Model is the concept of movement between processing grief and restoring one's identity and social roles, symbolized by an upward spiral. This continuous engagement facilitates the integration of loss into the individual's life narrative, promoting growth and resilience over time. The model acknowledges that the journey through grief is not uniform and involves oscillations, moments of stillness, and periods of forward movement and retreat.

The model is built upon four foundational principles:

1. Grief is a dynamic, nonlinear process, with diverse expressions.
2. Grief holds the potential for healing and growth.
3. Grief understanding and support should align with holistic and humanistic principles.
4. Grief is embedded within sociocultural structures and processes.

The Spiral Model's emphasis on social and cultural dimensions highlights that grief is not experienced in isolation but within a network of social relationships, cultural norms, and institutional systems. It argues that the forces of grief and healing arise not only from intrapersonal dimensions such as emotions. It also emerges from an intricate web of social and cultural factors that individuals embody and interact with. All of these factors interact to shape the individual's attitudes and experience toward death and grief, enabling or constraining the process of healing. This process is embedded in a matrix of four interconnected dimensions:

1. **Micro-level**, comprising physical, affective, cognitive, behavioral, social, and spiritual states.
2. **Social identity and positions**, such as age, gender, sexual orientation, race/ethnicity, nationality/immigration status, socioeconomic class, able-bodiedness, and marital status;
3. **Institutions** encompassing family, community, workplace, policies, law, and the overall care system.
4. **Broader macro dimensions**, including historical, economic, political, and geographical contexts.

[9] Refer to Fig. 1.1 for a graphic illustration of the Spiral Model.

Grieving persons are not defined by one dimension—such as emotion—but rather as holistic and cultural beings encompassing biological, psychological, social, and spiritual dimensions. This perspective highlights the importance of addressing all facets of the human experience during the grieving process, ensuring comprehensive and compassionate support.

The model proposes a "middle path" approach, balancing the passive nature found in stage-based theories with the intense activity of "grief work" models. For individuals, this balance lies between denial or repression and an overemphasis on active coping. The model validates diverse grief experiences while gently encouraging restoration-oriented actions that align with each person's unique journey.

For those who support grieving individuals—family, friends, and care providers—the "middle path" involves balancing respect for the individual's private experience and avoiding excessive intervention. This nuanced approach honors the natural flow of grief, acknowledging that healing is not about "moving on" or fully resolving grief but rather engaging with it in a way that allows for gradual integration and self-restoration.

This comprehensive framework supports the idea that grief involves continuous adaptation as individuals navigate both personal and collective elements of loss. The Spiral Model advocates a balanced approach, steering clear of extremes and encouraging professionals to create holistic and compassionate environments that honor the unique, evolving nature of grieving and healing.

4.10 Concluding Reflection

Understanding the bonds formed, the pain experienced, and the complex meanings attached to loss is a shared journey intertwined with social and cultural fabric. The evolution of grief theories reveals a shift from rigid, stage-based models to more individualized, nonlinear approaches that recognize the fluid and diverse nature of grief. Models such as Worden's task model and the dual process model emphasize active coping and the oscillation between grief and restoration. The concept of continuing bonds has redefined emotional ties, showing that maintaining a connection with the deceased can support healing. Contemporary perspectives also highlight the importance of cultural and spiritual influences, acknowledging grief as a deeply personal and context-dependent experience. Additionally, meaning reconstruction provides a valuable tool for resilience and healing. The Spiral Model of Grieving and Healing synthesizes and advances the major models and perspectives. This model portrays grieving as a dynamic, fluid, and socioculturally bound process in which individuals navigate loss-oriented and restoration-oriented tasks toward healing. The spiral metaphor captures the whirls, twirls, ups, and downs that characterize the grieving process as one integrates the loss into life, living, and self.

The historical recount and recent development serve as a reminder of the ever-growing nature of human inquiry, the complexities of human experience, and the collective commitment to relieving suffering.

References

Abraham, K. (1927). *Selected papers of Karl Abraham, M.D.* (A. Strachey & D. Bryan, Trans.). L. V. Woolf at the Hogarth Press.

American Psychological Association. (2018). *APA dictionary of psychology*. American Psychological Association. Retrieved from https://dictionary.apa.org/grief

Avis, K. A., Stroebe, M., & Schut, H. (2021). Stages of grief portrayed on the internet: A systematic analysis and critical appraisal. *Frontiers in Psychology, 12*. https://doi.org/10.3389/fpsyg.2021.772696

Biggs, A., Brough, P., & Drummond, S. (2017). Lazarus and Folkman's psychological stress and coping theory. In *The handbook of stress and health: A guide to research and practice* (pp. 349–364). Wiley.

Bowlby, J. (1969). *Attachment and loss* (No. 79). Random House.

Bowlby, J. (1979). Psychoanalysis as art and science. *International Review of Psycho-Analysis, 6*(1), 3–14.

Ciupak, Y. (2025). *Spiral model of grief and healing: An integrative sociological, psychological, and cultural framework* [Unpublished manuscript]. Northern Michigan University.

Corr, C. A., Corr, D. M., & Doka, K. J. (2019). *Death & dying, life & living*. Cengage.

Doka, K. J., & Martin, T. L. (2011). *Grieving beyond gender: Understanding the ways men and women mourn*. Routledge.

Fasse, L., & Zech, E. (2016). Dual process model of coping with bereavement in the test of the subjective experiences of bereaved spouses. *OMEGA - Journal of Death and Dying, 74*(2), 212–238. https://doi.org/10.1177/0030222815598668

Fiore, J. (2021). A systematic review of the dual process model of Coping with Bereavement (1999–2016). *OMEGA - Journal of Death and Dying, 84*(2), 414–458. https://doi.org/10.1177/0030222819893139

Folkman, S. (2001). Revised coping theory and the process of bereavement. In *Handbook of bereavement research: Consequences, coping, and care* (pp. 563–584). American Psychological Association. https://doi.org/10.1037/10436-024

Frankl, V. E. (1985). *Man's search for meaning*. Simon & Schuster.

Freud, S. (1917). *Mourning and Melancholia. The standard edition of the complete psychological works of Sigmund Freud, Volume XIV (1914-1916): On the history of the psycho-analytic movement, papers on metapsychology and other works*, pp. 237–258.

Harrington, J. A., & Neimeyer, R. A. (2020). *Superhero grief: The transformative power of loss* (Vol. 1, 1st ed.). https://doi.org/10.4324/9780429056666

Harris, D. L., Neimeyer, R. A., Thornton, G., & Winokuer, H. R. (2021). *Grief and bereavement in contemporary society: Bridging research and practice (classic)*. Routledge. https://doi.org/10.4324/9781003199762

Herman-Stahl, M. A., Stemmler, M., & Petersen, A. C. (1995). Approach and avoidant coping: Implications for adolescent mental health. *Journal of Youth and Adolescence, 24*(6), 649–665. https://doi.org/10.1007/BF01536949

Holland, J. M., & Neimeyer, R. A. (2010). An examination of stage theory of grief among individuals bereaved by natural and violent causes: A meaning-oriented contribution. *OMEGA - Journal of Death and Dying, 61*(2), 103–120. https://doi.org/10.2190/om.61.2.b

Hooyman, N. R., Kramer, B. J., & Sanders, S. (2021). *Living through loss: Interventions across the life span*. Columbia University Press.

Jacobs, S. (1993). *Pathologic grief: Maladaptation to loss*. American Psychiatric Association.

Janoff-Bulman, R. (1992). *Shattered assumptions: Toward a new psychology of trauma*. Free Press.

Khosravi, M. (2021, January 2). Worden's task-based approach for supporting people bereaved by COVID-19. *Current Psychology, 40*(11), 5735–5736.

Klass, D. (2006). Continuing conversation about continuing bonds. *Death Studies, 30*(9), 843–858.

Kosminsky, P. S., & Jordan, J. R. (2016). *Attachment-informed grief therapy: The clinician's guide to foundations and applications*. Routledge.

Kübler-Ross, E. (1969). *On death and dying*. Routledge.
Leichtentritt, R. D., Yerushalmi, A., & Barak, A. (2015). Characteristics of the ongoing bond. *The British Journal of Social Work, 45*(4), 1102–1118. https://doi.org/10.1093/bjsw/bct171
Maddrell, A. (2013). Living with the deceased: Absence, presence and absence-presence. *Cultural Geographies, 20*(4), 501–522. https://doi.org/10.1177/1474474013482806
Mallon, B. (2018). *Building continuing bonds for grieving and bereaved children: A guide for counsellors and practitioners*. Jessica Kingsley Publishers.
Milman, E., Neimeyer, R. A., Fitzpatrick, M., MacKinnon, C. J., Muis, K. R., & Cohen, S. R. (2019). Prolonged grief and the disruption of meaning: Establishing a mediation model. *Journal of Counseling Psychology, 66*(6), 714–725. https://doi.org/10.1037/cou0000370
Moos, R. H., & Schaefer, J. A. (1986). Life transitions and crises: A conceptual overview. In *Coping with life crises: An integrated approach* (pp. 3–28). Springer.
Neimeyer, R. A. (2020). What's new in meaning reconstruction?: Advancing grief theory and practice. *Grief Matters, 23*(1), 4–9. Retrieved from https://search.informit.com.au/documentSummary;dn=439384113866066;res=IELHEA
Neimeyer, R. A., & Burke, L. A. (2017). What makes grief complicated? Risk factors for complicated grief. In K. Doka & A. Tucci (Eds.), *Living with grief: When grief is complicated* (pp. 73–93). Hospice Foundation of America.
Piette, A. (2015). *Existence in the details: Theory and methodology in existential anthropology*. Duncker & Humblot.
Rando, T. A. (1993). The increasing prevalence of complicated mourning: The onslaught is just beginning. *OMEGA - Journal of Death and Dying, 26*(1), 43–59.
Sanders, C. M. (1999). *Grief: the mourning after: Dealing with adult bereavement* (2nd ed.). Wiley.
Shear, K., & Shair, H. (2005). Attachment, loss, and complicated grief. *Developmental Psychobiology, 47*(3), 253–267. https://doi.org/10.1002/dev.20091
Simpson, J. A., & Rholes, W. S. (2017). Adult attachment, stress, and romantic relationships. *Current Opinion in Psychology, 13*, 19. https://doi.org/10.1016/j.copsyc.2016.04.006
Stroebe, M., & Schut, H. (1999). The dual process model of coping with bereavement: Rationale and description. *Death Studies, 23*(3), 197–224. https://doi.org/10.1080/074811899201046
Stroebe, M., & Schut, H. (2016). Overload: A missing link in the dual process model? *Omega: Journal of Death and Dying, 74*(1), 96–109. https://doi.org/10.1177/0030222816666540
Stroebe, M., Schut, H., & Boerner, K. (2017). Cautioning health-care professionals: Bereaved persons are misguided through the stages of grief. *Omega: Journal of Death and Dying, 74*(4), 455–473. https://doi.org/10.1177/0030222817691870
Tang, S., & Chow, A. Y. M. (2017). How do risk factors affect bereavement outcomes in later life? An exploration of the mediating role of dual process coping. *Psychiatry Research, 255*, 297–303. https://doi.org/10.1016/j.psychres.2017.06.001
Worden, J. W. (2008). *Grief counseling and grief therapy: A handbook for the mental health practitioner* (4th ed.). Springer.

Chapter 5
Dying and End-of-Life Care

5.1 Introduction

Supporting individuals and their families through the end-of-life (EOL) process requires a compassionate, multifaceted approach that addresses the physical, emotional, social, and spiritual dimensions of care. Each dying trajectory—whether sudden, prolonged, or marked by terminal illness—demands tailored interventions that not only alleviate suffering but also provide comfort and dignity in one's final stages. Equally important is the support extended to family members, who face their own emotional and logistical challenges as they navigate the complexities of caregiving and grief. Ethical and legal considerations present delicate and challenging situations, including decisions about life-sustaining treatments, patient autonomy, and the role of advanced directives.[1]

This chapter examines the basic types of end-of-life (EOL) care. It emphasizes the importance of advance care planning in ensuring that care aligns with the values and preferences of the individual. It also explores the ethical and legal issues that arise for professionals and families, including decisions about life-sustaining treatments, patient autonomy, and the role of advance directives. The ultimate goal of EOL care is to alleviate suffering, enhance quality of life, and honor the person's dignity and values through collaborative efforts between families, patients, and care teams.

[1] Advanced directives are legal documents that outline a person's medical care preferences if they become unable to communicate their decisions. These include living wills, which specify treatment wishes, and healthcare power of attorney, which designates someone to make medical decisions on their behalf. Advanced directives ensure patient autonomy and communicate to healthcare providers and families about their preferences during critical situations.

Y. Z. Ciupak, D. C. Smith, *Death, Dying, and Grief*,
https://doi.org/10.1007/978-3-031-88467-2_5

5.2 End-of-Life Trajectories

End-of-life (EOL) is increasingly recognized as a distinct and often extended stage of life. During this period, the remaining time and quality of life become critical factors in planning care. Individuals approaching EOL may experience various trajectories, each marked by distinct patterns of change across physical, cognitive, and emotional domains. These trajectories affect both individuals and their loved ones, who often bear significant caregiving and decision-making responsibilities during this challenging period. Two primary approaches have emerged in EOL research: terminal decline (TD) and primary cause (Cohen et al., 2018; Lunney et al., 2003).

5.2.1 Terminal Decline Approach to EOL Trajectories

The terminal decline (TD) approach focuses on the overall process of mortality-related deterioration, which typically accelerates as death approaches. TD is often observed across various domains, such as cognitive function, emotional well-being, and physical health. During this period, individuals transition from a phase of relative stability to a rapid decline in their final years, months, or weeks. This pattern is often identified through longitudinal studies that track changes in these domains and correlate them with proximity to death (Cohen et al., 2018).

Cognitive decline Cognitive decline is the most extensively studied aspect of TD. Research shows that abilities, such as memory, perceptual speed, and semantic memory, often begin to decline several years before death. The onset of cognitive TD can vary, occurring anywhere from three years to over a decade before death, depending on the specific cognitive function being measured and the tools used for assessment. Factors like education, cognitive reserve, and the presence of conditions such as dementia influence this variation. These findings suggest that cognitive decline is a significant predictor of mortality, especially when specific cognitive functions, such as perceptual speed or episodic memory, are affected.

Subjective Well-Being Subjective well-being/life satisfaction also undergoes significant changes during the terminal phase. Studies have shown that positive affect tends to decrease gradually, whereas negative affect increases more sharply as death approaches. These changes are typically more closely related to proximity to death rather than chronological age, with significant shifts occurring approximately three to five years before death. A decline in well-being is often characterized by a decrease in life satisfaction and an increase in depressive symptoms. Research also indicates that a sense of personal control over life events can mitigate the steepness of this decline. This emphasizes the value of psychological and spiritual resilience during the end-of-life experience.

Physical Function Physical decline during the terminal phase is characterized by noticeable deterioration in motor function and, in many cases, significant weight loss. Research shows that motor function, assessed through tests of global motor abilities, typically begins to decline more rapidly two to three years before death. This physical decline often parallels cognitive decline, although the rates of deterioration in these domains are not always strongly correlated. Unintentional weight loss, particularly in the final years of life, is a common marker of impending death.

Variability and Models of TD The onset and rate of TD vary widely among individuals and are influenced by factors such as underlying health conditions, the presence of comorbidities, and individuals' cognitive and physical reserves. Researchers have proposed both single-phase and multiphase models to describe the TD process. Single-phase models depict a gradual decline leading to death, whereas multiphase models suggest a more complex process, where the decline starts slowly and then accelerates as death nears. The variability in the onset and progression of TD across different domains underscores the need for personalized approaches in EOL care, as each individual's experience may differ significantly on the basis of their unique circumstances.

Understanding TD across these diverse domains helps anticipate the needs of dying individuals and provide appropriate care. For example, early detection of cognitive decline may prompt interventions that focus on maintaining cognitive function and quality of life for as long as possible. Similarly, recognizing signs of emotional decline can lead to timely psychological support for both patients and their families. Physical decline, particularly in motor function and weight, may indicate the need for adjustments in care plans, such as increased assistance with daily activities or nutritional support.

5.2.2 *Primary Cause Approach*

The second approach examines EOL trajectories on the basis of the primary causes of death, offering a complementary and nuanced understanding of how different causes shape the varied process of functional decline (Lunney et al., 2003). This approach categorizes individuals into one of four main trajectories: sudden death, terminal illness, organ failure, and frailty. Each trajectory differs in the duration and shape of EOL, representing unique challenges, and requires tailored interventions to ensure that both the patient and their family receive appropriate care.

1. **Sudden death**: Individuals experiencing sudden death typically transition quickly from normal functioning to death, often without significant prior decline. This trajectory can be particularly challenging for families, as there is little time to prepare emotionally or practically. Providing immediate and compassionate support, including grief counseling and logistical assistance, is crucial for helping families cope with sudden loss.

2. **Terminal illness**: Terminal illnesses, such as cancer, often involve high functionality early in their final year but are markedly more disabling three months before death. Individuals on this trajectory may experience increasing physical symptoms, such as pain and fatigue, as well as emotional distress due to the awareness of impending death. Care for these individuals should focus on comprehensive palliative care that addresses not only physical symptoms but also psychological, social, and spiritual needs. For families, anticipatory grief can be significant. Providing support groups, counseling, and clear communication about the care plan can help them navigate this challenging time. Early integration of palliative care services can also help manage symptoms effectively and improve quality of life during the final months.
3. **Organ failure**: Individuals with chronic conditions such as heart failure or chronic obstructive pulmonary disease (COPD) often experience a trajectory characterized by a gradual decline with intermittent acute episodes. This unpredictable pattern includes periods of stability interrupted by sudden deterioration, with a marked decline during the last 3 months before death. Care for these patients should include regular monitoring and timely interventions to manage acute episodes, along with ongoing support to maintain the highest possible quality of life. Families may struggle with the uncertainty and frequent hospitalizations that characterize this trajectory, so providing them with education about the disease process, as well as respite care and emotional support, is essential. Ensuring that the family is involved in care planning and decision-making can also help them feel more in control and prepared for the eventual outcome.
4. **Frailty**: Frailty, often associated with advanced age and conditions such as dementia, is characterized by a slow and prolonged decline. Individuals in this trajectory experience increasing dependency over time, leading to a gradual loss of function and autonomy. Clinical research indicates that frail individuals are relatively more disabled in the final year and especially during the previous month. Care for frail individuals should focus on maintaining dignity and comfort, respecting their preferences and values. Given the extended nature of this trajectory, long-term care planning is crucial. Families may face significant caregiving burdens, often over many years, which can lead to physical, emotional, and financial strain. Providing access to community resources, caregiver support programs, and long-term care services can help alleviate some of these burdens and improve the overall well-being of both patients and their families.

Table 5.1 summarizes the primary causes, typical trajectories, and recommended support for different end-of-life experiences.

Table 5.1 Dying trajectory and support

Trajectory	Primary cause	Typical trajectory	Recommended support
Sudden death	Unexpected events (e.g., accidents, heart attack)	Quick transition from normal functioning to death without prior decline	Immediate, compassionate support for families, including grief counseling and logistical assistance
Terminal illness	Diseases like cancer	High function initially; significant decline 3 months before death, with physical and emotional symptoms	Comprehensive palliative care addressing physical, psychological, social, and spiritual needs; support groups, counseling, clear care plans
Organ failure	Chronic conditions (e.g., heart failure, COPD)	Gradual decline with intermittent acute episodes; marked decline in the final 3 months	Regular monitoring, timely interventions, education on disease, respite care, emotional support, family involvement in care planning
Frailty	Advanced age, conditions like dementia	Slow, prolonged decline with increasing dependency; significant disability in the final year and month	Long-term care planning focused on dignity and comfort, community resources, caregiver support programs, and emotional and financial assistance for families

5.2.3 Integrating Care Strategies

Understanding these EOL trajectories and their implications allows professionals to offer effective and compassionate care. By recognizing the specific trajectory an individual is on, services can be tailored to meet their evolving needs, whether through palliative care, acute interventions, or long-term support services. Furthermore, integrating these insights into care planning enables dying individuals and their families to prepare for the challenges they may face, ensuring that they receive the support and guidance necessary to navigate the end-of-life journey with resilience and grace.

In conclusion, recognizing and understanding the distinct trajectories of decline at the end of life helps deliver effective care that honors the dignity of the dying individual and provides meaningful support to their family. Through a combination of personalized care strategies, anticipatory guidance, and compassionate support, healthcare professionals can help ensure that the final phase of life is as comfortable and peaceful as possible for all involved individuals.

5.3 Theoretical Frameworks: Stage and Tasks

5.3.1 Stage Model: Cautions and Lesson

The five-stage model was introduced by Dr. Elisabeth Kübler-Ross in her seminal work *On Death and Dying* (1969). It had a profound and lasting impact on how society understands and discusses death, dying, and grief. Based on her work with terminally ill patients, she identified five psychological stages that individuals often experience when coping with dying: denial, anger, bargaining, depression, and acceptance. Table 5.2 summarizes each stage along with its key characteristics.

5.3.1.1 Criticisms and Limitations

The stage model provides a straightforward structure and vocabulary to make sense of the complex and often overwhelming emotions associated with death and grief. Its simplicity and accessibility resonated widely, embedding these stages into popular discourse. However, despite the model's popularity among the general public, it has faced significant criticism in research and clinical practice. Kastenbaum (2012) and Corr et al. (2019) summarized these critiques, highlighting several key issues:

1. **Lack of empirical evidence**: The existence of the five stages has not been consistently demonstrated through empirical research. There is insufficient evidence to support the idea that people universally progress through these stages in a linear fashion.
2. **Methodological limitations**: The original research that led to the model was based on a narrow study population, limiting its generalizability. The methods used to develop the model have been questioned because they do not adequately represent the diverse experiences of dying individuals.
3. **Blurred line between description and prescription**: The model has often been interpreted not only as a description of possible experiences but also as a

Table 5.2 Kübler-Ross's five-stage model for facing dying

Stage	Characteristics
Denial	Refusal to accept the reality of the situation. A temporary defense mechanism to manage overwhelming emotions. "Not me!"
Anger	Feelings of frustration, helplessness, and injustice; often directed at oneself, others, or a higher power. "Why me?"
Bargaining	Attempts to negotiate or change the situation; involves making promises or mental negotiations to delay or alter the outcome. "Yes me, but…"
Depression	Deep sadness and withdrawal as the reality of the loss sets in; marked by changes in behavior, sleep, and appetite.
Acceptance	Coming to terms with the situation; not devoid of emotional pain but characterized by a more peaceful acknowledgment of reality.

Note: Based on Kübler-Ross (1969). Death and Dying

prescriptive sequence that individuals are expected to follow. This has led to the misconception that there is a "right" and "normal" way to grieve.

4. **Narrow focus on emotional aspects**: Critics argue that the stage model overlooks the totality of a person's life, reducing the complexity of the dying experience to a series of intrapersonal emotional stages. This reductionist view fails to account for the rich, multifaceted nature of human life and identity, which includes social and spiritual aspects in addition to biopsychological aspects (WHO, 2020).
5. **Environmental and cultural context**: The model does not adequately consider the resources, pressures, and characteristics of the individual's immediate environment, nor does it account for the influence of social and cultural factors on the grieving process. This omission suggests that all humans respond to the stress of dying in similar ways, independent of their social or cultural background, which is not the case.

5.3.1.2 Legacy

Despite the limitations of the stage model, Dr. Elizabeth Kübler-Ross has made pioneering contributions to the conversation surrounding death and dying. Her work broke through cultural taboos and provided insights into caring for the dying persons:

1. **Recognition of life amidst dying**: One of the most profound legacies of Kübler-Ross is to recognize that individuals facing death are still living. They often have unfinished business, desires, goals, and the need for meaningful interactions. This perspective encourages caregivers to focus on enhancing the quality of the remaining time, ensuring that these needs are addressed with dignity and respect.
2. **Compassionate listening**: Kübler-Ross revolutionized patient care by emphasizing the significance of actively listening to individuals facing death. Rare interview footage showcases her compassionate and relatable communication with patients, including body orientation, empathetic eye contact, and gentle touch. In the interview, she humbly reflected that all she did was sit with the patients, listen to them, and truly *hear* them (Kübler-Ross, 1983).
3. **Humanistic patient-centered care:** Dr. Kübler-Ross advocated for a patient-centered approach that respects the autonomy and individual needs of each person. This lesson is essential in healthcare, reminding providers that effective care involves more than just treating symptoms—it requires understanding and responding to the unique experiences of each patient.
4. **Learning from the dying**: Throughout her career, Kübler-Ross emphasized the value of learning from those who are dying. She believed that their insights could lead to more compassionate and effective care practices. Her work emphasized the need to consider the emotional, spiritual, and relational aspects of dying, rather than simply focusing on clinical factors. By engaging with the

dying in honest and empathetic conversations, caregivers can provide better support and gain a deeper understanding of the human experience.

Kübler-Ross's work initiated a significant cultural change, promoting open discussions about death and improving end-of-life care awareness. While her stage model has limitations, the overall impact of her legacy has been transformative. This has led to improvements in caring for terminally ill patients, emphasizing the need for humane and holistic care that honors the dignity of each individual.

5.3.2 Corr's Task-Based Model

The task-based approach developed by Charles Corr (1992) provides a structured method for understanding how individuals cope with terminal illness. This model focuses on organizing daily tasks on the basis of their importance to the individual without adhering to a strict timeline. This approach emphasizes the proactive nature of coping, helping individuals manage their situation by prioritizing tasks that matter most to them (Corr, 1992).

Corr's model outlines four primary areas of task work in coping with dying, each addressing different dimensions of a person's experience:

1. **Physical dimension**: Lessening or managing physical pain and distress.
2. **Psychological dimension**: Addressing emotions such as anger, sadness, anxiety, and fear and helping individuals process these emotions to find comfort.
3. **Social dimension**: Connecting with important people and building a social network to provide security and comfort and address concerns about the family's future and unfinished projects.
4. **Spiritual dimension**: Facilitate patients' meaning-making and spiritual exploration as they integrate new experiences and reassess challenged beliefs due to illness, imminent death, and other life disruptions.

The task-based model acknowledges that each person copes differently and may shift priorities on a daily or even hourly basis. It encourages continuous engagement with these tasks, allowing them to be revisited and worked through over time (Corr, 1992). Those who assist them can use this model to identify the care receiver's priorities during each interaction, ensuring that the support provided is aligned with the individual's current needs and preferences. This model therefore aligns well with the Spiral Model of Grieving and Healing, addressing holistic and dynamic human experiences (Ciupak, 2025).

5.4 Four Pillars of Holistic End-of-Life Care (WHO)

The World Health Organization (WHO) defines palliative care as specialized medical care focused on improving quality of life and alleviating suffering for patients with serious illnesses. This care approach is holistic, addressing the physical, emotional, social, and spiritual dimensions of a patient's well-being (WHO, 2020). The WHO identifies four key pillars of holistic end-of-life care:

1. **Physical Support: Managing Pain and Symptoms**

The first pillar focuses on the identification and management of symptoms to alleviate physical suffering. Palliative care involves holistic treatment, ensuring that physical comfort is a priority. This includes the use of medications and technologies, such as pain relief measures and ventilation systems, to manage symptoms effectively. Ensuring the physical comfort of patients is a foundational aspect of holistic care.

2. **Psychological Support: Addressing Fears and Anxieties**

The second pillar addresses the emotional and psychological aspects of end-of-life care. This involves providing support to patients as they navigate the complex emotions associated with death and dying. To effectively deliver difficult news, the WHO recommends using the SPIKES metric:

- **Setting up the interview**: Arrange a meeting in a comfortable environment to discuss sensitive news.
- **Perception**: Use open-ended questions to gauge the patient's understanding of their condition.
- **Invitation**: Determine how much information the patient wishes to know about their condition.
- **Knowledge**: Deliver the news in a clear and compassionate manner, allowing the patient time to absorb the information.
- **Emotions**: Acknowledge and validate the patient's emotions, as well as those of their family.
- **Summarize and strategize**: Review the discussion and address any remaining questions, ensuring that the patient and family understand the next steps.

This communication approach helps create a supportive and empathetic environment, allowing patients to process their emotions with the guidance of healthcare professionals.

3. **Social Support: Maintaining Relationships**

The third pillar emphasizes the importance of social support in end-of-life care. Studies consistently show a strong association between perceived social support and improved emotional and physical quality of life, even during challenging times such as social isolation in the pandemic era (Grey et al., 2020). This includes support from family, friends, and healthcare personnel. Efforts that strengthen these support systems can significantly enhance the physical and psychosocial well-being of the person under care.

4. **Spiritual Support: Honoring Beliefs and Values**

The fourth pillar involves providing spiritual support. Practitioners should cultivate an understanding of diverse spiritual beliefs and integrate this awareness into care plans. Addressing spiritual needs not only reduces existential distress and provides profound comfort but also helps formulate care plans and decisions in alignment with the person's beliefs and values. This support goes beyond connecting patients with chaplains and spiritual care providers. *Improving the Quality of Spiritual Care as a Dimension of Palliative Care: The Report of the Consensus Conference* (Puchalski et al., 2009), a key and influential document, emphasizes that spiritual care must be integrated into all aspects of palliative care and carried out through the collaboration of the entire team. It recommends thorough spiritual assessments, training interdisciplinary teams to include spiritual care in treatment plans, and ensuring that chaplains are integral members of the care team. These practices create an environment where spiritual care is viewed as essential, fostering patient-centered and dignified care. For a detailed exploration of spiritual support practices, refer to Chap. 12.

The four pillars of palliative care recognize humans as simultaneously biological, psychosocial, and spiritual beings. Addressing each and every aspect of these needs ensures a holistic and humanistic approach that honors the last journey of life.

5.5 Major Types of End-of-Life Care

End-of-life care can be provided in various settings, such as hospitals and nursing homes, and through nonprofit or private organizations like home healthcare and hospice programs. End-of-life care generally falls into three main categories: hospice care, palliative care, and curative care.

Although there are variations across countries, hospice care is designed for individuals in the final stages of life, typically with a prognosis of six months or less, with a focus on comfort and quality of life rather than curative treatments. It is provided in various settings, including homes and hospice facilities.

Palliative care, on the other hand, can be administered at any stage of a serious illness, even alongside curative treatments, and aims to relieve symptoms and enhance the patient's quality of life.

Finally, curative care seeks to treat or cure the illness itself, often through interventions such as chemotherapy, surgery, or antibiotics and can be combined with palliative care to address both the disease and the patient's overall well-being.

Table 5.3 compares the critical differences between the three major care systems.

Table 5.3 Comparison of curative care, palliative care, and hospice care

Aspect	Curative care	Palliative care	Hospice care
Primary goal	Treat or cure the underlying illness or condition	Relieve symptoms and improve quality of life at any stage of serious illness	Provide comfort and improve quality of life in the final stages of life
Patient population	Patients with treatable conditions, not necessarily terminal	Patients with serious, potentially life-threatening illnesses	Patients with a life expectancy of six months or less
Treatment focus	Medical interventions aimed at curing or controlling the disease	Symptom management, pain relief, emotional and spiritual support, can be alongside curative treatments	Symptom management, pain relief, emotional and spiritual support
Care settings	Hospitals, clinics, specialized treatment centers	Hospitals, outpatient clinics, nursing homes, home care settings	Home, hospice facilities, nursing homes, hospitals
Involvement of curative treatments	Solely focused on curing the disease or condition	Can be provided alongside curative treatments	Curative treatments are generally stopped; focus shifts entirely to comfort care
Eligibility	No specific eligibility beyond the need for treatment of the illness	Available to anyone with a serious illness, at any stage	Usually, requires a prognosis of six months or less; typically, curative treatments have been stopped
Team composition	Primarily medical professionals focused on treatment (doctors, surgeons, specialists)	Interdisciplinary team including doctors, nurses, social workers, chaplains, and sometimes curative specialists	Interdisciplinary team including doctors, nurses, social workers, chaplains, volunteers

Curative Care

Curative care represents the starting point of treatment, with a focus on curing an illness or medical condition. When a cure is not possible, it may aim to slow disease progression. Examples include dialysis, antibiotics, chemotherapy, radiation, and setting a broken bone. Curative care is a crucial part of the healthcare system, particularly for conditions where recovery or prolonged life is possible.

Palliative Care

Palliative care, such as hospice, focuses on improving the quality of life by managing pain and symptoms. However, unlike hospice, palliative care can be provided at any stage of a severe illness. It aims to reduce suffering and support patients and their loved ones through an interdisciplinary, often hospital-based, team approach.

Since the 2000s, palliative care services have expanded significantly in the United States, reaching a wider range of patients, including children and young adults. Pediatric palliative care, for example, is tailored to provide compassionate care to children with chronic or life-threatening illnesses, enhancing their quality of life and minimizing suffering. However, a meta-analysis of palliative care durations across 23 countries revealed that care often begins too late to achieve the full benefits of a 3–4-month multidisciplinary approach. These findings also point to inequalities in access based on patient, service, and country factors (Jordan et al., 2020).

Hospice Care

Hospice care is one of the most highly utilized forms of end-of-life care worldwide. It provides holistic care to individuals in the final stages of life, typically during the last six months. The modern concept of hospice care is rooted in the work of Dame Cicely Saunders, who established St. Christopher's Hospice in London in 1967. This model of care emphasizes an interdisciplinary approach, addressing the physical, emotional, social, and spiritual needs of patients.

In the United States, hospice care is delivered through various organizational models, including independent agencies, hospital-based programs, and divisions of home health services. The availability and type of hospice care are often influenced by factors such as funding and patient needs. American hospice care has evolved to prioritize home-based care, reflecting cultural values of independence. Unlike inpatient-focused care in the United Kingdom, US hospice care programs emphasize providing services in patients' homes or through community-based settings. This model also relies heavily on volunteer work, with over 400,000 volunteers contributing millions of hours of service annually (Connor & Gwyther, 2018). The American model of hospice care requires that curative treatments stop and that the person has a life expectancy of six months or less.

The United States National Hospice and Palliative Care Organization has a set of four core philosophies (Table 5.4) and seven organizational values for hospice providers (Table 5.5).

Table 5.4 Core philosophical concepts of hospice care

Philosophical concepts	Summary
Dying as an experience	Emphasizes that dying is a process filled with meaning, encompassing emotional, spiritual, and relational aspects. It is more than a biological event.
Family-centered care	Recognizes the essential role of family relationships in supporting the personhood of the dying and treating the family as integral to the care process.
Nature and relief of suffering	Focuses on holistic care addressing "total pain" that affects physical, emotional, psychological, and spiritual aspects of the patient and family.
Restoring and supporting moral agency	Prioritizes enabling patients to maintain their sense of identity and integrity, allowing them to create meaning until death.

Note: Based on the National Hospice and Palliative Care Organization. (2023). *Guide to organizational ethics in hospice care* (Updated 2023). Alexandria, VA: National Hospice and Palliative Care Organization

Table 5.5 Key organizational values for hospice providers

Organizational values	Summary
Equitable access	Ensures transparent, fair, and appropriate criteria for providing care, emphasizing justice and removing barriers for underrepresented groups
Comfort and quality of life	Centers on symptom management and holistic well-being, respecting patient and family definitions of comfort and quality of life
Teamwork and collaboration	Promotes interdisciplinary coordination, ensuring team dynamics are supported for optimal patient and family care
Excellence	Involves striving beyond compliance to achieve the highest standards in care, integrating best practices, and continuous improvement
Stewardship	Advocates responsible resource use to align with the organization's mission, balancing financial health with patient care priorities
Transparency	Commits to clear, accurate, and accessible communication within the organization and with stakeholders to foster trust
Integrity	Embeds consistent, coherent values in practices and ensures alignment between stated principles and actual operations

Note: Based on: National Hospice and Palliative Care Organization. (2023). *Guide to organizational ethics in hospice care* (Updated 2023). Alexandria, VA: National Hospice and Palliative Care Organization

Evidence shows that hospice care greatly improves quality of life and reduces burdensome treatments and financial costs, especially when provided early, ideally 3–4 months before death. Research has shown that hospice care leads to better pain and symptom management, less emotional distress, and greater satisfaction with care for patients and their families than does standard medical care. Hospice patients often have fewer hospitalizations and emergency room visits, allowing them to spend their final days at home, surrounded by loved ones. Additionally, hospice care helps lower healthcare costs by reducing unnecessary medical interventions during the final stages of life. Families of hospice patients also report feeling more supported and better prepared for the death of their loved ones and often receive bereavement care (Jordan et al., 2020).

Despite the availability of hospice care and insurance coverage in Europe and North America, its use remains limited. While hospice care is intended for those with a prognosis of six months or less, the average length of stay is often much shorter. For example, the median duration of palliative care before death ranges from just 6 days in Australia to 69 days in Canada (Jordan et al., 2020). This short duration is often due to late referrals and the association of hospice with impending death, which can trigger anxiety for patients and families. Consequently, some individuals eligible for hospice may choose more expensive nursing homes instead.

In summary, end-of-life care offers a range of services to support the diverse needs of patients and their families during this critical time. Whether through hospice, palliative, or curative care, the focus is on improving quality of life. As the field evolves, expanding access and addressing disparities locally and globally are vital to providing equitable and meaningful support in the final stages of life.

5.6 Global Development of End-of-Life Care

End-of-life care, a critical aspect of healthcare that supports individuals in the final stages of life, has evolved significantly across different regions of the world. Its origins trace back to Europe, particularly in the United Kingdom, where the modern hospice movement began in the 1960s under the leadership of Dame Cicely Saunders. She founded St. Christopher's Hospice in London in 1967, pioneering an interdisciplinary approach to caring for the dying that focused on managing "total pain," which includes physical, emotional, social, and spiritual suffering. This model laid the foundation for what would become a global movement in palliative and hospice care.

The hospice philosophy soon spread to the United States, where it adapted to the local cultural context by focusing on home-based care and community involvement. The first hospice in the United States was established in 1974 in Branford, Connecticut, and was directly inspired by Saunders's work. By the 1990s, efforts to improve end-of-life care gained momentum, leading to the pivotal SUPPORT study (Study to Understand Prognoses and Preferences for Outcomes and Risks of Treatment), which was conducted from 1989 to 1995 (Gray & LeBlanc, 2018). This multicenter investigation, which included over 9000 seriously ill hospitalized patients, revealed significant deficiencies in end-of-life care. Key issues included poor communication between healthcare providers and patients, inadequate pain management, and a disconnect between patients' preferences and the treatments they received.

Despite the comprehensive implementation of interventions, the SUPPORT study demonstrated that merely providing more information or decision-making tools was not enough to improve outcomes or alleviate suffering. Many patients continue to receive invasive treatments that do not align with their wishes. These findings emphasized the need for systemic changes and a more patient-centered approach to palliative and end-of-life care in the United States.

The American model of hospice care has since evolved with a focus on maintaining patient autonomy and providing care in the home, reflecting cultural values of independence and a degree of skepticism toward institutionalized care. Lessons from studies such as SUPPORT have continued to shape the development of end-of-life care, highlighting the importance of compassionate and holistic approaches that honor the preferences of dying persons.

In Asia, end-of-life care has evolved through a blend of Western influences and local cultural traditions. For instance, in India, palliative care began to gain traction in the 1980s, focusing on holistic care and pain management for cancer patients. However, despite these advancements, palliative care services remain largely inaccessible to a significant portion of India's population, primarily because of economic barriers. Advocates suggest implementing community-based models, improving policy enforcement, and increasing funding to enhance accessibility throughout the country (Bag et al., 2020).

Countries like Japan and Singapore have made notable progress in incorporating palliative care into their health systems. However, challenges such as cultural perceptions, a lack of knowledge and skills, and issues with resource allocation persist (Martina et al., 2021).

Overall, the growth of palliative care in Asia has involved the integration of traditional practices with modern medicine, often tackling unique challenges such as limited healthcare access and prevailing cultural norms.

Across Africa and Latin America, the development of end-of-life care is still in its nascent stages and is often hindered by a lack of resources and infrastructure. However, there is growing recognition of the need for palliative care, especially in the context of the HIV/AIDS epidemic, which has highlighted the importance of pain management and compassionate care for terminally ill patients. International organizations and local initiatives are working to address these gaps, promoting education and advocacy to expand access to end-of-life care in these regions (Clark et al., 2020).

The World Health Organization (WHO) recognizes palliative care as an essential component of universal health coverage and advocates for its integration into health systems around the globe. The importance of providing quality end-of-life care is increasingly seen as a public health priority. Approximately 60 million people die each year worldwide, with the majority of these deaths occurring in low- and middle-income countries. However, only 14% of those in need of palliative care actually receive it. This gap highlights the moral and healthcare imperative to ensure access to compassionate and effective end-of-life care. Adequate national policies, programs, resources, and training on palliative care among health professionals are urgently needed to improve access. The WHO projects that the global need for palliative care will continue to grow due to the aging of populations and the increasing burden of noncommunicable diseases and some communicable diseases (WHO, 2020).

5.7 Advance Care Planning and Decision-Making

5.7.1 Introduction

Advance care planning (ACP) is an essential component of healthcare that ensures individuals receive medical treatment in alignment with their values when they are unable to communicate these preferences. It typically involves multiple discussions with healthcare professionals, potentially leading to the creation of an Advance Directive (AD). This legal document usually includes living wills and durable powers of attorney, guiding clinicians and family members in making informed medical decisions on behalf of an incapacitated individual.

While the principal elements of advance directives, such as living wills, are similar across the board, laws governing their use can vary significantly from state to state. These differences highlight the importance of ensuring that such documents comply with local legal requirements.

Many state legislatures, supported by major health institutions, recommend that competent adults over 18 years of age have an advance directive to ensure that their medical preferences are respected if they cannot communicate.[2] By taking this step early in life, individuals ensure that their medical preferences are documented and respected, regardless of age or health status. Once created, it is recommended to keep the document in an easily accessible place and inform loved ones where it is located. Sharing these preferences with loved ones before a medical crisis helps ensure that individuals receive the care they want.

Advance care planning often involves difficult and sensitive conversations with the person, family, and healthcare teams. However, involving family members in these discussions can strengthen relationships and reduce feelings of isolation for the dying person as well as many other positive outcomes (McMahan et al., 2020). The National Hospice and Palliative Care Organization (NHPCO) and other organizations offer free online resources to help facilitate these difficult but important conversations.[3]

5.7.2 Living Wills & Durable Power of Attorney

Advance directives often include living wills and durable powers of attorney, both essential tools in end-of-life planning, addressing essential aspects of "what I want and do not want" and "who can speak for me." A living will outline the types of medical interventions an individual does or does not want when facing terminal illness or incapacitation. These documents focus on avoiding unnecessary, life-prolonging measures when death is imminent, prioritizing comfort and palliative care instead. While living promotes individual autonomy, it may not cover every possible scenario, leading to potential debates among family members and healthcare providers.

Another crucial advance directive is the durable power of attorney for healthcare. This legal arrangement allows an individual to appoint a healthcare proxy or surrogate to make decisions on their behalf if they become incapacitated. The appointed person ensures that decisions align with the patient's values and wishes. The American Bar Association provides free online guides to help individuals understand this responsibility and make informed decisions.

---

[2] For example, Michigan Legislature (2021).

[3] For example, CaringInfo.org is a program of the National Hospice and Palliative Care Organization. It provides comprehensive resources and guidance for terminal ill patients and their family. This includes medical resources such as palliative care and hospice, financial resources such as insurance, legal resources such as advance directive, and personal resources. https://www.caringinfo.org/planning/

In addition to these directives, individuals may also include instructions related to organ and tissue donation, the disposition of their body, and the distribution of their estate. Although these aspects are sometimes not covered by medical advance directives, they are some common components of end-of-life planning.

5.7.3 Importance of Advance Care Planning

By outlining preferences for treatments and care in advance, patients increase the opportunity for end-of-life journeys to be in alignment with their preferences. For healthcare providers, having a clear understanding of a patient's wishes enables them to provide more personalized care. A scoping review of relevant studies highlights the importance of end-of-life conversations in improving the quality of care and reducing the emotional burden on families. Such discussions and planning are associated with lower healthcare costs, better quality of life in the final weeks, and reduced anxiety and fear surrounding death. Both patients and families of individuals with advanced directives report increased satisfaction with communication and decreased distress among family and physicians (McMahan et al., 2020).

The importance of advance directives is reinforced by key legal frameworks. For example, the Patient Self-Determination Act (1991) mandates that healthcare institutions receiving federal funding must inform individuals of their rights to accept or refuse treatment, execute an advance directive, and understand the options available to implement these rights. Furthermore, in 2016, Medicare began accepting billing from primary healthcare practitioners for engaging in advance care planning. This allows physicians and other healthcare professionals to dedicate face-to-face time with patients, family members, or surrogates to explain and discuss advance directives, ensuring that end-of-life care aligns with patient preferences.

5.7.4 Challenges and Strategies

Creating and executing an advance directive can present challenges. According to Michigan's 2021 guide on medical and legal decisions, some common problems include emotional and social factors, unclear language or lack of specifics in directives, and the potential for misinterpretation by healthcare providers or family members. Furthermore, some clinicians may find it challenging to reconcile the patient's expressed wishes with their medical judgment, notably if the advance directive lacks specificity or appears overly restrictive.

Addressing these challenges involves thoughtful discussions with healthcare providers, ensuring that the advance directive reflects specific and clear instructions, and revisiting the document periodically to ensure it remains aligned with the individual's current values and preferences.

The recommended strategies for creating an advance directive include several important steps:

Reflect on beliefs and values: Before drafting a living will or choosing a healthcare proxy, take time to consider beliefs, values, and what matters most. Think about what brings comfort or peace, including any spiritual or cultural factors that may guide decisions.

Define quality-of-life concerns: Clarify what quality-of-life means personally in the context of medical care. Reflect on questions like what makes life meaningful and under what circumstances life-sustaining treatments might be declined. These considerations help shape care preferences and provide clear direction.

Understand life-sustaining treatments: Learn about treatments like resuscitation, mechanical ventilation, feeding tubes, and dialysis. Think about when these interventions might or might not align with care goals. Providing clear preferences ensures that living wills offer useful guidance to healthcare providers and loved ones.

Consider a support network: Identify those who can provide support during critical times, such as family, friends, spiritual advisors, or healthcare professionals. Choosing a healthcare proxy who understands and respects these values is key to ensuring decisions reflect care preferences.

After reflecting on these preferences, they can be documented in a living will.

5.7.5 *What to Do Once You Have an Advance Directive*

The Michigan Legislature's 2021 guide recommends the following steps related to an advance directive:

- Everyone over 18 years should have an advance directive.
- Keep your advance directive in an easily accessible place and let loved ones know where it is.
- Sharing preferences before a medical crisis helps ensure that you receive the care you want.
- Update your directive as necessary: As your values, preferences, or health circumstances change, be sure to revisit and update your advance directive to reflect your current wishes.

5.8 Medically Assisted Death: Debate and Current State

Physician-assisted death (PAD), also known as "physician-assisted suicide" (PAS) or "medical aid in dying," remains an ethically and legally complex topic within modern healthcare. This issue intersects with debates on autonomy, the role of medicine and medical workers, and societal values. The practice usually involves mentally capable, terminally ill individuals ending their lives through the voluntary self-administration of a lethal dose of medication expressly prescribed by a physician for that purpose (Oregon Health Authority, n.d.). This option is primarily considered by patients enduring unrelievable suffering without hope of recovery, raising profound discussions about the limits of medical intervention, the sanctity of life, and the right to die with dignity. As attitudes toward death and dying evolve globally, different countries have approached this issue with varying degrees of acceptance, legality, and regulation, reflecting cultural, religious, and ethical differences across the world.

5.8.1 Legalization and Practices in the United States

Oregon became the first US state to PAD with the Death with Dignity Act in 1994, although its implementation was delayed until 1997 due to legal challenges. This law, and others such as it, stipulates criteria for eligibility, such as terminal illness with a prognosis of six months or less and the patient's capacity to make healthcare decisions. PAD has since been legalized in ten states and Washington, D.C., reflecting a growing acceptance of the practice within strict regulatory frameworks.

By 2024, ten US states—California, Colorado, Hawaii, Maine, Montana, New Jersey, New Mexico, Oregon, Vermont, and Washington—along with Washington, D.C., had legalized physician-assisted death (Mroz et al., 2021). In 2023, Oregon and Vermont removed residency requirements, allowing nonresidents to access this option (CNN, 2023). An increasing number of national and state medical societies have begun to endorse PAD or withdraw opposition to it in favor of neutrality. For example, the American Medical Association (AMA) affirms that physicians may participate in PAD on the basis of their conscience without violating professional ethical obligations (AMA, 2019). Meanwhile, a thorough review of 150 US medical and surgical society position statements on PAD and euthanasia revealed that only 8% of the participants had position statements (Barsness et al., 2020).

These developments reflect a broader national conversation about end-of-life care in the United States, but they are part of a global dialog that varies significantly across different cultural and legal frameworks.

5.8.2 International Perspectives on Physician-Assisted Death

Globally, attitudes toward physician-assisted death range from full legalization to outright prohibition. In countries such as Switzerland, Belgium, and the Netherlands, physician-assisted death is legal, and in some cases, euthanasia—where a physician directly administers the lethal dose—is also permitted (AMA, 2019). These countries have established strict protocols to ensure that patients' decisions are informed, voluntary, and consistent over time. In Switzerland, for example, the practice has been legal since 1942 and is available not only to Swiss citizens but also to foreigners, leading to the phenomenon of "suicide tourism"[4] (Carrigan, 2023).

Belgium and the Netherlands go further by allowing euthanasia for those suffering unbearable pain from both terminal and nonterminal conditions. This includes individuals with severe mental illnesses or disabilities, provided they meet strict criteria and have the agreement of multiple healthcare providers. These laws reflect a societal belief in the importance of individual autonomy and the right to die with dignity, a perspective shared by many who support physician-assisted death in the United States.

In contrast, many countries, including most nations in Africa and Asia, prohibit any form of assisted dying, often on religious or cultural grounds. For instance, in India, euthanasia and physician-assisted death remain illegal due to concerns about the sanctity of life as influenced by religious traditions such as Hinduism and Islam. However, passive euthanasia—where life-sustaining treatments are withheld or withdrawn—is legally permitted following a landmark Supreme Court decision in 2018, which upheld the right to die with dignity and introduced the use of Advanced Directives to guide end-of-life care (Mahajan, 2023).

The different approaches highlight the complex interplay of legal, ethical, and cultural factors that influence decisions about the end of life. These international examples demonstrate that physician-assisted death is not just a Western issue but is part of a global conversation on autonomy, dignity, and the limits of medical care.

5.8.3 Active vs. Passive Euthanasia

Within this broader debate, distinguishing between active euthanasia and passive euthanasia is critical. **Active euthanasia** involves directly causing a patient's death, such as administering a lethal injection. While this practice is legal in countries such as Belgium and the Netherlands, it is generally illegal in the United States and most other countries. Active euthanasia is often equated with homicide under US law and is treated separately from physician-assisted death, where the patient self-administers the medication.

Passive euthanasia, on the other hand, involves withholding or withdrawing life-sustaining treatments, allowing the patient to die naturally from their

[4]The way suicide tourism is portrayed in the media reveals a complex social construction shaped by cultural attitudes toward autonomy, death, and legal boundaries. In a recent mixed-methods study by Carrigan (2023) analyzing newspaper coverage of suicide tourism in four Western European countries from 2002 to 2021, four main themes were identified: (1) suicide tourism as an expression of autonomy and self-determination, (2) Dignitas as an 'emergency exit,' (3) laws on assisted suicide depicted as outdated and coercive, and (4) dying in Switzerland framed as a 'good death.' This study highlighted the consistent portrayal of this topic as a challenge to restrictive national laws and as a testament to modern desires for end-of-life choices.

underlying condition. This practice is more widely accepted and legal in many countries, including the United States. It typically involves decisions such as removing a ventilator or stopping feeding. Passive euthanasia is often seen as allowing nature to take its course, in contrast to the more active intervention involved in physician-assisted death.

5.8.4 Physician-Assisted Death Debates

Numerous scholars and organizations have examined the arguments for and against physician-assisted death (PAD). Some, such as the American Medical Association (AMA, 2019), have shifted their stance to allow physicians to provide PAD according to their conscience. In contrast, other institutions, such as the International Association for Hospice and Palliative Care (IAHPC), oppose PAD and emphasize the potential risks and ethical dilemmas associated with its practice. The IAHPC emphasizes the importance of ensuring universal access to palliative care while upholding professional standards. It asserts that palliative care units should not oversee or administer Physician-Assisted Dying (PAD), as these practices conflict with established professional ethics. Furthermore, the IAHPC supports the right of health professionals to conscientiously object to participating in PAD and encourages them to refer patients to a neutral advocate (De Lima et al., 2017). Based on these and other reviews, such as the comprehensive analysis by the National Academies of Sciences, Engineering, and Medicine (2018), the key points of arguments for and against PAD are outlined as follows:

5.8.4.1 Arguments in Favor of Physician-Assisted Death

1. **Autonomy and Control**: Supporters of physician-assisted death argue that it provides terminally ill patients with control over their end-of-life process. By giving patients the ability to choose the timing and manner of their death, physician-assisted death allows them to avoid prolonged suffering and maintain their dignity in the face of terminal illness. For many, the ability to make decisions about their own death is a fundamental aspect of personal autonomy.
2. **Reduction of Suffering**: Proponents also emphasize the compassionate aspect of physician-assisted death. When patients face intolerable suffering that cannot be alleviated by palliative care, physician-assisted death offers a humane option. This allows patients to avoid more painful or drawn-out methods of dying, such as refusing food or water. Research from Oregon shows that physician-assisted death has remained stable and accounts for only a small percentage of deaths, suggesting that it is a carefully considered choice that complements palliative care practices.
3. **Preventing Harmful Alternatives**: Supporters argue that without physician-assisted death as an option, some patients may resort to more harmful or

traumatic ways of ending their lives, such as self-inflicted harm or refusing basic sustenance. Physician-assisted death provides a more peaceful and controlled way to die, ensuring that patients can pass on their own terms without unnecessary trauma.

5.8.4.2 Arguments Against Physician-Assisted Death

1. **Ethical Concerns**: Critics argue that physician-assisted death conflicts with the core mission of medicine, which is to preserve life and alleviate suffering without directly causing death. The American College of Physicians, among other organizations, contends that doctors should focus on enhancing palliative care and supporting patients through their suffering rather than hastening death (Barsness et al., 2020). The ethical concern is that physician-assisted death could erode the trust between patients and healthcare providers and alter the fundamental nature of the medical profession.
2. **Potential for Abuse and Vulnerability**: Opponents also worry that legalizing physician-assisted death could disproportionately affect vulnerable populations, such as the elderly, disabled individuals, or those with limited access to healthcare. They fear that these groups may feel pressure to choose death due to financial or social burdens, rather than genuine personal desire. This concern has been echoed in court rulings, such as *Washington v. Glucksberg* (1997), which highlighted the state's interest in protecting vulnerable populations from potential coercion.
3. **Slippery Slope to Euthanasia**: Critics of physician-assisted death often express concerns about a slippery slope toward active euthanasia. While physician-assisted death requires the patient to self-administer the lethal medication, opponents worry that normalizing the practice could lead to further relaxation of safeguards, ultimately allowing medical professionals to administer life-ending treatments without the patient's direct involvement. This could undermine the sanctity of life and the ethical boundaries of medicine.
4. **Religious and Moral Objections**: Many religious and philosophical traditions uphold the sanctity of life and argue that intentionally ending a life, even to relieve suffering, is morally wrong. These perspectives view life as sacred and believe that only a higher power should determine the time of death. Opponents also argue that society should provide care and compassion to those who are suffering, rather than facilitating their death.

5.8.4.3 Inconclusive Conclusion: Future Prospects

While the social and political debate around PAD remains fierce, legislation for assisted dying has expanded significantly in Europe, America, and Australia over the past two decades. PAD and euthanasia practices are now legal in 18 jurisdictions, increasing the number of people with access to assisted dying to over 200 million (Mroz et al., 2021). The future of physician-assisted death (PAD) is likely to see continued efforts to broaden access and more in-depth research on its impacts and procedures. Honoring autonomy and relieving suffering gradually takes more priority than reserving life.

As societies grapple with legitimizing and seeking social approval for various forms of assisted death, key stakeholders—including individual citizens, elected representatives, and the judicial system—will be called upon to shape public policies and practices. However, these decisions are not made solely at the institutional level; they continue to occur in individual circumstances, raising critical questions about who should decide whether such assistance can, should, or will be provided. These decisions will need to account for the psychological and social impacts of PAD on patients, families, and communities.

For healthcare professionals and families faced with these decisions, it is crucial to carefully weigh both the legal and ethical dimensions alongside the personal values and beliefs of the patient. The arguments for and against physician-assisted death reflect profound philosophical differences about autonomy, the role of medicine, and the nature of suffering and a humane life. As more states and countries consider legislation, ongoing dialogue among patients, families, and healthcare providers will be essential in ensuring that end-of-life care remains compassionate, respectful, and aligned with the needs and wishes of the individual. The future of PAD lies not just in policy changes but also in the thoughtful and sensitive handling of each individual case.

5.9 Navigating the Complexities of EOL Care: Ethical and Legal Considerations

5.9.1 Overview

End-of-life care may sometimes present ethical dilemmas for healthcare professionals, patients, and their families. It requires balancing patient autonomy, clinical realities, and family dynamics. Key principles—autonomy, beneficence, nonmaleficence, and justice—serve as the foundation for decision-making, ensuring that care respects the patient's values and dignity (Akdeniz et al., 2021).

When patients lose the ability to make decisions, responsibility often shifts to family members, healthcare proxies, or physicians. This transition can impose significant emotional burdens on families, who may experience sadness, fear, and anxiety as they navigate complex choices. Disagreements among family members are common: some may advocate for aggressive life-prolonging measures, while others prioritize comfort and quality of life. These conflicts often place healthcare providers in challenging positions, requiring them to mediate family dynamics while adhering to ethical and clinical standards.

Advance directives, such as living wills and healthcare proxies, are essential tools for aligning care with patients' preferences. However, conflicts may still arise, even when advance directives exist, such as when family members oppose documented choices or when surrogates' decisions deviate from the patient's known wishes. In such cases, ethical committees or legal interventions may be necessary to resolve disputes and uphold the patient's dignity and values (Sedini et al., 2022).

In the absence of advance directives, families often rely on substituted judgment, making decisions based on the patient's known values and preferences rather than their own. While this approach can guide decision-making, it is not always straightforward and may lead to further disagreements, delaying critical care decisions.

Legal frameworks, such as those in the United Kingdom, provide guidance for acting in the patient's best interests and protect healthcare providers from liability when decisions align with ethical and clinical standards (Thorns, 2010). However, even with these protections, tensions between families and medical teams may persist. As illustrated in *Betancourt v. Trinitas Hospital* (2009) (see textbox), such cases highlight the challenges of reconciling medical judgments with family expectations.

The ultimate goals of end-of-life care are to alleviate suffering, enhance quality of life, and honor the person throughout the dying process. Achieving these goals depends on advance care planning, clear communication, and the effective use of ethical and legal resources. Collaboration among families, patients, and care teams is essential to addressing these challenges while upholding the patient's dignity and values.

Real-Life Case: Betancourt v. Trinitas Hospital (2009)

Ruben Betancourt's case is a widely cited example of ethical and legal challenges in end-of-life care. At 73, Ruben Betancourt underwent surgery at Trinitas Regional Medical Center in New Jersey to remove a thymus tumor. While the procedure was successful, complications during recovery left him with severe, irreversible brain damage after his breathing tube became dislodged. He was placed on mechanical ventilation and required kidney dialysis and a feeding tube to sustain life. When his family returned him to Trinitas after seeking care elsewhere, his doctors determined that further treatment was futile, as his condition would only deteriorate. They advised against prolonging interventions, considering it inhumane. However, his family believed he was still responsive and secured a court order to prevent the withdrawal of life support.

The hospital, citing futility, imposed a do-not-resuscitate (DNR) order. The family contested this in court and succeeded in having the DNR rescinded. In turn, the hospital sought legal permission to reinstate the DNR order and discontinue dialysis, but another court decision prevented them from stopping care. As the legal battle continued, Mr. Betancourt's health worsened, and he passed away in May 2009.

Source: Burkle and Benson (2012)

5.9.2 *End-of-Life Decision-Making for Families*

When deciding on end-of-life care, families often face difficult choices, especially if the patient has lost the capacity to make decisions and does not have an advance directive. In such cases, it is important for the healthcare practitioner to first determine the succession of responsibility—who is legally authorized to make decisions on behalf of the patient. Families should use substituted judgments, making decisions on the basis of the patient's known values and wishes rather than their own preferences. This can be emotionally challenging, particularly when family members hold differing views on the appropriate course of action (Akdeniz et al., 2021).

To navigate these challenges, families need a clear understanding of the patient's condition and prognosis, as well as the specific decisions they may need to make, such as whether to pursue artificial nutrition or hydration, cardiopulmonary resuscitation (CPR), or mechanical ventilation. These decisions require careful consideration, and families should prioritize the patient's best interests while working closely with healthcare providers to ensure informed and compassionate decision-making.

To help families stay focused during this difficult time, the following strategies are recommended:

1. **Clarify the patient's wishes**: Families should prioritize understanding and honoring the patient's values and preferences. If the patient has previously communicated their wishes, they should guide all decisions, even when they are difficult.
2. **Relying on advance directives**: If available, advance directives should be the primary reference for decision-making. These legal documents provide clear guidance on patients' wishes and alleviate the burden on families.
3. **Communication with healthcare providers**: Families should work closely with the patient's healthcare team to understand the medical options and consequences and align decisions with the patient's best interests. Healthcare providers can also help clarify any medical or ethical questions.
4. **Minimize conflicts**: Decisions should remain focused on the patient's well-being and wishes, avoiding power struggles or personal preferences. When disagreements arise, families could consider involving neutral mediators, such as the healthcare team or an ethics committee, to ensure patient-centered decisions.
5. **Respectful reflection**: Families should take the time to reflect on what the patient would want rather than rushing decisions or allowing emotional stress to dictate actions. By focusing on patients' dignity and quality of life, families can make more compassionate and informed decisions.

The above strategies help families make compassionate, patient-centered decisions that honor their loved one's wishes while also strengthening family bonds and reducing emotional strain during this challenging time.

5.9.3 Professionals' Roles in End-of-Life Care

End-of-life decision-making requires coordinated effort from an interdisciplinary team of professionals, including physicians, nurses, social workers, and chaplains. Each professional brings unique expertise to support the patient and their family, ensuring that care decisions are made with compassion and respect for their wishes.

5.9.3.1 Physicians: Balancing Ethical and Clinical Decision-Making

Physicians play a central role in end-of-life care, balancing clinical expertise with ethical decision-making to guide patients and families through this challenging phase. The American Medical Association (AMA) provides comprehensive guidance on end-of-life care in Chap. 5 of its Code of Medical Ethics. It emphasizes the physician's role to alleviate suffering and assisting patients in making informed decisions when cure is no longer possible. "Physicians have a responsibility to help patients define their goals for end of life care and to respect patients' preferences" (AMA, n.d.). The following outlines AMA opinions on some major EOL issues:

Advance Care Planning (Opinion 5.1)
Physicians are encouraged to engage *all* patients in conversations about their values and care preferences to ensure future medical decisions reflect their wishes. These discussions should be approached with cultural sensitivity, acknowledging that decision-making processes are influenced by factors such as faith, cultural traditions, and life experiences, tailoring these conversations to each person's unique situations and preferences.

Advance Directives (Opinion 5.2)
AMA emphasizes that "an advance directive never takes precedence over the contemporaneous wishes of a patient who has decision-making capacity." Physicians should assess the patient's decision-making capacity, confirm whether an advance directive reflects current preferences, and identify any designated surrogate decision-makers. Conversations about the patient's care goals and specific preferences should be documented in the medical record, incorporating any written directives for accessibility. When surrogates make decisions, physicians must guide them in honoring the patient's wishes, seeking ethics committee support for conflicts. In the absence of an advance directive or surrogate, physicians should consult institutional resources to determine the patient's best interests and document orders for treatments or limitations accordingly.

Withholding or Withdrawing Life-Sustaining Treatment (Opinion 5.3)
The AMA emphasizes that there is no ethical difference between withholding and withdrawing treatment. Physicians should elicit patient goals of care and preferences regarding life-sustaining interventions early in the course of care. Patients with decision-making capacity have the right to decline or discontinue such treatments, even if this results in death. When capacity is lacking, surrogates may decide

based on the patient's values or best interests. Physicians should document these preferences, provide relevant information, and seek ethics consultation if conflicts arise, ensuring decisions align with ethical and clinical standards.

Orders Not to Attempt Resuscitation (DNAR) (Opinion 5.4)
The AMA emphasizes the ethical obligation to respect patient autonomy, including decisions to refuse resuscitation, even if this leads to death. DNAR orders guide the healthcare team to withhold resuscitative measures as per the patient's wishes, applicable in any care setting and for any patient at risk of cardiopulmonary arrest. In the absence of a DNAR order, resuscitation should be initiated if medically appropriate but stopped if it is later confirmed that resuscitation contradicts the patient's preferences.

Medically Ineffective Interventions (Opinion 5.5)
Physicians should recommend and provide only medically appropriate interventions that are scientifically grounded and reflect their professional judgment of the risks and benefits in light of the patient's care goals. They are not obligated to offer interventions unlikely to achieve intended clinical benefits or agreed-upon goals, even if requested by the patient or surrogate. Respecting autonomy does not require fulfilling requests for interventions deemed ineffective.

Requests for medically ineffective care should be addressed through clear communication about the patient's goals and any misunderstandings. Physicians should reassure patients or surrogates that medically appropriate care, including symptom management, will continue, and work to negotiate a care plan aligned with clinical judgment and the patient's preferences. If disagreements persist, ethics committee involvement or transfer of care may be pursued, but physicians are not ethically obligated to provide interventions judged to lack clinical benefit.

Sedation to Unconsciousness in End-of-Life Care (Opinion 5.6)
Physicians have a duty to relieve pain and suffering, particularly for terminally ill patients experiencing severe, unrelieved distress despite aggressive palliative measures. In such cases, sedation to unconsciousness may be ethically appropriate as an intervention of last resort. However, this intervention must never be used with the intent to cause death.

Physician-Assisted Suicide (Opinion 5.7) & Exercise of Conscience (Opinion 1.1.7)
The AMA Code of Medical Ethics reflects the complex moral tension physicians face regarding assisted suicide, reflecting a divergent conclusion from a shared commitment to values of care, compassion, respect, and dignity.

Opinion 5.7 addresses the ethical concerns of those who oppose physician-assisted suicide, asserting that it is fundamentally incompatible with the physician's role as a healer. It emphasizes significant challenges, including the difficulty of regulation and societal risks. Instead, the AMA urges physicians not to abandon patients once it is determined that a cure is impossible, advising that physicians respect patient autonomy, provide clear communication and emotional support, and deliver appropriate comfort care and effective pain management.

While Opinion 1.1.7: Physician Exercise of Conscience does not explicitly address physician-assisted suicide, it emphasizes the importance of balancing personal moral integrity with professional ethical duties. Physicians are encouraged to act (or to refrain from acting) according to their consciousness while upholding professional principles.

5.9.3.2 Nurses: Providing Holistic Patient Care

Nurses play an essential role in managing end-of-life care, serving as primary points of contact and providing patient-centered support. The American Nurses Association (ANA) emphasizes that nurses are obligated to deliver comprehensive, compassionate care, which includes recognizing when death is near and communicating this to families or surrogates. Additionally, nurses should collaborate with healthcare teams to ensure optimal symptom management, support patients and families, and facilitate effective decision-making processes (American Nurses Association, 2024). The ANA outlines these roles and responsibilities in its recent position document to guide nurses in their critical work at the end of life. Key responsibilities include the following:

- **Symptom management**: Nurses are responsible for ensuring that patients receive effective symptom relief, which includes administering medications and implementing other measures within their scope of practice. This approach optimizes patient comfort and upholds the standards of holistic care by addressing both physical and emotional needs.
- **Patient advocacy and support**: Advocacy remains a crucial aspect of nursing care, particularly during end-of-life stages. Nurses play a vital role in guiding families through difficult decisions and providing consistent emotional support. The 2024 ANA position emphasizes the importance of educating families, preparing them for what to expect, and ensuring that they understand the progression of the patient's condition.
- **Interdisciplinary collaboration**: Effective end-of-life care requires seamless collaboration between nurses and the broader healthcare team. The 2024 ANA position calls for nurses to work with interdisciplinary teams to develop care plans that honor patient preferences while considering clinical realities. This collaboration involves consulting with palliative care specialists, ethics committees, and risk management teams, as needed, to align patient and family expectations with practical care strategies.

5.9.3.3 Social Workers: Delivering Comprehensive Support

The Standards for Palliative and End-of-Life Care developed by the National Association of Social Workers (NASW) emphasize the essential roles that social workers play in supporting individuals and their families facing life-limiting illnesses. These standards integrate professional ethics, cultural competence, interdisciplinary collaboration, and continued education to ensure holistic and equitable care. The framework assists social workers in addressing the biopsychosocial and spiritual dimensions of care. It enhances communication, advocates for client rights, and helps navigate complex ethical and legal considerations. This approach ensures that client dignity and self-determination are upheld throughout the palliative and end-of-life processes (National Association of Social Workers, 2004). Table 5.6 outlines the 11 NASW standards for palliative and end-of-life care, summarizing key areas that guide social work practices in delivering comprehensive support to patients and their families.

Table 5.6 National Association of Social Workers Standards for Palliative and End-of-Life Care

Standard no.	Standard	Summary
1	Ethics and values	Guided by professional ethics and bioethics, ensuring ethical decision-making in complex care settings
2	Knowledge	Demonstrates understanding of theoretical, biopsychosocial, and spiritual factors essential for effective practice
3	Assessment	Comprehensive client assessments that include biopsychosocial and spiritual factors for tailored care planning
4	Intervention/treatment planning	Develops intervention plans that empower client decision-making, considering biopsychosocial and spiritual needs
5	Attitude/self-awareness	Shows compassion, respects client dignity, and maintains self-awareness to manage personal beliefs in practice
6	Empowerment and advocacy	Advocates for client rights, linking them to resources and promoting equitable access to care while respecting spiritual beliefs
7	Documentation	Maintains accurate records to ensure continuity and quality of care
8	Interdisciplinary teamwork	Collaborates within interdisciplinary teams, integrating biopsychosocial and spiritual insights to advocate for client needs
9	Cultural competence	Develops an understanding of how cultural and spiritual values affect end-of-life care to provide sensitive support
10	Continuing education	Engages in ongoing professional development to maintain current knowledge of biopsychosocial and spiritual care practices
11	Supervision, leadership, and training	Provides mentorship and leads efforts that include the integration of biopsychosocial and spiritual practices

Note: Based on *NASW standards for palliative and end-of-life care* by the National Association of Social Workers (2004)

5.9.3.4 Chaplains: Ensuring Spiritual and Value Alignment

Spiritual care is one of the four pillars of palliative care, and chaplains play a crucial leadership role in embedding it as an essential part of holistic treatment and decision-making (Puchalski et al., 2009). They conduct spiritual assessments and guide interdisciplinary teams to identify and address the spiritual needs of people and their families. They facilitate meaningful conversations about values, beliefs, and end-of-life decisions, facilitating care that aligns with the patient's preferences.

Chaplains lead the education and training of healthcare professionals to address spiritual concerns effectively. This ensures that care remains patient-centered and respectful of individual beliefs. Their leadership builds trust and enhances compassionate, supportive care.

Practitioners must remain attentive to patients' belief systems when making end-of-life care decisions. This awareness fosters trust and supports compassionate, patient-focused care. When ethical dilemmas arise, such as conflicts between the values of the patient and those of the family or medical team, chaplains step in to mediate. They advocate for the patient's spiritual and existential needs, ensuring that care remains respectful and aligned with their beliefs and values.

The influential document *Improving the Quality of Spiritual Care as a Dimension of Palliative Care: The Report of the Consensus Conference* (Puchalski et al., 2009) highlighted the key roles Chaplains play in holistic palliative care:

- **Spiritual assessment and counseling**: Chaplains conduct thorough spiritual assessments to understand patients' beliefs and needs. They provide a supportive environment for patients to discuss concerns, such as fears of death or questions about the afterlife, and offer personalized guidance that aligns with their values.
- **Leading multidisciplinary teams in spiritual care**: Chaplains guide interdisciplinary teams to incorporate spiritual care into treatment plans, ensuring that all aspects of a patient's well-being are acknowledged and respected.
- **Education and professional training**: Chaplains train healthcare teams to recognize and include spiritual care in their practices. This leadership creates an environment where spiritual care is valued, leading to cohesive and patient-focused treatment.
- **Ensuring spiritual and value alignment**: Chaplains ensure that end-of-life care reflects the patient's values and beliefs. This can involve facilitating specific rituals, prayers, or practices that offer comfort to both the patient and their family.
- **Interfaith support**: Chaplains support individuals from diverse faith backgrounds, providing guidance that respects their beliefs. They work closely with the healthcare team to integrate spiritual care into the overall treatment plan.

5.9.4 *Conclusion on Ethical and Legal Complexity*

Legal and ethical considerations in end-of-life decision-making are complex and multifaceted. Ethical principles such as autonomy, beneficence, nonmaleficence, and justice are widely embraced in medical care. However, in real-world practices, social disparity, cultural differences, family system dynamics, practical obstacles, insufficient training, and more may pose various challenges (Schofield et al., 2021). End-of-life care, including advanced care planning, requires multistep, multidisciplinary collaboration with the person and their families. Cultural sensitivity and clear communication are essential for ensuring that decisions respect the dignity and wishes of the patient while upholding professional standards and legal obligations (Thorns, 2010; Akdeniz et al., 2021).

5.10 Concluding Reflection

Supporting individuals and families through the end-of-life journey calls for a compassionate, person-centered, and holistic approach that attends to physical, psychosocial, and spiritual needs. Meaningful conversations about end-of-life care and advance care planning empower individuals to make informed choices. These discussions alleviate uncertainty for families and ease the emotional and ethical challenges faced by healthcare teams, facilitating care that aligns with the person's wishes.

Effective end-of-life care extends beyond symptom management. It relies on the collaboration of interdisciplinary teams—including physicians, nurses, social workers, and spiritual care providers—to cultivate a cohesive and compassionate environment. Ultimately, end-of-life care is not merely about managing the process of dying. It is about honoring life, respecting the personal journey, and striving to shape their final chapter to reflect their values and aspirations.

References

Akdeniz, M., Yardımcı, B., & Kavukcu, E. (2021). Ethical considerations at the end-of-life care. *SAGE Open Medicine, 9*, 20503121211000918.

American Medical Association. (n.d.). *Caring for patients at the end of life.* AMA Code of Medical Ethics. Retrieved November 24, 2024, from https://code-medical-ethics.ama-assn.org/chapters/caring-patients-end-life

American Medical Association (AMA). (2019). *Proceedings of the 2019 annual meeting of the American Medical Association house of delegates: Council on ethical and judicial affairs (CEJA 2-A-19 report).* American Medical Association. Retrieved from https://www.ama-assn.org/delivering-care/ethics/physician-assisted-suicide

American Nurses Association. (2024). *Nurses' roles and responsibilities in providing care and support at the end of life [Position statement].* Retrieved from https://www.nursingworld.org/practice-policy/nursing-excellence/official-position-statements/id/nurses-roles-and-responsibilities-in-providing-care-and-support-at-the-end-of-life/

Bag, S., Mohanty, S., Deep, N., & Salins, N. (2020). Palliative and end-of-life care in India - Current scenario and the way forward. *Journal of the Association of Physicians of India*. Retrieved from https://www.researchgate.net/publication/347928990

Barsness, J. G., Regnier, C. R., Hook, C. C., et al. (2020). US medical and surgical society position statements on physician-assisted suicide and euthanasia: A review. *BMC Medical Ethics, 21*, 111. https://doi.org/10.1186/s12910-020-00556-5

Burkle, C. M., & Benson, J. J. (2012, November). End-of-life care decisions: Importance of reviewing systems and limitations after 2 recent North American cases. *Mayo Clinic Proceedings, 87*(11), 1098–1105.

Carrigan, K. (2023). One-way ticket to Zürich: Presentations of 'suicide tourism' in European news media. *Mortality*, 1–16.

Ciupak, Y. (2025). *Spiral model of grief and healing: An integrative sociological, psychological, and cultural framework* [Unpublished manuscript]. Northern Michigan University.

Clark, D., Baur, N., Clelland, D., Garralda, E., López-Fidalgo, J., Connor, S., & Centeno, C. (2020). Mapping levels of palliative care development in 198 countries: The situation in 2017. *Journal of Pain and Symptom Management, 59*(4), 794–807.

CNN Editorial Research. (2023, May 29). *Physician-assisted suicide fast facts*. CNN. Retrieved from https://www.cnn.com/2014/11/26/us/physician-assisted-suicide-fast-facts/index.html

Cohen-Mansfield, J., Skornick-Bouchbinder, M., & Brill, S. (2018). Trajectories of end of life: A systematic review. *The Journals of Gerontology: Series B, 73*(4), 564–572.

Connor, S. R., & Gwyther, E. (2018). The worldwide hospice palliative care alliance. *Journal of Pain and Symptom Management, 55*(2), 446–453. https://doi.org/10.1016/j.jpainsymman.2017.05.001

Corr, C. A. (1992). A task-based approach to coping with dying. *OMEGA-Journal of Death and Dying, 24*(2), 81–94.

Corr, C. A., Corr, D. M., & Doka, K. J. (2019). *Death & dying, life & living* (8th ed.). Cengage Learning.

De Lima, L., Woodruff, R., Pettus, K., Downing, J., Buitrago, R., Munyoro, E., Venkateswaran, C., Bhatnagar, S., & Radbruch, L. (2017). International association for hospice and palliative care position statement: Euthanasia and physician-assisted suicide. *Journal of Palliative Medicine, 20*(1), 8–14.

Gray, N. A., & LeBlanc, T. W. (2018). The study to understand prognoses and preferences for outcomes and risks of treatments (SUPPORT). In *50 studies every palliative care doctor should know* (online ed.). Oxford Academic. https://doi.org/10.1093/med/9780190658618.003.0030

Grey, I., Arora, T., Thomas, J., Saneh, A., Tohme, P., & Abi-Habib, R. (2020). The role of perceived social support on depression and sleep during the COVID-19 pandemic. *Psychiatry Research, 293*, 113452.

Jordan, R. I., Allsop, M. J., ElMokhallalati, Y., Jackson, C. E., Edwards, H. L., Chapman, E. J., Deliens, L., & Bennett, M. I. (2020). Duration of palliative care before death in international routine practice: A systematic review and meta-analysis. *BMC Medicine, 18*(1), 368. https://doi.org/10.1186/s12916-020-01829-x

Kastenbaum, R. (2012). *Death, society, and human experience* (11th ed.). Pearson.

Kübler-Ross, E. (1969). *On death and dying*. Macmillan.

Kübler-Ross, E. (1983). *Speaks to a dying patient [video]*. Nova Interview. Retrieved from https://www.youtube.com/watch?v=tIZ97OALEfE

Lunney, J. R., Lynn, J., Foley, D. J., Lipson, S., & Guralnik, J. M. (2003). Patterns of functional decline at the end of life. *JAMA, 289*(18), 2387–2392. https://doi.org/10.1001/jama.289.18.2387

Mahajan, R. (2023). *Validity of euthanasia in India: Constitutional and legal approach*. Retrieved from https://www.lexology.com/library/detail.aspx?g=247c8c66-b3ed-4179-bfe1-7df289a0cde5

Martina, D., Lin, C. P., Kristanti, M. S., Bramer, W. M., Mori, M., Korfage, I. J., van der Heide, A., van der Rijt, C. C. D., & Rietjens, J. A. (2021). Advance care planning in Asia: A systematic narrative review of healthcare professionals' knowledge, attitude, and experience. *Journal of the American Medical Directors Association, 22*(2), 349.e1–349.e28.

McMahan, R. D., Tellez, I., & Sudore, R. L. (2020). Deconstructing the complexities of advance care planning outcomes: What do we know and where do we go? A scoping review. *Journal of the American Geriatrics Society.* https://doi.org/10.1111/jgs.16801

Michigan Legislature. (2021). *Planning for your peace of mind: A guide to medical and legal decisions*. Retrieved from http://www.legislature.mi.gov/publications/peaceofmind.pdf

Mroz, S., Dierickx, S., Deliens, L., Cohen, J., & Chambaere, K. (2021). Assisted dying around the world: A status quaestionis. *Annals of Palliative Medicine, 10*(3), 3540–3553. https://doi.org/10.21037/apm-20-637

National Academies of Sciences, Engineering, and Medicine. (2018). *Physician-assisted death: Scanning the landscape: Proceedings of a workshop*. The National Academies Press. https://doi.org/10.17226/25131

National Association of Social Workers. (2004). *NASW standards for palliative and end of life care*. National Association of Social Workers. Retrieved from https://www.socialworkers.org/Practice/NASW-Practice-Standards-Guidelines/Standards-for-Palliative-and-End-of-Life-Care

National Hospice and Palliative Care Organization. (2023). *Guide to organizational ethics in hospice care (updated 2023)*. National Hospice and Palliative Care Organization.

Oregon Health Authority. (n.d.). *Death with dignity act*. Oregon Health Authority. Retrieved November 12, 2024, from https://www.oregon.gov/oha/PH/PROVIDERPARTNERRESOURCES/EVALUATIONRESEARCH/DEATHWITHDIGNITYACT/Pages/index.aspx

Patient Self-Determination Act, 42 U.S.C. § 1395 cc (1991).

Puchalski, C., Ferrell, B., Virani, R., Otis-Green, S., Baird, P., Bull, J., Chochinov, H., Handzo, G., Nelson-Becker, H., Prince-Paul, M., & Karen Pugliese Sulmasy, D. (2009). Improving the quality of spiritual care as a dimension of palliative care: The report of the consensus conference. *Journal of Palliative Medicine, 12*(10), 885–904. https://doi.org/10.1089/jpm.2009.0142

Schofield, G., Dittborn, M., Huxtable, R., Brangan, E., & Selman, L. E. (2021). Real-world ethics in palliative care: A systematic review of the ethical challenges reported by specialist palliative care practitioners in their clinical practice. *Palliative Medicine, 35*(2), 315–334. https://doi.org/10.1177/0269216320974277

Sedini, C., Biotto, M., Crespi Bel'skij, L. M., Moroni Grandini, R. E., & Cesari, M. (2022). Advance care planning and advance directives: An overview of the main critical issues. *Aging Clinical and Experimental Research, 34*, 325–330. https://doi.org/10.1007/s40520-021-02001-y

Thorns, A. (2010). Ethical and legal issues in end-of-life care. *Clinical Medicine, 10*(3), 282.

World Health Organization. (2020). *Palliative care*. Retrieved from https://www.who.int/news-room/fact-sheets/detail/palliative-care

Part III
Principles and Practices in End-of-Life and Grief Support

Chapter 6
Competencies and Principles in End-of-Life and Grief Support

6.1 Introduction

In essence, end-of-life and grief support is about utilizing the *self as an instrument* to accompany and assist individuals through their difficult journeys. This reflects the dual aspects of the unique essence of this line of work: professional yet personal.[1] Such an intertwined dual aspect brings out the most rewarding aspects and poses significant challenges.

Gamino and Ritter (2012) introduced the concept of "death competence" to describe the specialized skill of managing their own and clients' challenges related to dying, death, and bereavement. This competence is essential for helping professionals effectively support their clients while managing their work's profound emotional and existential impacts. Chan and Tin (2012) expand on this concept by introducing "self-competence in death work," which involves professionals possessing essential personal resources and the ability to cope with the emotions and existential issues that arise from their work. External professional resources, including professional training, peer support, and mentoring, are also crucial for helping professionals, particularly those relatively new to the field.

Research on the preparedness of counselors has revealed a significant gap between the needs and the education provided to professionals to support clients dealing with death, dying, and grief.[2] Many professionals are familiar only with stage models,

---

[1] See this chapter for a detailed discussion on the "self as an instrument" in end-of-life and grief support. This chapter explores how personal and professional roles intertwine, affecting how professionals approach care and support. It reinforces that self-care and personal growth are essential parts of professional development. Self-reflection and awareness are highlighted as ways to build resilience and provide effective care.

[2] Blueford et al. (2022) conducted a qualitative study highlighting gaps in counselor training and experiences related to grief counseling, revealing themes like inadequate preparation and systemic factors. The study calls for the integration of grief and loss education into course curricula and

Y. Z. Ciupak, D. C. Smith, *Death, Dying, and Grief*,
https://doi.org/10.1007/978-3-031-88467-2_6

which have received much criticism and may not be up-to-date with a more recent understanding of grief. The lack of adequate training affects their confidence and ability to deliver effective and compassionate care. In addition, frequent exposure to death, dying, and suffering can induce emotional and existential challenges (Hsiao et al., 2023). Therefore, there has been a widespread call in the past decade from nurses, college counselors, psychological therapists, and other professionals to enhance professional training on death and grief competency.[3] Many emphasize the incorporation of death and grief education within academic curricula and ongoing professional development. Despite many efforts, the gap and barrier persist.[4]

Because of the dual aspects of the human service profession, competency training and development should integrate both professional and personal development, incorporating experiential learning, self-reflection, and a more updated understanding of grief (Blueford et al., 2022; Hill et al., 2018). Programs should encourage professionals to reflect on their attitudes, beliefs, and experiences regarding death, dying, and grief. These programs should aim to deepen their conceptual understanding and provide practical tools to enhance their overall well-being. By doing so, professionals will be better equipped to model and integrate self-competence into their practice (Chan et al., 2016).

Integrating death and grief competence into professional practice helps professionals reduce their emotional burden and enhance the support they offer to their clients. By understanding and managing their own responses to death and grief, professionals can create a safe, compassionate environment that fosters effective grief work and meaningful end-of-life discussions. This holistic approach empowers both the professional and the client to navigate the complexities of death, dying, and grief with greater resilience and insight.

This chapter explores the skills and knowledge needed to support individuals and families during their profound journey. By understanding the principles of grief counseling, the goals of end-of-life care, and the ethical guidelines that govern these practices, professionals can deliver holistic and person-centered support. This chapter discusses the 4A4C competency framework and addresses strategies for self-care to provide sustainable and resilient service.

---

supervision to build a strong foundational understanding. Hill et al. (2018) conducted an analysis using the Grief Counseling Competency Scale to assess counseling students' self-perceived competency in handling grief-related issues. Findings indicated a significant need for additional training in grief counseling skills and theory, underscoring the importance of comprehensive education to support clients effectively (Wheat et al., 2022) advocate for embedding grief education in accredited counseling programs to address these training deficiencies.

[3] Calls for enhanced professional training on death and grief competencies come from various human service professions, including nursing as noted by Hsiao et al. (2023), college counseling by Jankauskaite et al. (2021), and psychological therapy by Ober et al. (2012).

[4] Integrating grief education into academic curricula has been emphasized by Hill et al. (2018), and Wheat et al. (2022), alongside continuing professional development as noted by Jankauskaite et al. (2021), and Ober et al. (2012), to improve training outcomes. However, persistent barriers to adequate training remain, including systematic and institutional issues such as saturated curricula, limited content expertise, training availability, and cost, as discussed by Chan et al. (2016), and Davis et al. (2021).

6.2 Grief Support, Counseling, and Therapy

Grief support is an integral part of daily life and occurs across all social settings. First responders, nurses, physicians, educators, family members, friends, spiritual leaders, and community members all play a crucial role in providing grief support to those experiencing loss. While their approaches may vary, the cumulative effect of these efforts fosters a compassionate culture and strengthens the fabric of society.

There are important distinctions between the terms "grief support," "grief counseling," and "grief therapy," although they are interconnected. **Grief support** is a broad concept that encompasses various services and actions from different sources that help individuals experiencing loss. This support can come from family, friends, communities, professionals, and organizations.

While not every person who is grieving requires counseling or therapy, everyone can benefit from some form of support to manage their grief. Similarly, although not everyone may be qualified to conduct grief therapy, anyone can and should offer some form of grief support, which plays a vital role in fostering resilience and healing. Enhancing the ability and confidence to provide such support contributes to a compassionate culture and a resilient society.

Grief support is adaptable and should be person-centered, addressing the diverse needs of individuals from various backgrounds and experiences. It acknowledges the multifaceted nature of grief, which can manifest emotionally, cognitively, behaviorally, physically, and spiritually. Effective grief support aims to create a safe and compassionate environment where individuals can express their feelings, share their experiences, and find comfort in knowing they are not alone. This support helps individuals adapt to their new life circumstances and promotes healing. Support can manifest in many forms, addressing the social, psychological, spiritual, and practical needs of those adapting to a changed world. Social support is essential for an individual's healing and general well-being.

At its core, grief support relies on two key principles: *validation* and *companionship*. Validation acknowledges and affirms the unique grief experience of each person, respecting the varied ways of grief styles, expressions, and processes. Companionship emphasizes the importance of showing up with genuine presence, empathy, and consistent support. Together, these principles form the foundation of meaningful grief support, helping individuals feel understood and less isolated in their journey.

6.2.1 Grief Counseling vs. Grief Therapy

Grief counseling and grief therapy are specialized forms of grief support conducted by trained professionals. In his comprehensive handbook, Worden (2009) makes an important distinction between the two:

- *Grief counseling:* This form of support assists individuals in coping with uncomplicated grief and mourning. It involves guiding and accompanying individuals through their grieving process, helping them acknowledge their loss, expressing their emotions, and adapting to life without their loved ones. Grief counseling focuses on facilitating the natural mourning process and providing emotional support to help individuals manage their grief (Worden, 2009).
- *Grief therapy:* Reserved for more specialized techniques, grief therapy helps people with complicated and prolonged grief reactions or those whose grief manifests as physical symptoms. It involves more advanced and intensive interventions aimed at resolving complex grief issues that significantly impair an individual's ability to function. Grief therapy often addresses underlying psychological issues and works to resolve deeply ingrained grief-related problems (Worden, 2009).

When individuals experience a significant loss in their lives, processing death and grief can be a difficult task. Counseling for individuals coping with death and grief provides a safe space and professional guidance as they navigate life after loss, especially when social support is lacking or insufficient. Grief counseling focuses on helping bereaved people who are coping with uncomplicated grief and is typically offered by psychologists, social workers, counselors, clergies, or other trained professionals. Grief counseling usually involves one-on-one sessions between a client and counselor, but it can also include couples, families, or groups who share the same or similar loss.

Effective grief counselors utilize their knowledge and experiences in bereavement and loss to help individuals understand loss and grief, identify and process emotions, examine and improve coping mechanisms and problem-solving strategies, and find meaning amid the loss. Grief counselors facilitate reframing the situation for clients and shape how the interaction takes place by guiding them to understand their grieving reactions and processes (Rosenblatt, 2019). When grief counselors are working with clients, it is important to assess each distinct client's needs, experiences, and goals in their journey with grief. A collaborative approach to forming a *therapeutic alliance* between counselors and clients helps mitigate differences, formulate person-centered care plans, and provide compassionate service (Harris & Winokuer, 2021).

6.2.2 Principles and Goals of Grief Counseling

Worden (2009) outlines ten principles essential for effective grief counseling. These principles offer a structured approach for counselors to support individuals in navigating the complexities of grief and loss. The following summary integrates insights from Worden (2009) and other scholars such as Corr et al. (2019).

1. *Help the survivor actualize the loss:* Counselors assist clients in understanding and accepting that a loss has occurred and that the deceased will not return. This helps acknowledge the reality of the loss.
2. *Help the survivor identify and experience feelings:* Counselors facilitate the expression and identification of emotions related to the loss, including anger, guilt, anxiety, helplessness, and sadness. This process may involve helping clients recognize feelings they are unaware of or have difficulty naming. Recent counseling modalities, such as Somatic Experiencing Therapy, developed by Peter Levine, and Compassionate Inquiry developed by Gabor Maté,[5] emphasize the somatic connection of emotions. This approach encourages clients to identify bodily sensations to process and release emotions.
3. *Assist living without the deceased:* Counselors support clients in adapting to life without their loved one, encouraging the development of effective coping strategies and validating their unique methods of managing the loss.
4. *Help meaning reconstruction in loss:* Counselors aid clients in discovering personal meaning in their loss and help them rebuild their assumed world. Dr. Robert Neimeyer's Grief Therapy as Meaning Reconstruction is an exemplary model that focuses on rebuilding meaning around one's loss, relationship, and identity.[6]
5. *Facilitate emotional relocation while carrying on life:* This principle involves helping clients find a new place for the deceased in their emotional lives, enabling them to continue living and forming new relationships while honoring and maintaining a connection (continuing bond) with the deceased.
6. *Provide time to grieve:* Recognizing that grieving takes time, counselors offer continuous support, assisting clients in navigating and processing their grief over time.
7. *Interpreting and validating "normal" behavior:* Counselors provide education about the common variations in grieving among individuals, normalizing the grieving process, validating the range of emotions and behaviors that clients experience, and reassuring them that their reactions are not indicative of mental instability.
8. *Allow for individual differences:* Grief manifests differently in each person. Counselors respect these differences and help clients understand and accept that others may grieve differently from them.
9. *Examine defenses and coping styles:* Counselors help clients identify, evaluate, and, if necessary, modify their coping behaviors and strategies to facilitate healthier ways of dealing with their grief.
10. *Identify prolonged grief disorder and refer:* Counselors should assess and identify cases of complicated or prolonged grief that may require specialized intervention and refer clients to appropriate resources or professionals.

---

[5] https://compassionateinquiry.com/the-approach/

[6] For information about Grief Therapy as Meaning Reconstruction: https://www.portlandinstitute.org/

In addition to the specific principles and goals of grief counseling, it is important to emphasize the core philosophy of counseling, which acknowledges the inherent strengths and resilience of humans that can be utilized during challenging times and crises. Counseling serves as a means to empower individuals, enabling them to tap into their internal resources to navigate difficult situations. Therefore, additional objectives of counseling based on the principle of compassion and empowerment also include the following (Harris & Winokuer, 2021):

11. *Engaging clients to recognize their innate strengths in coping with and adapting to significant changes.*
12. *Enhancing clients' skills in managing distressing situations.*
13. *Empowering clients to become their own most potent advocates.*

The above goals were primarily discussed in the context of bereavement. However, grief counseling increasingly extends to supporting individuals through various transitions and losses, such as the ending of a relationship, a social role, employment, and physical ability. These principles are largely applicable or adaptable to nonfinite losses.

6.2.3 Couple and Family Counseling

Although grief counseling is typically conducted on an individual basis, couple and family counseling can sometimes serve as alternatives or supplements. There has been a recent rise in the family-centered care model in medicine, which has developed most notably in pediatrics but has emerged in cancer, aging, palliative, and end-of-life care (Kovacs et al., 2006).

Couples and families who share a significant loss may encounter incongruent grief, leading to disruptions and conflicts within the family system. After prolonged caregiving and managing logistics related to death, family members might be depleted of energy to address underlying family dynamics and accumulated stress, which often surface following a family member's death. These challenges can be compounded by different grieving styles (Doka & Martin, 2010). Counselors trained in couple and family therapy, with a deep understanding of the complexities of grief within family systems, can assist in alleviating strain in these family dynamics (Harris & Winokuer, 2021).

6.2.3.1 Couple and Family Counseling in Grief Support

Significant loss and grief can shake the foundations of intimate relationships, often leading to emotional disconnection and conflicts. The most common cases are after the death of a child (Finkbeiber, 2012). The significant stress of losing a child may sometimes trigger other relationship issues to surface. Additionally, partners may process their grief differently, and these varied responses can create empathy gaps.

For example, some individuals might express their grief openly (expressive grievers), whereas others may internalize their emotions and apply cognitive or behavioral coping strategies (instrumental grievers). Nevertheless, others may experience delayed grief, all of which can cause misunderstanding and further emotional distance.

Couple counseling aims to improve communication and empathy between partners. Counselors can help provide information and education about grief, help partners develop open dialog and emotional regulation skills, and facilitate mutual support during the grieving process. By addressing defensive patterns and validating vulnerability, couples can work through their grief together, leading to growth and a renewed connection.

Family counseling provides a platform for all family members to express their grief in a supportive environment. It helps families navigate the complexities of shared loss, enabling them to cope individually and collectively. Family sessions can also address relational conflicts and help members understand each other's grieving processes, explore unfinished businesses, encourage adapted family traditions, and foster a sense of unity and mutual support.

Additionally, strong social support can help bereaved individuals cope better with psychological distress, although the quality and consistency of this support are crucial. Therefore, integrating family and community support systems into counseling increases effectiveness.

6.2.3.2 Practical Guidance for Implementing Couple and Family Counseling

Counselors may employ various techniques, such as guided imagery, role-playing, an empty chair, and other therapeutic interventions, to help families and couples process their grief and strengthen their relationships. These methods aim to facilitate emotional expression, improve communication, and rebuild trust and respect within relationships. Effective grief counseling acknowledges the unique needs of each family member while promoting collective healing and resilience:

1. *Creating a safe environment*: Counselors should create a safe, confidential space where every family member can express their feelings without fear of judgment. This involves setting clear boundaries and guidelines for respectful communication.
2. *Facilitating open communication*: Encouraging family members to share their grief experiences openly. Techniques such as reflective listening, empathetic responses, and turn-taking can help individuals validate their feelings and promote understanding.
3. *Addressing defensive patterns*: Identify and address defensive behaviors that family members may use to protect themselves from pain. Teaching emotional regulation techniques and improved mindfulness can help family members express their emotions more constructively.

4. *Promoting empathy and understanding*: Use exercises that foster empathy, such as role-playing and perspective-taking activities. This can help family members appreciate each other's unique grieving processes and build stronger emotional connections.
5. *Incorporating meaning-centered approaches*: Meaning-Centered therapy helps families find meaning in their loss, which can aid in the healing process. This involves meaning restrictions and exploring spiritual beliefs and practices that provide comfort and understanding during grief.
6. *Support groups*: Participating in bereavement groups can provide additional support and validation. These groups offer a community of individuals who understand the grieving process. When care is taken to screen the members and monitor the group dynamic, support groups can be particularly beneficial for those experiencing disenfranchised grief and those who lack support from the immediate social network.
7. *Techniques for emotional expression*: Techniques such as guided imagery and role-playing can facilitate emotional expression and help family members process their grief. For example, role-playing allows individuals to express thoughts and emotions that they may find difficult to share, helping to resolve unspoken issues, and promote healing.
8. *Creating memory books, new traditions, family alter, and rituals*: Encouraging families to create memory books with photos, letters, and memorabilia can help them reminisce and keep the memory of their loved one alive. Modified or new family traditions can be explored and encouraged. Establishing rituals, whether continuing old rituals or creating new rituals, provides a sense of continuity and connection. These practices help families honor the deceased while adapting to their new reality. Part III of this book provides a comprehensive list of tools and activities for individuals and families to process their grief, aid in healing, and strengthen the family fabric.

The above techniques, coupled with classical counseling modalities such as cognitive-behavioral therapy (CBT) and acceptance and commitment therapy (ACT), help address the intricate and complex dynamics of the disrupted family system after significant loss. These modalities provide structured approaches to identify and change negative thought patterns, promote acceptance of difficult emotions, help break the destructive cycle of blame, and encourage behaviors that align with the family's values and goals.

6.2.4 Grief Counseling and Therapy Techniques

Over the past two decades, there has been an encouraging increase in the development of techniques and modalities specialized for grief counseling and therapy. Robert Neimeyer has edited a series of four books (2012, 2016, 2018, 2021) that provide a comprehensive collection of contributions from various authors, offering hundreds of assessments, interventions, and techniques used in the field. These techniques can be broadly categorized as follows:

1. Emotional and Psychological Interventions

Emotional processing and support: Addressing the emotional aspects of grief through techniques such as mindfulness, the use of psychotropic medication and managing multiple losses. These approaches help individuals process their grief and find emotional balance.

Complicated grief and trauma: Methods to manage trauma-related grief, such as Eye Movement Desensitization and Reprocessing (EMDR) and trauma dialogs, which are designed to address and alleviate the symptoms of complicated grief and trauma.

2. Physical and Somatic Approaches

Body-centered exercises: Leveraging mental-somatic connections to promote overall well-being, including yoga, tai chi, qigong, uninhibited dances or movements, allowing emotions to be released without judgment. Other techniques include progressive muscle relaxation, which involves tensing and relaxing muscle groups while breathing deeply, and guided movement therapy with a practitioner to explore emotions through body awareness.

Somatic therapies of grief: Somatic Experiencing Therapy, developed by Peter Levine, and Compassionate Inquiry, developed by Gabor Maté, guide clients to identify bodily sensations to process and release emotions.

3. Cognitive and Behavioral Interventions

Cognitive and meaning restructuring: Techniques such as cognitive restructuring help individuals address catastrophic thoughts and develop improved responses. Meaning-reconstruction therapies guide people in reframing the loss, relationship, and sense of identity. These approaches help change negative thought patterns and enable individuals to find new meaning in their experiences.

Behavioral activation: Interventions to change behavior and manage grief through assertiveness training and interventions. These methods encourage proactive behaviors that support coping and adaptation.

4. Narrative and Writing Therapies

Storytelling and journaling: Techniques such as life review, directed journaling, and virtual dream stories help individuals recompose their narrative after loss. These methods provide a structured way to explore and express grief.

Rewriting life narratives: Using narrative therapy to process and integrate grief, including metaphorical reframing and documenting life stories. These techniques help individuals reframe their experiences and create coherent narratives.

Uninhibited writing: Setting a time for free and uninhibited writing without worrying about grammar, allowing individuals to freely express their thoughts and emotions.

5. Art, Music, and Creative Expression

Creative techniques: Methods such as drawing, labyrinth walking, and figurative sand tray therapy to process grief through artistic means. These approaches encourage expression through various forms of art.

Improvisational music and dance: Improvisational music and uninhibited dances process grief, allowing individuals to explore and express their emotions through movement and sound. In one particularly moving workshop, three musicians guided participants to create harmonies using their own name or a loved one's name. This exercise fostered connection, healing, and a sense of affirmation.

6. Rituals and Spiritual Practices

Therapeutic rituals: Rituals to support grief, such as therapeutic rituals, barefoot walkabouts, and memory boats, provide structured ways to honor and process loss.

Spiritual and symbolic acts: Methods to incorporate spiritual practices in grief therapy, including spiritual devotionals and metaphorical reframing. These techniques offer spiritual comfort and meaning during the grieving process.

7. Mindfulness Practices

Mindfulness techniques: Techniques such as mindfulness meditation, body scans, and breathing exercises can help individuals stay present and manage their grief. These could be used during therapy sessions.

Integrating mindfulness in daily life: Encouraging the incorporation of mindfulness in everyday activities to promote awareness and connection to the present. This includes mindful walking, mindful eating, and mindful listening.

8. Technology-Assisted Interventions for Grief and Trauma

Innovative technologies have been developed to support individuals dealing with grief and trauma. One such method is Eye Movement Desensitization and Reprocessing (EMDR), which uses guided eye movements to help reprocess traumatic memories, thereby reducing their emotional impact. Another approach is Virtual Reality Exposure Therapy (VRET), which immerses individuals in controlled virtual environments. This allows them to gradually confront and desensitize themselves to traumatic triggers. Additionally, biofeedback and neurofeedback tools monitor physiological responses, such as heart rate and brain activity, enabling individuals to better regulate their emotions and manage stress more effectively.

9. Social Support and Group Work

Facilitating group support: Approaches for group therapy and social support, including orchestrating social support and bereavement support groups. These methods foster community and shared understanding among those grieving. Group and community-based rituals and activities are especially valuable to address collective grief.

Family and systemic approaches: Techniques for working with families and systemic grief, such as discussing grief with couples and families. These approaches recognize the impact of grief on family systems and promote collective healing.

In summary, the diverse techniques of grief counseling and therapy aim to enhance coping strategies and resilience while addressing the affective, cognitive, behavioral, spiritual, and practical dimensions of grief. While this section outlines many key approaches, it is important to acknowledge that numerous other valuable methods and contributors in the field may not be listed here owing to the broad nature of the topic. Parts III and IV of the book include tools and exercises that are adaptable to various needs.

6.3 End-of-Life Support

End-of-life support encompasses a variety of services and care strategies aimed at ensuring comfort, dignity, and quality of life for individuals in their final stages of life. As detailed in Chap. 5: Dying and End of Life Care, various services and care systems—such as palliative care, hospice care, and other specialized programs—play critical roles in delivering comprehensive support. Successful end-of-life support engages multidisciplinary teams and resources, including healthcare professionals, clergy, social workers, and volunteers, to provide holistic care. End-of-life support also extends to the needs of the family.

The growing emphasis on family-centered care (FCC) in end-of-life and palliative settings recognizes families as a critical unit of care, advocating for collaboration between healthcare providers and families to align care decisions with their values, beliefs, and cultural backgrounds. Studies have shown that FCC enhances patient and family satisfaction, improves health outcomes, and optimizes healthcare resource use (Kovacs et al., 2006).

Objectives of End-of-Life support include:

Comfort: Prioritizing the person's comfort and well-being through effective pain and symptom management.

Dignity: Ensuring the person's dignity is maintained through respectful and compassionate care.

Quality of life: Enhancing the remaining quality of life based on the unique values and preferences of the person.

Family support: Providing continuous support and resources to family members and caregivers to help them cope with the end-of-life process.

Holistic person-centered care: Honor persons as holistic biological, psychological, social, and spiritual beings. Take a holistic approach to meet the needs of the dying person and family (WHO, 2020).

6.4 Ethics and Guidelines

Various professional associations have established ethical codes and practice guidelines relevant to grief support, education, and counseling. For example, the Association for Death Education and Counseling (ADEC) outlined nine basic tenets for death education and grief counseling, which can be summarized as follows (ADEC, 2010):

1. *Knowledge of current thanatological literature*: Staying informed about current data, methodology, and theory in the field of thanatology.
2. *Self-awareness*: Strive to understand their death-related feelings and experiences and the ways in which these feelings and experiences may impact their thinking and work in the field.
3. *Client understanding*: Obtaining a deep understanding of, and respect for, the client's cultural background, developmental status, perceptions, and individual differences and needs.
4. *Professional integrity*: Neither exploiting nor deceiving clients. Strive to improve the health and well-being of individuals and society, charge fair fees, and conduct research ethically.
5. *Advocacy*: Serve as advocates, helping individuals and society cope with death-related issues. Prevent exploitation and provide education on rights, responsibilities, and options.
6. *Presentation of diverse perspectives*: Present various views on death-related questions, respect the client's choices, and, when appropriate, share their own values.
7. *Conflict recognition*: Recognize potential conflicts of interest and discuss confidentiality and responsibilities to individuals, families, institutions, communities, and society.
8. *Referral and consultation*: Acknowledge limitations and have access to adequate consultation and referral resources, assessing the effectiveness of these systems through feedback.
9. *Public education*: Work to enhance the understanding of dying and death among laypersons and professionals, promoting a more satisfying life and personal acceptance of death.

Gamino and Ritter (2009) expand on ADEC's ethical standards, emphasizing death competence, consent, and confidentiality in grief counseling. They assert that well-rounded death competence is crucial for practitioners working with grieving clients. This competence includes using one's understanding of grief and life experiences to enrich and inform the counseling process. Ensuring fully informed consent and maintaining confidentiality is paramount, allowing clients to express and process their thoughts and feelings around loss and grief freely.

Additionally, Gamino and Ritter highlight two other key ethical principles for grief therapy practitioners: individuality and pluralism. Individuality involves respecting each client's unique experience and processing of death and grief, providing them with autonomy to process their feelings in a way that best suits them. Pluralism allows clients to express a variety of beliefs related to their experience of death and grief, acknowledging and respecting diverse perspectives (Gamino & Ritter, 2009).

6.5 4A4C Competency Framework in End-of-Life and Grief Support

End-of-life and grief support essentially involve using *oneself as an instrument* to accompany and facilitate others' difficult journeys. Strengthening our ability to provide such support promotes a compassionate and resilient society and contributes to our own professional and personal growth. The 4A4C Competency and Healing Framework provides a holistic model to facilitate this process. This framework was developed with the input of several student cohorts who assisted in reviewing codes of ethics, principles, guidelines, and best practices in various human services fields. The material was synthesized and conceptualized into eight key components to ensure that the 4A4C competency and healing framework aligns with the standards and missions of various professional associations and scholarly work within the human services field. These associations, along with the years of their most relevant guidelines or publications that were reviewed, include but are not limited to:

American Counseling Association (ACA) (2014)
American Psychological Association (APA) (2015)
Association for death education and counseling (ADEC) (2010)
American Nurses Association (ANA) (2015)
National Association of Social Workers (NASW) (2021)
Hospice and Palliative Nurses Association (HPNA) (2022)
National Education Association (NEA) (2020)

Many international organizations provide essential guidelines and resources for professionals, ensuring adherence to international standards and best practices.

- *International Federation of Social Workers (IFSW)* (2018): This global organization promotes social justice, human rights, and social development through best practices in social work and international cooperation.
- *International Council of Nurses (ICN)* (2002): Represents nurses worldwide, advocating for the profession and advancing health policies.
- *World Federation of Mental Health (WFMH)* (n.d.): Promotion of mental health awareness, prevention of mental disorders, and best practices globally.
- *International Association of Schools of Social Work (IASSW)* (2020): Enhances the quality of social work education globally through research and scholarship.
- *International Association for Hospice and Palliative Care (IAHPC)* (2013): Advances hospice and palliative care services worldwide through education, advocacy, and research.

The 4A4C framework encapsulates eight interrelated core components that form a dynamic and holistic structure, which is particularly relevant for human service professionals specializing in end-of-life and grief support.

The first component, *awareness*, lays the foundation for *acceptance*, which cultivates *affirmation*—validating life, innate human value, and diverse experiences. This progression leads to *actualization*, where individuals realize their potential and enable the healing and growth of others. Actualization deepens awareness, creating a continuous loop of growth benefiting both the professional and those they support.

Similarly, within 4Cs, *compassion* serves as a powerful catalyst for forging connections and understanding. These *connections*, in turn, facilitate *composure,* instilling a sense of calm and stability through genuine connections with oneself, the client, and other sources of strength. Composure, with its grounding effect, encourages *commitment*, empowering professionals to navigate challenges with resilience, determination, and advocacy for the client's benefit and social justice. Conversely, commitment fuels compassion, as unwavering dedication to supporting and uplifting others drives meaningful action and empathy. This intricate web of interconnectedness underscores the holistic nature of the framework, where the components synergize to provide robust guidance not only for grief counselors and grief support personnel but also for human service professionals at large.

The 4As primarily focus on self-development and subsequently extend toward interactions with others. For instance, self-awareness paves the foundation for extending awareness toward others, which in turn expands to encompass social-cultural awareness. Similarly, self-acceptance lays the groundwork for fostering nonjudgmental acceptance of others, paralleled by how self-affirmation naturally extends to affirming others. Furthermore, self-actualization not only facilitates personal growth but also empowers individuals to support others in their own journey toward actualization.

On the other hand, the 4Cs predominantly emphasize an outward orientation toward others, while holding relevance for self-application. Compassion for those being supported is enhanced by cultivating self-compassion. Establishing connections with others forms the basis of supportive relationships and effective communication while fostering a deeper connection with oneself enriches these interactions. Additionally, while commitment to others' well-being is a fundamental value in helping professions, commitment to one's own authenticity and well-being is equally vital, as it ensures congruency and fosters sustainability in our efforts to assist others. The following section explores these concepts and their application in the context of healing, as well as supports dying and grieving persons. Figure 6.1 illustrates these aspects.

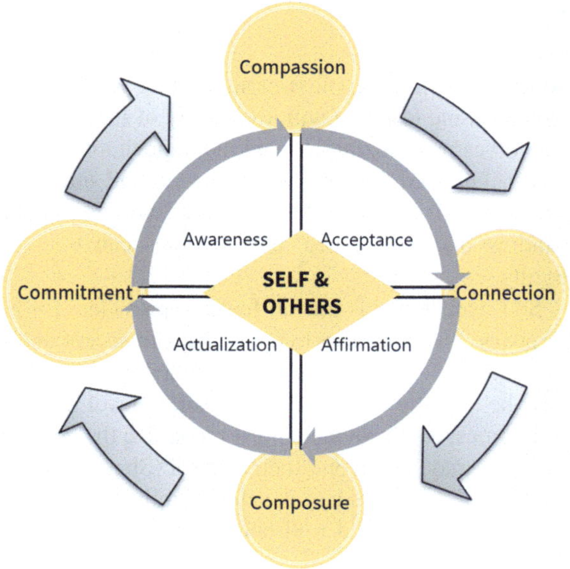

Fig. 6.1 4A4C

6.5.1 Awareness

Awareness in supporting dying and grieving individuals means being fully present, emotionally attuned, and empathetic. It enables caregivers to offer person-centered care, recognize cultural and social influences, and acknowledge every person's journey in transitions or grieving. This involves mindful listening and cultural sensitivity, being aware of cultural nuances in expressing grief, and supporting clients in a manner that honors their cultural background.

Self-awareness includes recognizing personal triggers, understanding one's own background, strengths, and limitations, and knowing how these factors might influence interactions. Professionals should engage in self-reflection to understand their own attitudes, experiences, and feelings related to death and grief (Chan & Tin, 2012). This self-awareness is crucial for maintaining emotional resilience and providing unbiased support (Wheat et al., 2022).

When professionals address their anxieties about death and grief, it benefits both themselves and their clients. Professionals with a positive attitude and low death anxiety are more likely to initiate end-of-life conversations (Chan & Tin, 2012). This positive attitude can help ease clients when discussing stressful topics such as grief and associated experiences.

6.5.2 Acceptance

Acceptance, in the context of supporting death, dying, and grief, involves helping persons come to terms with the reality of loss and the emotions that accompany it. It involves recognizing humankind's inevitable mortality and natural grieving process, acknowledging the depth of pain and unique journey experienced by those grieving, and validating their emotions without judgment. Based on this deep understanding and acceptance, professionals can treat every individual with holistic dignity.

Self-acceptance is crucial for care providers for both professional and personal purposes. It is important to recognize and accept one's own limitations, vulnerabilities, and triggers. This means acknowledging that everyone has flaws and that there may be situations where the desired level of outcomes cannot be achieved. Sometimes, care providers must recognize that certain aspects of their professional practices may be beyond their control (Shapiro et al., 2011). By embracing acceptance, care providers can develop humility and resilience, which in turn enhances their effectiveness and well-being in both challenging and rewarding situations.

6.5.3 Affirmation

Affirmation in end-of-life and grief support involves recognizing and validating the inherent worth, dignity, and potential for growth in each individual. Caregivers ensure that individuals are heard and respected, forming a therapeutic alliance to formulate goals and care plans congruent with the person's values and priorities. While it is crucial to validate genuine emotions and intrinsic worth, caregivers should gently guide individuals to challenge cognitive narratives that hinder their healing process.

Equally crucial to affirming the client is the professional's ability to affirm their own worth, good intentions, and righteous actions without becoming overly attached to outcomes. This enhances professional resilience and sustainable compassion.

6.5.4 Actualization

Actualization in end-of-life and grief support involves helping individuals realize their potential for personal growth, fulfillment, and healing. Based on Maslow's hierarchy of needs, self-actualization represents fulfilling one's unique potential, a principle of human motivation (Maslow, 1943). It reflects the human tendency to find meaning and purpose even in the face of adversity, echoing Viktor Frankl's *Man's search for meaning* (1985). Caregivers support individuals in identifying and leveraging their strengths to navigate their grief journey effectively.

By facilitating clients' reflection, expression, and personal development, caregivers enable individuals to take active steps toward self-discovery, fulfillment, and healing. In the process, caregivers also progress on their own journey of self-actualization.

6.5.5 Compassion

Compassion in end-of-life and grief support goes beyond empathy; it indicates the intention and action to alleviate suffering—be it physical, psychosocial, or spiritual. Compassion recognizes the shared human experiences of mortality and vulnerability, fostering connections and humanity. Compassionate presence, both verbal and nonverbal, is therapeutic and fosters healing. In addition, counselors can use compassionate reframing to help clients feel more comfortable within themselves by taking a noncritical approach and reconstruct their narratives (Harris & Winokuer, 2021).

Sometimes, it is easier to be compassionate toward others but not the self. It is crucial for caregivers to cultivate self-compassion to manage the challenges of confronting others' suffering. This includes understanding "vicarious grief" and preventing "compassion fatigue," which are common in professions that involve frequent exposure to others' pain (Rando, 1997; Woolhouse et al., 2012). Recognizing and addressing these challenges is crucial for maintaining personal well-being and professional effectiveness. In addition, it is essential to integrate compassion with wisdom and skillful means for sustainable support. Please refer to the section on self-care and prevention of compassion fatigue.

6.5.6 Connection

Connection is vital in end-of-life and grief support, encompassing connections to the client and the authentic self.

First and foremost, connection lies at the heart of effective communication and relationships. Although communication is an acquired skill, connection requires genuine intention. A compassionate intention to care for and learn from those we serve sets the foundation to connect. Creating a confidential, safe, and comfortable environment to allow others to express themselves freely is essential (Blueford & Adams, 2021). Empathy is conveyed through tone, eye contact, body language, facial expressions, and allowing for pauses or silences, which creates a supportive presence. Research shows that strong connections with health care providers and support networks improve the quality of life and well-being of individuals facing terminal illness (Breen, 2019; Koopmans et al., 2020).

Continuing bonds have been shown to facilitate the grieving process and provide comfort (Hewson et al., 2023). Supporting a grieving person through rituals, traditions, and memories helps them reconnect with loved ones who have passed away, promoting healing.

Additionally, spiritual or transcendental connections, such as faith, spirituality, and a sense of connectedness with nature or the universe, offer solace and meaning during times of death and loss (MacKinlay & Trevitt, 2010; Klass, 2014). Engaging in nature, rituals, prayer, or other spiritual practices fosters peace and healing, promoting personal growth and resilience.

The connection to one's authentic self is equally vital. While helping professionals often prioritize the needs of those they serve, they are also psychosocial and spiritual beings shaped by diverse cultural, religious, and philosophical traditions. For many, their professional calling reflects foundational personal beliefs (AMA, n.d.). Therefore, professionals preserve the opportunity to align their actions with the dictates of their conscience when fulfilling professional obligations and upholding ethical principles (AMA, Opinion 1.1.7, n.d.).

6.5.7 Composure

Cultivating composure is crucial in providing effective support to individuals facing death and grief. It involves maintaining emotional stability, resilience, and the presence of the mind in challenging situations. By remaining calm and composed, professionals create a safe environment for clients to explore their emotions and work toward healing. Furthermore, composure enables professionals to model healthy coping strategies and emotional regulation techniques.

Any professional conducting grief or death work should also acquire a level of comfort in discussing death, grief, and loss to effectively assist clientele (Blueford et al., 2022). This ability to manage the impact of death on themselves, as well as emotions, is considered to be the most essential "death competency," a term proposed by Gamino and Ritter (2012). They use "death competence" to describe "specialized skill in tolerating and managing a client's problems related to dying, death, and bereavement" (p. 23).

Lingering trauma or sensitivity to death or grief could impact professionals' composure and the efficacy of counseling and support. Therefore, addressing one's unresolved grief and healing is not just self-care but also enhances professional competence.

Maintaining emotional and mental balance is essential for helping professionals. It is beneficial for balancing empathy and composure, somewhat detaching from clients' experiences, emotional responses, and care outcomes. This ability to detach from overbearing emotions helps protect professionals from vicarious trauma. Achieving composure is not about becoming indifferent but about managing one's emotional responses and behaviors to provide consistent support.

6.5.8 Commitment

Commitment denotes unwavering dedication to supporting people through their journey. This includes being consistently present both physically and emotionally and providing sustained support and follow-up care. Professionals committed to end-of-life care and grief support uphold ethical principles and standards of practice, promoting the dignity, autonomy, and holistic well-being of those they serve. Commitment also involves advocacy and empowerment, ensuring that individuals' needs and preferences are respected and honored, particularly in interactions with various social systems and institutions (NASW, 2021).

The commitment extends to lifelong learning. Professionals engage in continuing education and professional development to stay informed about grief theories and models, best practices, emerging research, and innovative tools in end-of-life care and grief support (ADEC, 2010). This commitment to professional growth enhances their ability to provide effective support (Ober et al., 2012).

Equally important is the dedication to personal growth and well-being. When professionals address their own needs and unprocessed grief, they enhance their capacity to support others effectively. Practices like self-reflection, peer groups, seeking professional help, and engaging in personal development and self-care strengthen their resilience and ability to provide sustainable care.

6.5.9 Summary

The 4A4C competency and healing framework provides a holistic approach for human service professionals, highlighting the connection between self-development and serving others, especially in the context of end-of-life and grief support. Chan and Tin introduced the concept of "self-competence in death work" (Chan & Tin, 2012) to highlight this connection, advocating for the development and enhancement of one's inner resources to achieve both professional and personal growth.

By promoting awareness, acceptance, affirmation, actualization, compassion, connection, composure, and commitment, professionals can provide holistic and empathetic care that honors the dignity and unique experiences of individuals undergoing life transitions or experiencing grief. This approach not only improves the quality of care but also supports the personal and professional growth, ensuring sustainability and resilience in their essential roles.

Tables 6.1 and 6.2 illustrate how the 4A4C components can be practically implemented. They summarize the key points of each element, which can be divided into self-oriented and other-oriented dimensions:

Table 6.1 Awareness, acceptance, affirmation, and actualization (4A)

Components	Self	Other
Awareness	– Be aware of one's reactions and personal triggers – Acknowledging one's own background, strengths, and limitations, and understand how they influence interactions – Mindfulness practices – Learn about diverse cultural perspectives	– Being fully present, emotionally attuned, and empathetic – Mindful listening – Noticing and identifying the clients' preferences, tasks, coping styles, etc. – Incorporating cultural sensitivity into interaction, aware of and respecting cultural and social influences on individual experiences
Acceptance	– Recognizing and accepting personal limitations and vulnerabilities – Cultivating humility and resilience Utilize cognitive-behavioral techniques to manage personal biases and stressors. – Accepting the limits of control in professional practice	– Helping come to terms with the reality of loss and their experiences – Acknowledging and validating the pain and unique journey of those grieving or dying
Affirmation	– Affirming one's own worth, good intentions, and actions – Enhancing professional resilience and self-care – Identify and challenge one's own cognitive distortions – Engaging in cultural humility and lifelong learning about diverse cultures and perspectives to affirm our shared humanity	– Recognizing and validating the inherent worth, dignity, and potential for growth in each individual – Validating genuine emotions and experiences while gently challenging cognitive distortions – Providing person-centered culturally responsive care
Actualization	– Engaging in personal and professional growth, fulfillment, and healing – Progressing on their own journey of self-actualization	– Helping individuals realize their potential and navigate their grief journey – Supporting clients in reflection, expression, and personal development

6.6 Communication in End-of-Life and Grief Support

Effective communication is essential for providing meaningful support. It involves more than just spoken words; its true essence lies in the compassionate presence conveyed through nonverbal cues, such as tone, body language, and personal space. This section delves into the nuances of communication in these sensitive contexts, with the goal of fostering a deeper understanding and connection.

Table 6.2 Compassion, connection, composure, and commitment (4C)

Components	Self	Other
Compassion	– Cultivating self-compassion to manage challenges – Preventing compassion fatigue and addressing vicarious grief	– Alleviating physical, emotional, and spiritual pain – Creating a supportive environment and using compassionate reframing
Connection	– Connecting to the true self beneath social conditioning and past experiences – Form and maintain strong social support and allies – Explore and strengthen connection with nature, meaning, and spirituality	– Forming therapeutic alliances and using effective communication – Facilitating continuing bonds with loved ones who have passed away – Support connecting to the true self and nature – Supporting spiritual or existential connections
Composure	– Maintaining emotional stability and presence of mind – Develop equanimity – Mindfulness practices	– Providing a safe and supportive environment for clients – Demonstrating emotional regulation, resilience, and adaptive coping mechanisms to inspire clients – Strengthening the ability to handle crisis
Commitment	– Committing to one's own healing and self-development – Engaging in continuous learning and professional growth – Receiving regular supervision and support	– Providing consistent support, guidance, and companionship – Advocating for and empowering clients to make informed decisions aligned with their values

6.6.1 *Nature of Communication*

Communication is essentially an encoding and decoding process. McLean (2005) identified the following key components in interpersonal communication:

- *Sender:* The originator of the message who encodes and transmits information.
- *Message:* The content or information being conveyed.
- *Medium:* The channel used to transmit the message, such as spoken words, written text, or nonverbal gestures.
- *Receiver:* The person or group who decodes and interprets the message.
- *Feedback:* The response from the receiver, indicating whether the message was understood.
- *Context:* The environment or situation that influences communication.
- *Interference:* Any barrier that can distort or hinder the communication process, such as noise or emotional distress.

The medium, context, and internal and semantic noises all potentially interfere with the transmission of the messages; the communication is often likened to an iceberg: what is visible above the surface is only a small fraction of the whole. The words, tone of voice, facial expressions, body language, and eye contact constitute visible aspects. However, much lies beneath the surface, including our history, motives, past experiences, values, education, assumptions, profession, emotional state, beliefs, and biases.

In end-of-life and grief support, understanding this iceberg is crucial. The bereaved or dying person's reactions are shaped by their unique experiences and background. Effective communication requires sensitivity to these underlying factors and an awareness that what is unspoken can be as significant as what is spoken.

6.6.2 *Validating and Invalidating Statements*

One of the core elements of supportive communication is validation—the validation of emotions and a person's inherent worth. Validating statements acknowledge and affirm the person's feelings and experiences, creating a sense of being heard and understood. Conversely, invalidating statements, sometimes out of good intentions, can dismiss or undermine a person's feelings, leading to further distress.

6.6.2.1 Validating Statements

Acknowledging feelings and importance: "I can see how upset this makes you feel. I understand that this is important to you."

Offering support and presence: "Please know I'm here for you. I'm here to listen if you want to talk more."

Expressing gratitude and empathy: Thank you for sharing this with me. I would feel the exact same way."

Recognizing hurt and stress: "It sounds like you were truly hurt by this. What a stressful situation."

Clarifying and providing practical help: "Therefore, I heard you are feeling overwhelmed. Is there anything I could do for you?"; "I'm a phone call away if you would like someone to help run some errands for you"; "Would you like me to walk your dog? I need to walk mine anyways!"

6.6.2.2 Invalidating Statements

Labeling actions: "You did the right thing" or "You did the wrong thing."

Dismissing emotions: "You can be so sensitive/dramatic/emotional," or "You need to calm down"; "Aren't you over him yet; he has been dead for years!"

Shifting focus to yourself: "This reminds me of the time that I got fired. Remember how rude my old boss was? …"

Forcing positivity: "You should feel lucky/blessed/fortunate that you have a family that cares about you." "Be strong."

Minimizing: "It could have been worse"; "At least she lived a long life"; "It's just a dog."

Generalizing: "Life's not fair."
Blaming: "If you had only listened to my advice before." Or "If you had only dumped him the first time he cheated on you…"
Playing devil's advocate: "Maybe they didn't mean it that way."

The appropriateness of certain statements often depends on the role, relationship, and context involved. For example, "I am sorry for your loss" may be seen as offensive by some but accepted as a conventional expression of condolence by others. Similarly, asking "How are you, truly?" with an emphasis on "truly" can be supportive in a close relationship and intruding among acquaintances. Meanwhile, if probing for more detail and authentic replies, be prepared to offer practical help.

6.6.3 Effective Communication Strategies in End-of-Life and Grief Support

Rosenblatt (2019) outlined several strategies for effective communication in grief counseling: active listening, respecting the client, allowing pauses of silence, normalizing the processing of emotions, and creating a nonjudgmental space.

Clients may be reluctant to share their stories, experiences, and emotions with counselors who operate on rigid, sterile principles. Blueford and Adams (2021) emphasize the importance of creating a space where clients feel heard and empowered to take ownership of their grief journey. They argue that bereaved clients are particularly vulnerable and that enabling their autonomy can lead to more effective assessment and communication. For example, counselors can provide a safe space by asking clients' permission to begin the session, co-creating goals to guide the clients' grief journey, seeking clients' consent before introducing new care plans, and regularly evaluating the counseling experience from the client's perspective. These practices not only foster a supportive environment but also enhance the therapeutic alliance and facilitate more meaningful progress in grief counseling.

The following lists some essential strategies to strengthen the effectiveness of communication in end-of-life and grief support:

1. *Active listening:* Show attentiveness and understanding through eye contact, nodding, and reflective responses.
2. *Open-ended questions:* Encourage detailed responses (e.g., "Can you tell me more about …?").
3. *Reflective responses:* Mirror the speaker's words and emotions to validate their feelings (e.g., "It sounds like you're feeling very overwhelmed right now").
4. *Validation:* Validate the emotions and the person's inherent value.
5. *Providing silence:* Allow moments of silence to give individuals time to process their thoughts and emotions.
6. *Cultural sensitivity and humility:* Be aware of and respect cultural differences in communication styles and grieving practices; showing willingness to learn.

7. *Compassionate presence:* Offer a calm, consistent, and compassionate presence, maintaining mindfulness, composure, and compassionate listening through all stages of communication.

Communication is more than a technique. Genuine, albeit awkwardly expressed, kindness and care often work better than polished superficial words. Sometimes, a hug speaks louder than eloquent speech, and kind gestures or actions, like helping with daily chores, speak more profoundly than general statements.

The key to effective communication is "to connect," and the key to building a relationship is "to relate." Genuine connection and support stem from a sincere interest in the other person's well-being. A compassionate presence is inherently therapeutic, demonstrating empathy, a willingness to listen without judgment, and a commitment to alleviating suffering. This involves showing consistency in presence and readiness to take meaningful action. Maintaining a compassionate presence provides a stable, supportive environment that fosters connection and healing through genuine, heartfelt interactions.

6.7 Self-Care for Professionals and Prevention of Compassion Fatigue

Self-care is vital for helping professionals because it directly impacts their ability to be fully present and provide quality support. Many professional associations recommend self-care. For example, the Council on Social Work Education (CSWE) Educational Policy and Accreditation Standards (EPAS) explicitly states in Competency 1 that social workers take measures to care for themselves professionally and personally and that self-care is paramount for competent and ethical social work practices. Without proper self-care and attention to their needs, practitioners risk not effectively fulfilling their duties and responsibilities to clients (CSWE, 2022, p. 8).

Based on CSWE (2022) and the American Association of Colleges of Nursing (AACN) (n.d.), as well as other literature, *self-care* can be generally defined as the *intentional actions and choices individuals make to maintain and improve their health and well-being.*

Self-care helps prevent compassion fatigue and vicarious grief. Working with dying patients and grieving families can sometimes pose existential and emotional challenges (Gamino & Ritter, 2012). By prioritizing self-care and adopting effective strategies, professionals can maintain their well-being and continue to provide high-quality care to their clients. Practitioners can achieve *compassion satisfaction*, a positive state defined as the pleasure derived from helping others. This leads to resilience, optimism, good health, and a balanced lifestyle. Additionally, it creates a positive work environment and fosters a better therapeutic relationship for the client (Stamm, 2013).

6.7.1 Understanding Compassion Fatigue and Vicarious Grief

Compassion fatigue refers to a phenomenon common among care professionals, resulting from prolonged exposure to client suffering, which is often compounded by a lack of support in the workplace and at home. Figley (2002) identified four primary contributors to compassion fatigue: poor self-care routines, unresolved personal trauma, inability to manage workplace stressors, and dissatisfaction with work. This condition can lead to burnout, which is characterized by emotional exhaustion, depersonalization, and a diminished sense of accomplishment (Rotenstein et al., 2018). Additionally, practitioners experiencing compassion fatigue are at risk of developing secondary or vicarious trauma, as they absorb their clients' trauma and stress. The risk decreases when professionals encounter traumas they have personally faced, when they are dealing with unresolved trauma, or when they handle trauma endured by children.

Vicarious grief is the sorrow one feels for a loss suffered by another person. There are two major types. The first type is exclusively based on empathy, whereas the second type occurs when unprocessed grief from personal loss is reactivated by another's loss (Rando, 1997). In type I vicarious grief, the secondary griever may not know the deceased very well, and there is no loss of attachment. The feelings come directly from empathy for the primary mourner. In type II vicarious grief, there is a continuation of grief from a primary loss reactivated by another's loss. The secondary griever is reminded of their own unresolved grief triggered by the primary griever's condition. Therefore, in type II vicarious grief, in addition to the vicarious losses being identified, there are "personally experienced losses (Rando, 1997, p. 261)" associated with relatively intense reactions to the actual mourner's loss and may challenge one's foundational beliefs about the self or the world.

The intensity of vicarious grief is influenced by the degree of distance between the primary and secondary grievers, which can be physical, psychological, or social. The closer the secondary griever is to the primary griever, the greater the probability of increased empathy and vicarious grief. The media also play a role in vicarious grieving by creating narratives during community tragedies that people can empathize with (Sullender, 2010).

During the COVID-19 pandemic, healthcare workers experienced heightened levels of vicarious grief due to the unprecedented number of deaths they encountered daily. This phenomenon also affects hospice staff, faith-based workers, and mental health professionals. These professionals regularly interact with grieving individuals in their roles, and the pandemic intensified these encounters. Many workers reported difficulties in handling the grief-related aspects of their jobs, experiencing high levels of depression and fatigue, as well as shifts in their worldviews coinciding with their increased exposure to grief (Sera Jose et al., 2023).

Although vicarious grief and vicarious trauma have traditionally focused mainly on adverse effects, increasing attention has been given to positive and life-affirming aspects in recent years. Vicarious posttraumatic growth is similar but not identical to posttraumatic growth, such as becoming a more compassionate and effective professional (Ogińska-Bulik & Juczyński, 2024). This concept reinforces grief's collective nature and human resilience.

6.7.2 Warning Signs and Prevention Strategies

Recognizing early warning signs of compassion fatigue facilitates implementing timely self-care strategies. These signs can include emotional exhaustion, reduced empathy, depersonalization, and physical symptoms such as headaches or fatigue. The development of a personal "early warning system" can help practitioners monitor their emotional and physical depletion levels and take corrective actions before reaching a critical state.

The *Compassion Fatigue Workbook* (Mathieu, 2012*)* provides several practical strategies and exercises to help professionals mitigate compassion fatigue and vicarious trauma:

Creating a self-care plan: A personalized self-care plan involves identifying realistic self-care goals and specific activities and regularly reviewing and adjusting the plan as needed.

Mindfulness and relaxation techniques: Incorporating mindfulness practices and relaxation techniques, such as deep breathing exercises, progressive muscle relaxation, and guided imagery, can help reduce stress and improve emotional regulation.

Building resilience: The workbook suggests building resilience through activities that foster a sense of purpose and meaning. This includes hobbies, volunteering, and connecting with a supportive community.

Professional support: Seeking supervision, mentorship, or therapy can provide space for professionals to process their experiences and gain insights into managing compassion fatigue. Peer support groups can also offer a platform for sharing experiences and strategies.

Setting boundaries: Establishing clear professional boundaries helps prevent overextending oneself. This involves learning to say no, delegating tasks when possible, and ensuring a healthy work-life balance.

6.7.3 Self-Care and Resilience

Self-care is essential for preventing compassion fatigue. Zastrow and Hessenauer (2019) emphasized five areas of self-care to build resilience: physical, psychological, social, spiritual, and professional care.

Physical Care

- Focus on a balanced diet and better sleep habits.
- Incorporate regular physical exercise.

- Use stress management techniques.
- Limit or avoid alcohol and drugs.

Psychological Care
- Practice mindfulness and build a positive self-concept.
- Set short- and long-term life goals.
- Explore strategies to manage anxiety and depression.
- Clarify personal values and the characteristics of the person you aspire to be.

Social Care
- Strengthen relationships with family and friends.
- Cultivate new friendships and end unfulfilling or harmful relationships.
- Develop assertiveness in social interactions.

Spiritual Care
- Reflect on and engage with your religious or spiritual beliefs.
- Participate in ceremonies, rituals, or spiritual practices, individually or in a community.
- Seek guidance from a spiritual mentor or spend time in prayer or other personal practices.

Professional and Academic Care
- Define career goals and focus on time management.
- Improve study habits and explore volunteer opportunities.
- Strive for a fulfilling career while maintaining a balance between work, academics, and family life.

In addition to self-care, building resilience involves the ability to adapt to and recover from adversity, access necessary resources, and maintain well-being in challenging situations. Combating compassion fatigue is not solely an individual concern; it is often influenced by the work environment and the level of social support available. Resilience is a dynamic and multilayered capacity that encompasses not just individuals but also families, communities, institutions, and society as a whole.

Family resilience involves collective efforts to respect, appreciate, and support each member, fostering a sense of belonging.

Community resilience includes social networks and structures that provide resources and support, enabling individuals and families to thrive despite challenges.

Institutional resilience refers to the capacity of organizations, such as schools, workplaces, and healthcare systems, to withstand and adapt to external pressures and continue to function effectively. Organizations play crucial roles in preventing burnout and compassion fatigue among employees. They can achieve this by fostering an inclusive culture and implementing supportive policies. This includes ensuring fair labor practices, avoiding role overload and internal role conflict, and providing resources for self-care, mental health, and professional development.

Societal resilience encompasses broader social, economic, and cultural systems supporting communities and institutions, ensuring they can adapt to and recover from large-scale disruptions (Koh et al., 2011; Lebid et al., 2023).

In addition to individual self-care, practitioners can enhance resilience by strengthening institutional, community, cultural, and societal resilience. This involves promoting policies and practices that support equitable access to resources, fostering inclusive and supportive community environments, and building strong social networks. By doing so, professionals help create a resilient society where individuals, communities, institutions, and society can support each other in times of crisis and beyond (Cacciatore et al., 2021; Health.gov, 2021). Therefore, resilience is not merely an individual trait but also a collective capacity nurtured and sustained across different levels of society. Integrating personal, institutional, community, and societal resilience practices leads to a more robust and sustainable support system for all.

6.7.4 Integrating Compassion and "Skillful Means" for Sustainable Support

In addition to the general recommendations discussed above, insights from Eastern philosophies, such as Buddhist and yogic thoughts, provide valuable perspectives for preventing compassion fatigue. While rooted in specific traditions, these thoughts may benefit anyone regardless of their faith or beliefs.

Buddhism, particularly within the Mahayana tradition, emphasizes compassion on the basis of the principles of interconnectedness, wisdom, and "*skillful means*."

Interconnectedness refers to the understanding that all things and experiences are interconnected and depend on other factors. This is often referred to as dependent origination or dependent arising. It underscores the idea that nothing and no one exist in isolation and that all is contingent upon other factors for their existence.

Wisdom (prajna) in Buddhism involves developing insights into reality, seeing things as they are, and transcending ignorance to recognize the true nature of the self and mind. One essential teaching of the Buddha is the impermanent nature of all phenomena, as everything arises from a collection of causes and conditions that continuously change. This understanding reduces grasping and suffering, allowing for a more compassionate response to one's own and others' suffering.

Skillful means (upaya) require Bodhisattvas to accept others as they are and meet them where they are when helping. It indicates a personalized approach to education, guidance, and support. This approach ensures that the helping methods are accessible and relevant to a diverse audience, congruent with the particular needs, capacities, values, and circumstances of different individuals. Skillful means also require an awareness of and respect for one's own limitations and capacities.

The *Bodhisattva* path represents the ideal of striving for enlightenment not only for oneself but also for all beings. A Bodhisattva vows to benefit others and help them achieve liberation from suffering. This path involves cultivating and practicing the six *paramitas*, or transcendent perfections, which include generosity, ethical conduct, patience, joyful effort, a clear and focused mind through meditation, and wisdom. Bodhisattvas are motivated by great compassion (mahakaruna) and are committed to helping others attain enlightenment, believing that their own liberation is intertwined with the liberation of all beings.

In the yogic tradition, particularly within the practice of *Karma Yoga*, the concept of Seva (selfless service) is integral. Seva involves performing actions to serve others without attachment to the outcome or the sense of being a "doer." This practice helps individuals avoid tying their self-worth to specific results, fostering a sense of selflessness and sustainability in their service. The *Bhagavad Gita* (1995), a key text in yogic philosophy, emphasizes acting without attachment to the fruits of one's actions as a path to spiritual growth and liberation.

Nonattachment is a core principle in both Buddhism and Yoga. This does not mean maintaining a cold psychological distance; rather, it means performing one's duties and actions without grasping their outcomes and the need to fulfill a self-serving ego. Nonattachment helps practitioners transcend the ego, attain composure in adversity, and remain humble in success. Professionals act as companions, facilitators, and enablers to explore and enable the healing process. This practice helps maintain composure, serve others, and accompany them on their journey without being swayed by immediate outcomes. By focusing on intention and action, practitioners can cultivate inner peace and resilience.

These Eastern perspectives enhance the self-care strategies concepts commonly found in professional literature. They emphasize the importance of a holistic approach to personal and professional well-being. The principles of wisdom, skillful means, and nonattachment complement compassion and help prevent "fatigue." As a result, compassion becomes self-sustaining, providing satisfaction and reinforcing dedication to service. These multicultural-inspired principles can be applied without requiring adherence to any specific religious beliefs, promoting a comprehensive approach to foster both personal growth and the well-being of those being served. This integration ensures that the service remains effective, fulfilling, and sustainable.

6.8 Concluding Reflection

Supporting people during their vulnerable time of transition and grieving can be simultaneously rewarding and demanding. End-of-life support addresses the physical, emotional, psychological, spiritual, and practical needs of individuals and their families.

Ethical principles and effective communication are integral to ensure that the end-of-life and grief support provided is compassionate, culturally sensitive, and person-centered. It is important for helping professionals to prevent compassion fatigue and address vicarious grief. This can be facilitated by combining compassion with wisdom and skillful means, recognizing signs of emotional exhaustion, and establishing strong self-care practices. These measures help care providers continue to provide empathetic and effective support while also strengthening their own well-being and resilience.

The 4A4C competency framework integrates these essential competencies, providing a structured approach for human service professionals. By emphasizing awareness, acceptance, affirmation, actualization, compassion, connection, composure, and commitment, the framework guides professionals in delivering holistic and compassionate care. Implementing the 4A4C framework ensures that care providers can support others effectively while fostering their own professional and personal growth.

Ultimately, the core philosophy of end-of-life and grief support focuses on recognizing and harnessing individuals' inherent strengths and resilience. By empowering individuals to access their resources and enhancing their coping skills, care professionals can facilitate meaningful progress in their challenging journeys. In this process, helping professionals not only support others' healing but also foster their own professional and personal growth.

Bhagavad Gita states, "You have the right to work, but never to the fruit of work" (Sivananda, 1995, Chapter 2, Verse 47). The statement reflects the principle of *karma yoga*. By focusing on the intentions and acts of service, end-of-life and grief support can enrich both their own path and the lives they touch.

References

American Association of Colleges of Nursing. (n.d.). Self-care concept. In *Developing nurse well-being and leadership tool kit*. https://www.aacnnursing.org/developing-nurse-well-being-and-leadership-tool-kit/tool-kit/self-care-concept

American Counseling Association. (2014). *ACA code of ethics*. Author. https://www.counseling.org/docs/default-source/default-document-library/ethics/2014-aca-code-of-ethics.pdf?sfvrsn=55ab73d0_1

American Medical Association. (n.d.). *Caring for patients at the end of life: AMA Code of Medical Ethics*. https://code-medical-ethics.ama-assn.org/chapters/caring-patients-end-life

American Nurses Association. (2015). *Nursing: Scope and standards of practice* (3rd ed.). Author.

American Psychological Association. (2015). *Standards of accreditation for health service psychology*. Author. https://www.apa.org/ed/accreditation/about/policies/standards-of-accreditation.pdf

Association for Death Education and Counseling (ADEC). (2010). *ADEC code of ethics*. https://www.adec.org/page/code_of_ethics#Tenets

Blueford, J., & Adams, C. (2021). Creating empowering spaces in grief counseling. *Journal of Counseling and Development, 99*(2), 145–153. https://doi.org/10.1002/jcad.12361

Blueford, J. M., Diambra, J. F., & Wheat, L. S. (2022). Counselor preparedness to counsel grieving clients: Insights and implications. *Death Studies, 46*(10), 2413–2423. https://doi.org/10.1080/07481187.2021.1956644

Breen, E. G. (2019). Capacity is only one aspect of decision-making at life's end. *The British Journal of Psychiatry, 214*(3), 171–172.

Cacciatore, J., Thieleman, K., Fretts, R., & Jackson, L. B. (2021). What is good grief support? Exploring the actors and actions in social support after traumatic grief. *PLoS One, 16*(5), e0252324. https://doi.org/10.1371/journal.pone.0252324

Chan, W. C. H., & Tin, A. F. (2012). Beyond knowledge and skills: Self-competence in working with death, dying, and bereavement. *Death Studies, 36*, 899–913.
Chan, W. C. H., Fong, A., Wong, K. L. Y., Tse, D. M. W., Lau, K. S., & Chan, L. N. (2016). Impact of death work on self: Existential and emotional challenges and coping of palliative care professionals. *Health & Social Work, 41*(1), 33–41.
Corr, C. A., Corr, D. M., & Doka, K. J. (2019). *Death & dying, life & living* (8th ed.). Cengage Learning.
Council on Social Work Education. (2022). *Educational policy and accreditation standards for baccalaureate and master's social work programs*. https://www.cswe.org/getmedia/bb5d8afe-7680-42dc-a332-a6e6103f4998/2022-EPAS.pdf
Davis, A., Lippe, M., Glover, T. L., McLeskey, N., Shillam, C., & Mazanec, P. (2021). Integrating the ELNEC undergraduate curriculum into nursing education: Lessons learned. *Journal of Professional Nursing, 37*(2), 286–290.
Doka, K. J., & Martin, T. L. (2010). *Grieving beyond gender: Understanding the ways men and women mourn* (2nd ed.). Routledge.
Figley, C. R. (2002). Compassion fatigue: Psychotherapists' chronic lack of self care. *Journal of Clinical Psychology, 58*(11), 1433–1441.
Finkbeiner, A. K. (2012). *After the death of a child: Living with the loss through the years*. Simon and Schuster.
Frankl, V. E. (1985). *Man's search for meaning*. Simon and Schuster.
Gamino, L. A., & Ritter, R. H. (2009). *Ethical practice in grief counseling*. Springer Publishing.
Gamino, L. A., & Ritter, R. H., Jr. (2012). Death competence: An ethical imperative. *Death Studies, 36*, 23–40.
Harris, D. L., & Winokuer, H. R. (2021). *Principles and practice of grief counseling* (3rd ed.). Springer Publishing.
Health.gov. (2021). *Equity and enhanced individual and community resilience are integral to a meaningful recovery*. https://health.gov/news/202107/equity-and-enhanced-individual-and-community-resilience-are-integral-meaningful-recovery
Hewson, H., Galbraith, N., Jones, C., & Heath, G. (2023). The impact of continuing bonds following bereavement: A systematic review. *Death Studies*, 1–14. ahead-of-print. https://doi.org/10.1080/07481187.2023.2223593
Hill, J. E., Cicchetti, R. J., Jackson, S. A., & Szirony, G. M. (2018). Perceptions of grief education in accredited counseling programs: Recommendations for counselor education. *Journal of Social, Behavioral, and Health Sciences, 12*(1), 74–83. https://doi.org/10.5590/JSBHS.2018.12.1.05
Hospice and Palliative Nurses Association. (2022). *Guiding principles*. https://www.advancingexpertcare.org/get-involved/advocacy/guiding-principles/
Hsiao, et al. (2023). Researched nurses' readiness to provide grief counseling for family caregivers of terminally ill cancer patients. *Journal of Clinical Nursing, 32*(7–8), 1053–1064. https://doi.org/10.1111/jocn.16335
International Association for Hospice and Palliative Care (IAHPC). (2013). *The IAHPC manual of palliative care* (3rd ed.). IAHPC Press. ISBN 978-0-9834597-6-7.
International Association of Schools of Social Work. (2020). *The updated global standards for social work education and training*. https://www.iassw-aiets.org
International Council of Nurses. (2002). *Nursing definitions*. https://www.icn.ch/resources/nursing-definitions
International Federation of Social Workers. (2018). *Global social work statement of ethical principles*. https://www.ifsw.org/global-social-work-statement-of-ethical-principles/
Jankauskaite, G., O'Brien, K. M., & Yang, N. (2021). Assessing knowledge and predicting grief counseling skills among university counseling center therapists. *The Counseling Psychologist, 49*(3), 458–484.
Klass, D. (2014). Spirituality. In *The A–Z of death and dying: Social, medical, and cultural aspects* (pp. 390–391).

Koopmans, R., Sampson, E. L., Van den Block, L., & Peisah, C. (2020). Providing quality end-of-life care to older people in the era of COVID-19: Perspectives from five countries. *International Psychogeriatrics, 32*(11), 1345–1352.
Koh, H. K., Piotrowski, J. J., Kumanyika, S., & Fielding, J. E. (2011). Healthy people: A 2020 vision for the social determinants approach. *Health Education & Behavior, 38*(6), 551–557. https://doi.org/10.1177/1090198111428646
Kovacs, P. J., Bellin, M. H., & Fauri, D. P. (2006). Family-centered care: A resource for social work in end-of-life and palliative care. *Journal of Social Work in End-of-Life & Palliative Care, 2*(1), 13–27.
Lebid, A. E., Stepanov, V. V., & Nazarov, M. S. (2023). The informational components of social resilience within realization of the UN sustainable development goals. *International Journal of Media and Information Literacy, 8*(2), 324–338. https://doi.org/10.13187/ijmil.2023.2.324
MacKinlay, E., & Trevitt, C. (2010). Living in aged care: Using spiritual reminiscence to enhance meaning in life for those with dementia. *International Journal of Mental Health Nursing, 19*(6), 394–401. https://doi.org/10.1111/j.1447-0349.2010.00684.x
Maslow, A. H. (1943). A theory of human motivation. *Psychological Review, 50*(4), 370–396. https://doi.org/10.1037/h0054346
Mathieu, F. (2012). *The compassion fatigue workbook: Creative tools for transforming compassion fatigue and vicarious traumatization*. Routledge.
McLean, S. (2005). *The basics of interpersonal communication*. Pearson/Allyn and Bacon.
National Association of Social Workers. (2021). *Code of ethics*. https://www.socialworkers.org/About/Ethics/Code-of-Ethics/Code-of-Ethics-English
National Education Association. (2020). *Code of ethics for educators*. https://www.nea.org/resource-library/code-ethics-educators
Neimeyer, R. A. (Ed.). (2012, 2016, 2018, 2021). *Techniques of grief therapy series*. Routledge.
Ober, A. M., Granello, D. H., & Wheaton, J. E. (2012). Grief counseling: An investigation of counselor' training, experience, and competencies. *Journal of Counseling & Development, 90*(2), 150–159. https://doi.org/10.1111/j.1556-6676.2012.00020.x
Ogińska-Bulik, N., & Juczyński, Z. (2024). Vicarious posttraumatic growth: The benefits of indirect exposure to trauma. In *Routledge International Handbook of Posttraumatic Growth* (pp. 445–457). Routledge.
Rando, T. A. (1997). Vicarious bereavement. In S. Strack (Ed.), *Death and the quest for meaning: Essays in honor of Herman Feifel* (pp. 257–274). Jason Aronson.
Rosenblatt, P. C. (2019). Effective communication in grief counseling. In *The art of grief: The use of expressive arts in a grief support group*. Routledge.
Rotenstein, L. S., et al. (2018). Prevalence of burnout among physicians. *JAMA, 320*(11), 1131–1150. https://doi.org/10.1001/jama.2018.12777
Sera Jose, K. M. C., Navarro, A. J., Pomida, A. N., & Hechanova-Alampay, M. R. (2023). Bereaved in me: Understanding the vicarious grief experiences among helping professionals during the COVID-19 pandemic. *OMEGA-Journal of Death and Dying, 00302228221150870*.
Shapiro, J., Astin, J., Shapiro, S. L., Robitshek, D., & Shapiro, D. H. (2011). Coping with loss of control in the practice of medicine. *Families, Systems, & Health, 29*(1), 15.
Sivananda, S. (1995). *The Bhagavad Gita*. The Divine Life Society. (Original work published ca. 400 BCE)
Stamm, B. H. (2013). Measuring compassion satisfaction as well as fatigue: Developmental history of the compassion satisfaction and fatigue test. In *Treating Compassion Fatigue* (pp. 107–119). Routledge.
Sullender, R. S. (2010). Vicarious grieving and the media. *Pastoral Psychology, 59*, 191–200. https://doi.org/10.1007/s11089-009-0227-5
Wheat, L. S., Matthews, J. J., & Whiting, P. P. (2022). Grief content inclusion in CACREP-accredited counselor education programs. *Journal of Counselor Preparation and Supervision, 15*(2), Article 14. https://digitalcommons.sacredheart.edu/jcps/vol15/iss2/14
Worden, J. W. (2009). *Grief counseling and grief therapy: A handbook for the mental health practitioner* (4th ed.). Springer Publishing.

Woolhouse, S., Brown, J. B., & Thind, A. (2012). "Building through the grief": Vicarious trauma in a group of inner-city family physicians. *Journal of the American Board of Family Medicine, 25*(6), 840–846.

World Federation of Mental Health. (n.d.). *About us.* https://wfmh.global

World Health Organization. (2020). *Palliative care.* https://www.who.int/news-room/fact-sheets/detail/palliative-care

Zastrow, C., & Hessenauer, S. (2019). *Social work with groups: Comprehensive practice and self-care* (10th ed.). Cengage Learning.

Chapter 7
Assessments and Care Plans in End-of-Life and Grief Support

7.1 Introduction: Strength-Based Approach

The primary goal of end-of-life and grief assessments is to guide person-centered care that eases suffering and improves quality of life. While identifying problems is necessary, strength-based assessments are equally vital. They focus on coping styles and resources—both internal and external—that empower individuals and promote independence.

Strength assessments are especially valuable for those facing terminal illness and grief. Unlike problems, which may fluctuate daily, strengths like coping styles often remain stable. By focusing on these strengths, care providers can uncover lasting resources to address various needs.

Focusing solely on problems risks disempowering individuals and can create a harmful dynamic: "You have all the problems, and we hold all the solutions." This approach may lead individuals to exaggerate their struggles to justify care, increasing feelings of anxiety or depression. In contrast, strength-based assessments foster collaboration, mutual respect, and empowerment, emphasizing resilience and independence.

Recognizing and nurturing the strengths of both care providers and recipients creates powerful tools for addressing even the most demanding situations. This approach fosters growth and connection within the caregiving relationship.

This chapter emphasizes practical tools and real-life examples to identify strengths and create care plans rooted in empowerment and collaboration.

Y. Z. Ciupak, D. C. Smith, *Death, Dying, and Grief*,
https://doi.org/10.1007/978-3-031-88467-2_7

7.2 Assessments in Hospice and Palliative Care

Assessments in hospice, terminal illness, and palliative care involve various factors, reflecting the four pillars of palliative care: biological, psychological, social, and spiritual (WHO, 2020).

1. **Physical Symptom Evaluation:**

   Pain and symptom management: Discomfort at the end of life may come from various sources, such as pain, breathing problems, skin irritation, digestive issues, temperature sensitivity, or fatigue. Tools such as the Edmonton Symptom Assessment System (ESAS) help quantify symptom severity and monitor changes over time, allowing timely adjustments to care plans (Hui & Bruera, 2017).

   Functional status: This type of assessment examines a person's ability to perform daily activities. Instruments such as the Karnofsky Performance Status (KPS) scale or the Palliative Performance Scale (PPS) are commonly used to evaluate functional abilities and guide care decisions (Anderson et al., 1996).
2. **Emotional and Psychological Well-Being:**

   Anxiety and depression screening and quality of life: Various tools are available to identify psychological distress, such as the Hospital Anxiety and Depression Scale (HADS) or the Patient Health Questionnaire (PHQ-9). These assessments help identify mental health issues, ensuring that patients receive the necessary psychological support (Kroenke et al., 2001; Bjelland et al., 2002).
3. **Social and Support Networks:**

   Family and caregiver support: Assessments often include evaluating caregiver burden and the adequacy of support systems to ensure that both individuals under care and their caregivers receive necessary assistance.

   Social needs: Identifying a person's social needs, such as companionship and social interaction, helps address potential feelings of isolation and loneliness, contributing to a more supportive care environment (World Health Organization, 2020).
4. **Spiritual and Existential Considerations:**

   Spiritual distress: Addressing spiritual needs and existential concerns is crucial in providing holistic end-of-life care. Tools such as the FICA Spiritual History Tool guide conversations around spiritual beliefs and practices, ensuring that care respects and incorporates the person's spiritual needs (Puchalski & Romer, 2000).

   Meaning and purpose: Supporting individuals in finding meaning and purpose in their experiences can greatly enhance their well-being. Assessments that explore these aspects help ensure that spiritual care interventions align with their values and beliefs.

   Refer to Chap. 11 for detailed discussions about spiritual assessment and tools to address spiritual needs.
5. **Advance Care Planning:**

   Goals of care: Clarifying and documenting goals of care, including preferences for medical treatments and interventions, is an essential part of end-of-life assessments. This practice ensures that care plans align with the person's wishes and values, fostering a sense of control and dignity.

Legal and ethical issues: Addressing legal and ethical considerations, such as advance directives and decision-making capacities, safeguards patients' rights and autonomy, ensuring that care aligns with their desires and legal requirements. Refer to Chap. 5, for detailed discussions about advanced care planning, decisions, and ethical considerations.

Some comprehensive tools and methods have been developed to assess end-of-life care needs and outcomes, such as the Comprehensive Geriatric Assessment (CGA) (Parker et al., 2018), which evaluates the medical, psychological, and functional capabilities of elderly patients to develop a coordinated care plan. The Palliative Care Outcome Scale (POS) measures outcomes in palliative care, including physical symptoms and emotional and spiritual needs.

7.3 Bereavement Assessment

A bereavement assessment is a systematic approach used by healthcare professionals to evaluate the emotional, psychological, social, and spiritual needs of individuals who have experienced significant loss. This process identifies those at risk for prolonged grief disorder and tailors appropriate care plans to support them through their grieving process. The level of intervention can vary from grief support to grief counseling and grief therapy. There are a number of structured and quantifiable measures of grief severity that are often used by researchers and can assist some assessments. In practice, open-ended interviews with bereaved individuals offer valuable holistic insights into their personal experience, coping mechanisms, and specific needs, ensuring a more personalized and nuanced understanding of their situation. Personalized interviews combined with selected standardized tools can ensure effective person-centered care. The goal is to use insights from different methods in feedback sessions to develop personalized care plans that meet each individual's unique needs.

Generally, the key components of a bereavement assessment include the following:

1. **Emotional and psychological evaluation**: This involves assessing the individual's emotional response to the loss, including feelings of sadness, anger, guilt, and despair. The prolonged grief disorder (PGD) assessment, specified in the Diagnostic and Statistical Manual of Mental Disorders, Fifth Edition (DSM-5) (American Psychiatric Association, 2022), outlines criteria for diagnosing PGD. It distinguishes this condition from common grief, posttraumatic stress disorder (PTSD), and major depressive disorder (MDD) by focusing on persistent and intense grief that significantly impairs daily functioning.
2. **Behavioral and functional impact**: This dimension includes changes in sleep patterns, appetite, energy levels, and the ability to perform daily activities.

3. **Social networks**: This involves evaluating the support systems available to the bereaved person, including family, friends, and community resources. The assessment may involve questions about the availability and effectiveness of these support networks in providing emotional and practical help.
4. **Cultural and spiritual considerations**: Understanding the cultural and spiritual background of a bereaved person is important for providing culturally sensitive care. This includes acknowledging and respecting cultural rituals and practices related to death and mourning, as well as values, meanings, and purpose.
5. **Physical health assessment**: Grief can significantly impact physical health, leading to symptoms such as headaches, gastrointestinal issues, cognitive decline, and increased susceptibility to illnesses. A comprehensive bereavement assessment also considers these physical health aspects.

The above assessment is based on a holistic view of humans—simultaneously physical, social, psychological, and spiritual, cultural beings. A supplemental framework to the above dimensions is the Mourning Task model developed by the renowned grief therapy expert William Worden (2009). This model assesses which of the four mourning tasks the patient is struggling with, and the tasks do not necessarily appear in a sequential stage:

Task I: To accept the reality of the loss
Task II: To process the pain of grief
Task III: To adjust to a world without the deceased
Task IV: To find a connection with the deceased while carrying on with life.

7.4 Strength-Based Assessments

A strength-based assessment can guide healing better than focusing only on problems, as it identifies both direction and actionable steps. The following questions may guide this process to explore a person's strengths:

- Please tell me your three strengths.
- What compliments have you received from family and friends?
- When family and friends have turned to you for help, what kind of help have they usually sought?
- What have you done in your life that makes you proud?
- Tell me about some moments in your past when you felt you were at your best. What qualities did you show at those times?
- When your life is over, what things are people going to miss the most about you?

7.4.1 *Case Example: The Preacher*

Rick's[1] powerful sermons filled his church every Sunday, where he felt most alive. Preaching is his way of serving others and connecting with something greater than himself. However, outside the pulpit, Rick was different. His interpersonal skills were limited. When his wife passed away, Rick's grief was immense, yet he did not feel drawn to counseling or support groups. His associates and friends, concerned for him, suggested that he take a break to rest and grieve. However, for Rick, stepping away from preaching felt like a loss of its own.

Therefore, Rick made a decision. Instead of taking a break, he chose to keep preaching, but with a deeper purpose. He decided to weave his grief into his sermons, not only as a way to process his pain but also to connect it to the spiritual lessons he wanted to share with his congregation. Rick realized that his journey through loss could offer insights to others who were struggling with their own challenges. Every now and then, he would reference his wife or their relationship, using their experiences to illustrate larger truths about love, faith, and resilience. These moments were not just for his healing—they were meant to inspire and comfort his congregation as well.

In this way, Rick found that standing at the pulpit allowed him to work through his grief while continuing to serve his community. His sermons became a blend of personal reflection and spiritual teaching, helping him and those who listened to navigate the pain of loss with hope and understanding.

Reflection Rick's story highlights the power of integrating personal experience into public service. Rather than seeing his grief as something to be hidden or handled privately, Rick chose to use it as a tool for teaching and connection. His decision to keep preaching while grieving not only allowed him to heal in his way but also offered his congregation valuable insights into the human condition.

It is essential to respect the autonomy of those we try to help. Rick's associates and friends encouraged him to take a break, but Rick's choice to continue preaching allowed him to honor his grief in a way that was meaningful both to him and his community. By using his sermons to process his loss, Rick was able to offer his congregation lessons concerning vulnerability, strength, and healing.

Dale Larson highlights the importance of stepping back, "*We must resist our impulses to provide them with all the answers, to point out what they are doing wrong, and to single-handedly meet all their needs*" (Larson, 1993, *p. 152*). Rick's decision to use his sermons to work through his grief shows healing does not always follow a prescribed path. By allowing Rick the space to find his own way, his friends supported his growth and his continued ability to serve.

Ultimately, Rick's experience shows grief can become a source of resilience and wisdom, not only for the individual but also for those around them. His sermons

[1] All stories are based on real-life cases. However, all names in this text except the authors are pseudonyms, and identifying details have been removed to protect the confidentiality of individuals.

helped his congregation see that grief, though deeply personal, can also be shared and used as a bridge to deeper understanding and connection.

7.4.2 Case Example: The Dancer

Kira's life has always centered around dance. She started dance lessons at 4 years of age, majored in dance in college, and led dance workshops around the country, usually accompanied by her adopted daughter, Tamara.

One Saturday, between trips with her mom, Tamara rode her bicycle into the street, was struck by a car, and she died instantly. Kira was devastated. She canceled a couple of months of workshops and seriously questioned how she could be motivated enough to ever dance again.

Kira's therapist suggested that she continues dancing and that her dances be an ongoing expression of her love and grief for Tamara. When expressing joy, she dances to the joy she felt with Tamara and the joy she saw in Tamara. When expressing sadness, she dances her grief over losing her daughter. When expressing love, she imagines herself dancing with or before Tamara. Through this, Kira's therapist helped her grieve by nurturing her strength: her ability to dance.

Reflection While it can be helpful for care providers to draw on their strengths and resources, the true focus of caregiving should be on discovering and building upon the strengths of those being supported. For example, when working with a terminally ill person who finds strength in their faith, reminding them of this resource can help them reconnect with their inner resilience, fostering a sense of control and meaning even amidst pain and suffering.

Similarly, supporting someone who draws on their humor can empower them to feel more self-reliant and capable. Highlighting these strengths helps individuals realize they have resources within themselves, nurturing a sense of autonomy and dignity even in the face of ongoing challenges.

7.4.3 Case Example: Discovering Jane's Inner Peace

Jane, a hospice patient, was experiencing significant anxiety. Initially, the intervention guided her into imagining herself on a peaceful beach in Hawaii, feeling the breeze, and smelling the salt air, encouraging her to match her breathing with the gentle rhythm of the ocean waves.

However, rather than relaxing, Jane's anxiety visibly escalated. Her breathing became rapid, her fists clenched, and her neck strained. When gently asked what was happening, Jane explained that the imagery of the waves frightened her—she had nearly drowned as a child. It became clear that focusing on Jane's own resources, rather than external relaxation techniques, was essential.

Jane was encouraged to recall a moment from her own life that brought her peace. She immediately described the day her last child left home—a moment filled her with a deep sense of tranquility. She had celebrated the occasion with her husband at bed and breakfast, where she spent the afternoon being absorbed in a long-awaited book. It was, in her words, "heavenly."

The next time Jane felt anxious, she was invited to close her eyes and return to that peaceful memory. By guiding her to relive the experience—remembering the setting, the book, and the feeling of calm—Jane was able to ease her anxiety, one page at a time.

Reflection Effective caregiving emphasizes the client's inner strengths and resources. By staying observant, adaptable, and responsive, care providers can guide clients to find paths to peace. As Walker (2015) states, *"Caregiving often calls us to lean into love we didn't know possible"* (p. 12). This reflection emphasizes the transformative power of providing care when approached with empathy and a deep respect for the unique experiences and capacities of each individual. Ultimately, it is through sensitivity and attunement that care providers can empower others to navigate their challenges in a way that feels authentic and healing to them.

7.4.4 Tool: Assessing Personal Strength, Peace, and Security

Exploring, understanding, and leveraging individuals' inner resources and personal strengths can significantly enhance the care's effectiveness and overall well-being. Ask the person to write down or verbalize answers to the following questions to explore psychological resources.

Strength:

1. What is "strength" for you?
2. Where can you go to get it?
3. Who gives it to you?
4. How can you get more?

Peace:

1. What is "peace" for you?
2. Where can you go to get it?
3. Who gives it to you?
4. How can you get more?

Security:

1. What is "security" for you?
2. Where can you go to get it?
3. Who gives it to you?
4. How can you get more?

7.4.5 Tool: Glue of My Life

This exercise works well for both individual and group activities. Ask the participants to bring two to five objects to the activity and place them on a small table. These objects should symbolize what holds the most meaning in their life, what gives them purpose, and what they cherish most. Refer to these items as "the glue" or "safety net" that holds their life together.

Once the objects are chosen, ask questions to explore the strengths and resources they represent. Possible objects might include.

- A book
- Photographs
- Religious objects
- Mementos
- Artwork
- Materials gathered from nature
- A letter, letters, or other personal documents
- A record, CD, or tape of a musical piece

7.4.6 Case Example: Gertrude

Doug was working with Gertrude, who had recently experienced significant loss and isolation following a messy divorce. Before the next meeting, Gertrude was invited to place two to five objects on a table representing her beliefs, values, strengths, and resources—the things that held her world together.

When Doug returned, there was only one object: a photograph of a German shepherd. Initially, it seemed that the instructions might not have been fully understood, but when asked why she chose just that picture, Gertrude shared her story. During her divorce, all her friends had distanced themselves, except for her dog.

"If you want to talk about my beliefs, values, or strengths, it's that unconditional love my dog had for me, when no one else did," she said.

It was clear then that Gertrude understood the assignment perfectly. Her choice spoke deeply to the loyalty and love she experienced from her dog, providing her with the support when she needed it most.

Reflection Gertrude's choice of the dog's photograph highlights her deep need for unconditional love and loyalty. This assessment suggested that her care plan should focus on offering consistent, nonjudgmental support. Regular check-ins could provide a stable and understanding presence and would help Gertrude feel emotionally safe, allowing her to explore her feelings without fear of rejection. What Gertrude values most is not just care but consistency and acceptance—mirroring her bond with her dog—guiding her through the grieving process with compassion and patience.

7.4.7 Case Example: Scott's Strength

Scott was a patient with Alzheimer's and a very difficult one. In fact, he was thought to be the most unmanageable patient in a facility with 40 patients with Alzheimer's. What made Scott so unmanageable was a particular habit. Whenever Scott had a mess in his diaper, he would immediately stick his hand into the diaper, take out what was there, and smear it on the walls.

This was obviously a significant problem! The staff would try their best to stop Scott, rushing to him as soon as they saw him grunting, holding him down on his back, and changing his diapers before he could reach into them. However, more often than not, the staff was unable to anticipate Scott's bowel movements, leaving them with the terrible task of cleaning the walls.

One of Scott's care providers was so imaginative that she perceived Scott's supposed problem as a strength; she saw Scott's problem as a strength in disguise. She came to the conclusion that Scott was a great artist, a truly great artist: he literally could take an unpleasant situation and turn it into art.

Once this caregiver discovered Scott's strength, she nurtured it. Each morning, she supplied Scott with finger paintings and a newsprint. Scott never reached into his diapers again.

Reflection Care providers may encounter individuals unaware of their own strengths, such as those unknowingly holding a golden bowl while begging. In Scott's case, what appeared to be a behavioral problem was actually a hidden artistic inclination and an expressive desire. It takes an attentive and open heart to recognize these hidden strengths and nurture them. Everyone has untapped potential, and through compassionate care, these inner resources can be revealed, allowing individuals to find dignity and express themselves even in difficult circumstances.

7.4.8 Case Example: Using Some Detective Work

Hank was a patient with Alzheimer's in a nursing home. Almost every night, he would get up in the middle of the night, take off his pajamas, and start to walk around his unit, often walking into women's rooms, which understandably caused distress and screaming.

What desires was Hank trying to fulfill? What were his wishes, needs, concerns, expectations, and priorities? Was he trying to be a nudist? Was he attempting to turn the entire nursing home into a nudist colony? Or could he pose a real danger, potentially being a threat? What was happening? Why was he walking around without any clothes on? What was he trying to achieve? What was his care plan?

In a conference with Hank's family, a counselor from the nursing home learned that Hank used to sleep in the nude. In fact, there were several family jokes about it.

Based on this information, the counselor advised Hank's care providers to stop putting pajamas on him at night. Sure enough, Hank slept through the night without incident.

Hank's care plan was simple: He just didn't want to wear pajamas. Apparently, Hank used to get up in the middle of the night because he felt uncomfortable in them. He would take them off, and since he was already up, he might as well go for a walk.

Reflection Sometimes, individuals are unable to clearly express their care needs. Whether due to confusion, intellectual impairment, or an inability to communicate, it becomes the caregiver's responsibility to uncover those needs with patience and care. In Hank's case, understanding his past habits led to a simple but effective solution. Rather than imposing external expectations, it took some detective work to reveal that Hank's discomfort with pajamas was driving his behavior. By respecting personal history and preferences, care providers were able to provide more compassionate and effective care.

7.4.9 Tool: Psychosocial Comfort Assessment Form

When assessing strengths and challenges, it is helpful to use an assessment form that combines positively and negatively worded statements or questions. This balanced approach can provide a more accurate and unbiased picture of a person's emotional and social well-being:[2]

A = Never
B = Rarely (less than 1 day per week)
C = Occasionally (1–2 days per week)
D = Frequently (3–5 days per week)
E = Always or almost always (6 or more days per week)

1. I am comfortable with my emotional self. A B C D E
2. People perceive me as having a positive attitude. A B C D E
3. I get depressed. A B C D E
4. I get angry. A B C D E
5. I hold in my feelings. A B C D E
6. I feel comfortable in social situations. A B C D E
7. I laugh. A B C D E
8. I cry. A B C D E
9. I like touching people and being touched. A B C D E
10. I feel I have a sense of purpose. A B C D E

[2] This Psycho-Social Comfort Assessment Form was developed by the authors and has been applied in clinical practice to assess both strengths and challenges. Although this tool has been successfully applied in practice, it has not been formally tested for validity or reliability through formal research studies.

11. I feel that my family and friends need me. A B C D E
12. I look forward to my future. A B C D E

7.5 Family Strength Assessment

In caregiving, it is essential to recognize that an individual's well-being is often deeply influenced by their family dynamics. From a family systems perspective, the strengths of each family member are interconnected, shaping the overall functioning of the family unit. Understanding and nurturing these collective strengths not only supports the individual but also empowers the entire family to navigate challenges more effectively.

This section introduces questions and techniques to explore and nurture a family's collective strengths. These questions are designed to assess the family's structure, communication patterns, and coping strategies, helping to identify areas of support and growth. Drawing from family assessment models, such as the Calgary Family Assessment Model (Wright & Leahey, 2009) and the Friedman Family Assessment Model (Friedman et al., 2003), the approach evaluates family culture, structure, and function to identify strengths and needs. Collaborative strategies from other family-strengthening frameworks have also been adapted to provide a holistic view of family resilience.

A. Family Strengths

1. What are the three greatest strengths of your family?
2. How do members of your family complement one another, making you stronger collectively than individuals?
3. What are some key moments in your family history that have brought joy or fond memories?
4. How might members of your community admire the strengths of your family?
5. If your family were to change or separate, what aspects of your family unit would be missed the most?

B. Complementary Strengths

1. How do family members support each other during difficult times?
2. What are some ways your family collaborates to solve problems?
3. Describe a time when your family works together to achieve a common goal.

C. Family Dynamics

1. How does your family address conflicts or disagreements?
2. What traditions or rituals does your family practice that strengthen your bonds?
3. How do family members communicate their needs and emotions to one another?

D. External Support

1. How do friends and the community contribute to supporting your family?
2. Are there external resources (e.g., community centers, religious institutions) that your family relies on for support?

3. How does your family engage with these external resources?

E. Resilience and Adaptability
1. Describe a time when your family faced a significant challenge. How did you overcome it?
2. What changes has your family had to adapt to, and how have you managed these changes?
3. How does your family maintain resilience in the face of adversity?

F. Emotional and Social Well-Being
1. How does your family express love and appreciation for one another?
2. What activities do you enjoy doing together as a family?
3. How do you ensure that each family member feels valued and heard?

7.6 Grieving Style Assessment

People receiving care can have different grieving styles, which may be primarily feeling-centered, thought-centered, or action-centered. Understanding and assessing these styles is important for providing appropriate tools tailored to each individual's needs. Offering a thought-centered tool to a feeling-centered person, for example, would not be effective. Integrating Ken Doka's work on intuitive vs. instrumental grieving styles can further refine this assessment. According to Doka and Martin (2010), intuitive grievers experience and express emotions intensely, whereas instrumental grievers focus on thinking and doing to manage their grief. These are not gender-specific and can display a spectrum. In addition, people may display dissonance in how they publicly mourn versus how they authentically experience and process grief (Doka & Martin, 2010).

The following multiple-choice questions, where the individual responds with the answer that feels closest to the truth, can give us some idea of that person's adapting style.

A. Most people who know me would describe me as
1. Primarily feeling-centered (intuitive).
2. Primarily thought-centered (instrumental).
3. Primarily action-centered (instrumental).

B. I would describe myself as
1. Primarily feeling-centered (intuitive).
2. Primarily thought-centered (instrumental).
3. Primarily action-centered (instrumental).

C. In highly emotional situations where others express their emotion
1. My emotions come right out (intuitive).
2. I will sometimes express my emotions.
3. I will rarely, if ever, express my emotions (instrumental).

D. When confronted with difficult situations

1. I will immediately try to think of a way to make the situation less difficult (instrumental).
2. I will sometimes choose a rational way out of the situation.
3. I often find it very difficult to concentrate on anything (intuitive).

E. When I am under a great deal of stress or tension

1. I cannot stand still; I need to do something (instrumental).
2. I will sometimes do something to end the stress and sometimes just wait it out.
3. I am often immobilized.

7.6.1 Case Example: Wally's and Djuna's Grieving Styles

Wally and Djuna lost their daughter of 8 weeks old. She had been born quite premature and had died due to several complications with her heart and lungs.

After death, Djuna returned immediately to her work as a college professor, determined to make this the best year of her teaching career. Her evenings and weekends, if not laboriously preparing for class, were spent gardening. Gardening had always been her favorite pastime. However, after the death of her daughter, gardening took on an intensity it never had before: she would dig in the ground with strong determination, pull out weeds with a fervor, and ever-so-gently and lovingly nurture each individual plant as it grew.

Wally could not return to his work as an accountant because his emotions were pouring out all the time. He could not focus on anything. Often, he would take himself into the basement and cry for hours. Sometimes, he would go out in his car to some deserted place and just yell at the horizon. He sometimes becomes so depressed that he cannot communicate and is unable to speak or hear anything.

Djuna thought that Wally was much too emotional and believed that he needed to return to work to "do something" to "get over" what she saw as his emotional quagmire. Wally felt that Djuna was not emotional enough, thinking she was "avoiding" her grief by always "doing" things, and he felt she would eventually "crash" due to her failure to address her emotions.

They were both fully grieving but processing their grief in different ways. Djuna was a cognitively centered and action-centered griever; she processed her grief intellectually and through physical activities. Wally was more of a feeling-centered griever; he processed his grief emotionally.

Reflection Understanding the different grieving styles is crucial for care providers. Djuna's instrumental (action-centered) grieving style and Wally's intuitive (feeling-centered) grieving style highlight the diversity in how people process loss and the necessity of validating the various styles. Recognizing and respecting these differences allows for effective support and patience toward others and the self.

7.7 Physical Dimension Assessment

Emotions such as sadness, anger, anxiety, and depression often manifest through physical symptoms. As Bessel van der Kolk (2014) noted in *The Body Keeps the Score*, there are strong psychosomatic connections, meaning that emotions, thoughts, and experiences are deeply intertwined with the physical state. When assessing care needs, it is helpful to gather information about the physical dimensions of a person's emotional and psychological experiences. This helps to address pain and suffering and establish comfort. The following four-part assessment form provides a practical tool for achieving this goal.

1. **Where do you feel most of your pain/suffering?**

   (Or, where is your sadness/pain showing up in your body?)

   Mark the areas where your pain/suffering is most felt. If there is more than one site, label each site with the letters A, B, C, and D, from the most intense to the least intense, using these same letters in steps 2, 3, and 4 of this form.

   - ____ head
   - ____ neck
   - ____ back
   - ____ shoulders
   - ____ chest
   - ____ arms
   - ____ hands
   - ____ stomach
   - ____ groin
   - ____ buttocks
   - ____ legs
   - ____ feet
   - ____ joints
   - ____ other ______________________________

2. **Describe how the pain/suffering feels**

   (Or: Can you describe what it is like?)

   Place the corresponding site letters in the blanks that most appropriately describe the feeling.

   - ____ sharp
   - ____ dull, aching, or diffuse
   - ____ radiating or shooting
   - ____ pressing or tight
   - ____ burning
   - ____ pulling
   - ____ other ______________________________

3. **Describe the intensity of the pain/suffering on a scale of 0 to 5, with 5 representing the most intense in the various sites. How intense? How frequent?**

4. **Additional Questions**
   A. What makes your pain/suffering worse?
   B. Are there times of day or night when your pain/suffering is worse?
   C. What has helped in the past control the physical symptoms of your pain/suffering?
   D. What does the pain/suffering prevent you from doing?

It is important to identify several aspects of pain/suffering because they are often interrelated. Understanding each aspect and its possible connections to others enhances the ability to alleviate pain and suffering. Assessing these issues should include recommended steps that empower individuals and their loved ones to manage their care actively.

7.8 Developing Personalized Care Plans

Once thorough assessments have been conducted to identify the unique needs and strengths of a person, these insights serve as the foundation for developing tailored care strategies. Personalized care plans are designed not only to alleviate distress and improve comfort but also to enhance the overall quality of life for both individuals and their families. A key component in this process is the **therapeutic alliance**, a multidimensional concept involving emotional, cognitive, and behavioral connections between the client and the professional. By collaboratively setting goals and committing to the care process, a strong therapeutic alliance enhances client engagement, motivation, and openness, ultimately improving outcomes (Flückiger et al., 2018). For a more detailed discussion of the therapeutic alliance and its importance in forming meaningful client relationships, refer to Chap. 1.

This section explores the development of empowering person-centered care plans, starting with understanding the individual's expectations and clearly defining the caregiver's role. The use of one-question care plans is discussed as a method to set clear, achievable goals, with practical case studies to illustrate these concepts. Interactive tools and activities facilitate meaningful conversations and the achievement of care objectives. Through these strength-based personalized care plans, care can draw upon and strengthen the individual's internal and external resources, fostering healing during the end-of-life and grieving processes.

7.8.1 *Allowing Our Roles to Be Defined*

Rather than assuming a care plan, it is essential to first explore person's hopes and expectations and develop a care plan collaboratively. This first step builds rapport and trust, form a foundation for a therapeutic alliance. The following forms can be provided during intake to discover these expectations, allowing individuals the opportunity to exercise choice and control.

7.8.1.1 Social Worker or Counselor Role Definition

Please indicate your preferences from the list of potential services below. Place an "X" beside those that best complete the statement: "I would like my social worker or counselor to help me ..." Cross out any item you feel you will never want from a caregiver. Place a question mark next to any items you are unsure about. Use the blank space for anything else you wish to say.

I would like my social worker or counselor to help me...

____ explore nonmedical ways of relieving pain or anxiety;
____ address some emotional problems I'm having;
____ explore some issues related to my purpose and self-worth;
____ address some problems I'm having with my social life;
____ explore religious or spiritual issues;
____ address financial issues;
____ make some decisions about my future;
____ put some more fun and humor into my life;
____ communicate feelings toward one particular person (____);
____ finish a project (______________________________);
____ do the following (______________________________).

7.8.1.2 Chaplain Role Definition

Please review the list of potential services below and indicate your preferences. Place an "X" beside those that best complete the statement: "I would like my chaplain to help me..." Cross out any item you feel you will never need from a chaplain. Place a question mark next to any items you are unsure about. Use the blank space for anything else you wish to say.

I would like my chaplain to help me ...

____ maintain contact with my congregation, minister, rabbi, or priest;
____ strengthen my life with prayer and/or meditation;
____ explore some of my spiritual concerns;
____ feel a sense of worth and dignity;
____ settle some religious differences within my family;
____ address some emotional problems I'm having;
____ help a particular member of my family;
____ find some good study materials for my struggles;
____ address some of my doubts, fears, and/or anger;
____ do the following (____).

7.8.1.3 Volunteer Role Definition

Please consider the list of potential tasks below and indicate your preferences. Place an "X" beside those that best complete the statement: "I would like my volunteer to help me…" Cross out any item you feel you will never need from a volunteer. Place a question mark next to any items you are unsure about. Use the blank space for anything else you wish to say.

I would like my volunteer to …

____ give me some occasional companionship;
____ help me with housekeeping matters;
____ run some errands outside the home;
____ help me do some "handyman" projects;
____ help me with my social life;
____ relieve some of my other care providers of their duties;
____ put some more fun and humor into my life;
____ address some emotional problems I'm having;
____ explore religious/spiritual issues;
____ help me finish a project (______________________________);
____ do the following (___________________________________).

7.8.1.4 Nursing Role Definition

Please review the following list of potential tasks and indicate your preferences. Place an "X" beside those that best complete the statement: "I would like my nurse to help me …" Cross out any item you feel you will never need from a nurse. Place a question mark next to any items you are unsure about. Use the blank space for anything else you wish to say.

I would like my nurse to help me …

____ find medication for pain relief;
____ find medication for other physical problems;
____ find medication for some emotional issues;
____ learn more about alternatives to medication;
____ learn about ways to put more quality into my life;
____ communicate with my physician(s);
____ make more decisions regarding my own well-being;
____ communicate my concerns and wishes to my family and friends;
____ communicate feelings toward a particular person ();
____ finish a project (____________________);
____ do the following (___________________________________).

7.8.1.5 Home Health Aide Role Definition

Please review the list of potential tasks below and indicate your preferences. Place an "X" beside those that best complete the statement: "I would like my home health aide to help me …" Cross out any item you feel you will never need from a home health aide. Place a question mark next to any items you are unsure about. Use the blank space for anything else you wish to say.

I would like my home health aide to help me …

____ bathe and clean myself;
____ dress myself;
____ maintain a clean and safe environment;
____ achieve some mobility;
____ use and exercise my muscle groups;
____ massage away soreness and tension;
____ purchase, prepare, and/or serve meals;
____ do light housekeeping;
____ finish a project (______________________);
____ do the following (____________________________).

7.9 One Question Care Plan for End-of-Life

Traditional care plans are often designed to cover an array of potential problems that any patient might encounter. However, many governing and reviewing bodies, such as the Joint Commission on Accreditation of Healthcare Organizations (JCAHO), emphasize the need for care plans that focus on the specific needs, concerns, and priorities of individual patients (The Joint Commission, n.d.). This shift highlights the importance of personalized care in a way that makes it meaningful to the individual rather than applying a one-size-fits-all approach.

One-question care plans allow for a focus on the patient's individual goals and preferences without getting overwhelmed by complex or time-consuming paperwork processes.

As renowned psychiatrist Dr. Elisabeth Kübler-Ross (1969) and grief expert Therese Rando (1993) emphasize, individuals facing the end of life often experience a profound loss of control. They are unable to prevent physical deterioration or death, which can lead to a sense of powerlessness. To help counteract these overwhelming emotions, one of the most potent interventions that care providers can provide is offering the person a sense of dignity and autonomy. The following carefully crafted questions aim to restore that autonomy by focusing on what truly matters to the individual, ensuring that care is guided by their own wishes and priorities.

- Given your current situation, how would you most like to spend your remaining time?
- What do you hope will be the most meaningful outcome of our time together?

- If I want to do my best to help you achieve three wishes for your future, what would they be?
- Over the next few weeks, what are your most important needs, concerns, expectations, and priorities?
- Do you feel comfortable sharing your greatest worries and concerns right now, let us see how we can work on that?
- Who would you like to be involved in your care, and how can we best support their involvement?
- Are there any specific cultural or spiritual practices you would like us to incorporate into your care?
- How do you define quality of life at this stage, and what can we do to help you maintain it?
- What gives you the most comfort right now, and how can we ensure that comfort continues?
- What legacy or message, if any, would you like to leave for your loved ones?
- Is there anything that brings you peace or joy that we can incorporate into your daily care?
- How would you like to be remembered, and how can we help honor that?

These person-centered questions are designed to ensure that care plans reflect the individual's values and aspirations, allowing for personalization and adaptability. They facilitate open dialog between the caregiver and the individual, helping to clarify expectations and focus on what truly matters during the last journey of life.

In professional caregiving, balancing the requirements of governing agencies with the unique needs of the person is crucial. Rather than forcing patients to fit into predefined frameworks, care should be adapted to the individual, ensuring that it remains personal and meaningful. While governing agencies frequently call for "measurable outcomes," it is possible to track patient care in meaningful ways without unnecessary complexity. By breaking down a patient's care plan into three to six measurable outcomes—whether focused on physical, emotional, or spiritual aspects—care progress can be recorded and reviewed periodically. This process ensures that regulatory standards are met while keeping care individualized, effective, and manageable.

7.9.1 Case Example: The Fishing Trip

Herb and Floyd were residents in a life-care community in Florida, both nearing the end of their lives. They had always been avid fishermen and loved to share their fish stories with each other. Despite their poor health, they told the activities director at the community that they wanted to go on one last fishing trip to Minnesota. Given that this trip was impossible, the activities director developed a creative solution.

He grabbed two fishing poles and took Herb and Floyd to the man-made lake on the facility's property. The sight of the Activities Director pushing two wheelchairs, each occupied by a feeble old man holding a fishing pole, was quite a scene. They spent two hours by the lake, casting their lines and enjoying each other's company.

After the trip, Floyd said, "I had never thought I would ever go fishing again. And this was probably the best fishing trip I ever had."

Although they did not catch any fish or travel to Minnesota, they still had a wonderful time. Their wish was honored, and some people cared enough to make their dreams come true, even in a modified way. The joy and satisfaction they felt were genuine, showing that oftentimes, genuine intention and effort matter the most.

Reflection In some cases, individuals may express goals or care plans that seem unattainable or unrealistic. Their desires, concerns, and expectations may be shaped by emotions and hopes that are difficult to fulfill literally. However, even when these wishes cannot be fully realized, it remains crucial to honor them by getting as close to their intent as possible, sometimes using creativity and imagination. Knowing one's wishes and desires are honored is validating and comforting.

H. Frederick Reisz's (1992) emphasis that *"A dying person is a living person"* reminds care providers that those at the end of life are still fully alive. Despite life-limiting circumstances, and sometimes because of them, individuals continue to have desires, memories, and emotional needs. Caregiving should focus on fulfilling these goals in meaningful and creative ways. Those who are facing death often have a profound wish to feel connected to the world of the living and to find a sense of peace and fulfillment about their life. Whether it involves recreating a dream experience, engaging in a beloved hobby, or addressing unfinished business, ensure they feel heard and valued.

7.9.2 Case Example: Trevor's Campfire

Trevor was spending his final days in a hospice facility. He had one last wish tied to a cherished family tradition. Every summer, his family—including aunts, uncles, cousins, brothers, and sisters—would gather for a weekend reunion at a campsite in northern Wisconsin. On the first night, they would build a campfire and sit around it, sharing stories from the past year. As part of this tradition, everyone over the age of 21 years would sip a beer while recounting their tales.

Trevor's wish was to stay alive until summer, go to Wisconsin, sit around a campfire, tell his last story, and sip his beer. However, the hospice workers knew that Trevor was unlikely to survive until summer, and even if he did, he would not be able to endure the trip to northern Wisconsin. However, that was Trevor's last wish, his personal care plan, his one goal, and we wanted to make it as real as possible.

The staff set a date for the following week and called as many relatives as they could. They came to the hospice house and built a fire in the fireplace. The staff wheeled Trevor out of his bed in front of the fire. His brother brought beer and straw. Trevor sipped that beer and told his last story to his family.

7.9.3 *Case Example: One Last Christmas*

Becky wanted to have one more Christmas, her favorite holiday. However, it was August, and her care providers were fairly sure that she would not make it through September. Therefore, the care providers decided to bring Christmas to August. One Sunday, they cut down an evergreen tree, brought it to her room, and decorated it with ornaments and lights. They spent the entire afternoon decorating, laughing, and sharing stories of past Christmases.

That evening, a small child's choir came to Becky's room and sang several Christmas carols. The last song they sang was "Silent Night," and tears could be seen in many people's eyes. The next morning, Becky was found peacefully lying in her bed, having spent her last day on the earth celebrating her favorite holiday.

7.10 One Question Care Plans for Grieving

Ask any or a combination of the questions to explore the grieving person's goals and needs for support.

(1) For you, what is the best thing that can come from us working together?
(2) When we lose a loved one, we can feel as though we have lost our "other half." Describe the half of you that is now missing: what did you previously have that you do not have now? What parts of you are crying out for replacement?
(3) Are there any desires you have that you now think will not be fulfilled because of this death?
(4) How has the death of your loved one impacted your everyday life and routines?
(5) How do you feel about your current support system/resources? Is there anyone you wish to lean on more?
(6) What are some things that bring you comfort or peace right now?

7.10.1 *Case Example: Kayak Trip*

Tim was referred to a grief specialist by his physician. He had been experiencing many symptoms, including trouble sleeping, frequent headaches, and increased substance use since his teenage son, Michael, tragically died in an accident.

During his first meeting with the counselor, Tim said, "I don't know why we are wasting each other's time. You can't help me. All I want is to have Michael back and take him on the kayak trip we planned."

His voice broke as he continued, "We had been planning it for years. We spent a lot of time working out a great route and bought gear. We were going to do it this summer after his high school graduation." He could not continue. He kept repeating, "I want to take Michael on that kayak trip."

The counselor listened patiently without interruption. Eventually, they began working together on a care plan honoring Tim's seemingly impossible goal. The counselor asked, "Would you be able to take time off work?"

Tim responded, "I could, but work helps me stay busy. Without it, I'd go crazy." Tim worked a hands-on manufacturing job and was clearly an instrumental griever, finding solace in activity and work.

Based on the care plans they formulated, Tim took a 3-month leave from work. During the first 6 weeks, he spent his entire waking hours building a beautiful kayak from a kit. Rather than working in a numb and mechanical way at his job, Tim poured his heart and soul into shaping this meaningful piece of art. When the kayak was finally completed, stroke by stroke, he carefully painted on both sides of the kayak: "*MICHAEL*."

The next 6 weeks Tim spent paddling the kayak through Minnesota, following the exact route he and Michael had planned together. The trip was filled with a range of emotions—tears, anger, and love. Each evening, Tim wrote in a journal, pouring his thoughts and feelings into letters addressed to Michael. He wrote about their past, reflected on his relationship with Michael, and thought about his relationship with his family and work. On some peaceful moonlit nights on the river, he felt Michael was with him, providing soothing warmth and comfort.

By the end of the trip, Tim had gained new clarity. Through his writing and reflection, he had set new priorities for his life, placing his remaining family at the top of the list. His job, once a place of distraction, had fallen ninth in importance. His reliance on substances also lessened as he was more comfortable processing his pain.

Tim's seemingly impossible wish had been fulfilled through this care plan: he had taken Michael on the kayak trip they had planned.

Reflection Care plans do not always focus on the caregiver meeting the desires of those they support. Often, they can be designed as a way for the person to help themselves. In this case, Tim's care plan was less about external support and more about empowering him to find healing through his own actions and reflection. Tim exhibited an *instrumental grieving style*, where he processed his grief through activity and problem-solving rather than through overt emotional expression and talking. The process of building and paddling the kayak became a powerful *behavior-based ritual*, allowing him to symbolically honor his son and work through his grief. By engaging in this meaningful ritual, Tim was able to reduce his reliance on substances and focus on the deep connection he had with Michael. This journey of action and ritual allowed him to grieve and heal in his way, ultimately finding peace and continuing his bond with his son while carrying on life.

7.10.2 *Case Example: Personalized Ritual and Spaces*

Pat was grieving the loss of a spouse, Marjorie. In response to this grief, Pat created a quiet space in the home library—a private sanctuary to grieve in a personal way. Whenever overwhelmed with pain, Pat would retreat there to spend a little time.

In the library, Pat kept a scrapbook titled "Marjorie" on a small table. Next to it was a CD with Neil Sedaka's "Calendar Girl" ready to play—a song that held a special place in their relationship. Before settling in, Pat would light a scented candle, its soft fragrance filling the room and creating a calm, comforting atmosphere.

Pat's routine was straightforward but meaningful. Sitting in a favorite recliner, Pat would open the scrapbook, turning the pages slowly and pausing at photos and mementos. Each moment brought back vivid memories—shared laughter, simple joys, or quiet moments together. Afterward, Pat would sit back and listen to the music, letting it carry them back to those times. The candlelight and familiar scent added a sense of peace, grounding Pat in the present while honoring the past.

After spending time in this space, Pat would blow out the candle and return to daily life. The library became a place to hold and revisit grief on their own terms—a boundary where emotions could be processed in a way that felt safe and manageable.

Reflections For many grievers, their care plan can be practiced only in some space: a time and place where they can extract themselves from the rest of the world and fully center upon their necessary agenda. This provides a safe environment where individuals can process their emotions without external pressures or distractions. Encouraging patients to find or create such space can be a valuable part of their care plan. It might be a physical room, such as Pat's library, or a specific time or date dedicated to reflection and remembrance.

7.10.3 *Tool: Self-Care Plan for a Grieving Person*

Step One: Choose Four Words

Choose four words from the right column that you would most like to describe you in 6 months. Circle those four words and mark an "X" on the scale (1-5) to represent how you feel now.

1	3	5
hopeless		hopeful
1	3	5
fragmented		whole
1	3	5
sad		happy
1	3	5
constrained		free
1	3	5
tense		relaxed
1	3	5
spent		energized
1	3	5
resentful		grateful
1	3	5
troubled		peaceful
1	3	5
socially alienated		socially integrated

Step Two: Plan to Achieve Your Desired States

Take each of the four words you chose in Step One and fill them into the first blanks of the following sentences. Then, fill in the second and third blanks with how you plan to achieve each of those states.

A. I plan to make my life more ______ by ____and by ________.
B. I plan to make my life more ______ by ____and by ________.
C. I plan to make my life more ______ by ____and by ________.
D. I plan to make my life more ______ by ____and by ________.

The above self-care plan facilitates actionable steps toward healing and transformation over a certain period of time. Reflecting on where individuals are now and where they want to be can help them set clear goals and find meaningful ways to cope with their grief and track progress.

7.10.4 Tool: From "I Need" to "I Can Get"

This activity is designed to enhance a sense of control using a technique from the rational emotive therapy approach. It empowers individuals facing terminal illness or grief to recognize choices they may not have realized were available.

1. **Homework Assignment:**
   Ask the individual to complete 12 sentences beginning with "I need…". Examples include
   - "I need people to touch and hold me."
   - "I need some private time."
2. **Select Care Plan Goals:**
   From the list of 12 needs, ask them to choose three to five that could become actionable goals. Transform each "I need…" statement into "I can get…" statements. For example:
   - "I can get people to touch and hold me."
   - "I can get some private time."
3. **Develop Strategies:**
   For each "I can get …" statement, create a plan to make it a reality. Write the statement at the top of a separate sheet of paper, followed by practical strategies. For example:
   - To gain private time, set aside 45 minutes each afternoon and use a sign such as "PLEASE DO NOT DISTURB UNTIL 4:30" to avoid interruptions.

7.10.5 Tool: My Ideal Death Story

Approaching the end of life often brings a mix of emotions, reflections, and hopes about what matters most. This activity offers an opportunity to imagine and describe an ideal passing—not as a fixed outcome, but as a personal vision grounded in one's values, beliefs, and cultural traditions. Reflecting on this vision can provide clarity while also guiding loved ones and care providers to honor these wishes as fully as possible.

Recognizing that cultural, spiritual, and personal values shape each person's view of a meaningful death, this activity respects and embraces those differences. Some individuals may prioritize family presence, specific rituals, or spiritual practices, while others may focus on a quiet, private experience. Each choice reflects what feels most comforting and authentic.

Ask these questions thoughtfully and at appropriate timing. This activity should be approached at the individual's own pace. These questions are meant to serve as a gentle starting point for crafting a vision of what a meaningful end-of-life experience might look like:

- Where would you feel most at peace in your final moments?
- What kind of setting would you like? Is there particular music you want to play?
- Who or what would you like to have near you?
- What rituals, traditions, or practices would bring you comfort?
- How would you like to spend your last few days and hours?
- What is the last thing you would like to do or say?

This process is not about setting rigid expectations but about exploring possibilities that reflect personal and cultural values. Care providers and loved ones can use these reflections to support an end-of-life experience that is meaningful and aligned with the person's wishes.

7.11 Games and Activities to Start the Conversation

Games and activities can provide a non-threatening way to discuss thoughts and values related to death and life. Here are some examples:

1. **Hello Game**: The Hello Game is designed to start conversations about end-of-life values in a comfortable and engaging way. It involves question booklets and thank-you chips to facilitate discussions on what matters most to the participants through life and death. https://commonpractice.com/products/hello-game
2. **Heart-to-Heart Cards**: Heart-to-Heart Cards help family members understand each other's wishes for end-of-life care. Originally designed for the Chinese-speaking community, these cards can be used by anyone to discuss various end-of-life scenarios and preferences.
3. **The death deck**: The death deck is a party game that prompts players to answer thought-provoking questions about death in a group setting. It is a way to explore personal preferences and beliefs about dying in a light-hearted yet meaningful manner.
4. **Go Wish**: Go Wish cards help individuals articulate what is most important to them if their life is shortened by illness. This game encourages participants to prioritize their wishes and discuss them with family members. https://gowish.com/
5. **Now and Then board game**: Now and then guide players through their past, present, and future, prompting discussions on significant life decisions and end-of-life preparations through a mix of fun and deep challenges.

These activities facilitate open communication surrounding end-of-life by incorporating elements of play and reflection. They are also beneficial for community workshops and events.

7.12 Tool: Guided Imagery/Visualization: The Medicine Man

Guided imagery/visualization is versatile for addressing various issues. This exercise can help discover a dying person's desires and care plan. Script:

Close your eyes when you feel comfortable. Take a deep breath, feeling your chest and abdomen expand. Hold the breath for a moment, then slowly exhale, letting go of any tension. Repeat this deep breathing a few times until you feel a sense of calm wash over you.

Now, imagine you have heard about a great medicine man who knows the secret to finding purpose in his final years. You decide to talk to him to discover your main purpose for the time you have left …

Imagine flying by helicopter to the top of a mountain in New Mexico. You find yourself seated at a campfire, with the medicine man sitting across from you. You can barely make out his features. Picture what he is wearing… How does his body appear? … Examine his face closely… Look into his all-knowing eyes…

Now, ask him what important task you are to accomplish between now and the end of your life. What do your priorities need to be for the rest of your life? … At first, he stares at you in silence … His eyes penetrate into the depths of your being. You watch him watching you … Finally, he speaks, telling you what to do. What does he say about your purpose during the remainder of your life? What is your goal during your final days? What are you supposed to do? …

Now, respond to the medicine man. How do you react to what has been said to you?… What feelings do you have toward him?…

Get ready to leave the medicine man. There is nothing more you need here. You know what your purpose is for the rest of your life. You know the task set for you. You know what your priorities now need to be … Say goodbye to the medicine man in whatever manner seems most fitting to you … Slowly open your eyes….”

After the exercise, discuss the following:

- What did the medicine man say you're supposed to do?
- How do you feel about what was said?
- If you were to do what the medicine man suggested, how would you best go about doing it?

7.13 Concluding Reflection

The effectiveness of any care plan depends on its ability to be truly person-centered. This requires consistently addressing three fundamental questions: What are the person's needs? What do they want? What are their wishes? When these questions are not clearly reflected in the care plan, its purpose is diminished, and the individual's well-being is overshadowed by external priorities. When external concerns take precedence, the essence of care is lost.

Ira Byock (2012) observed in *The Best Care Possible* that while it may not always be possible to fix the situation, it is always possible to care. This insight captures the heart of caregiving: even when the course of illness or grief cannot be changed, the care experience can still be profoundly meaningful. Care that prioritizes a person's unique needs, preferences, and values honors their humanity and dignity. Even when certain wishes seem unattainable, care providers can creatively adapt plans to offer meaningful support. Ensuring that individuals feel heard, respected, and valued is most essential.

When care is rooted in compassion and person-centered principles, it fosters peace, comfort, and a sense of control for both individuals and their families, even in the most challenging and vulnerable moments.

References

American Psychiatric Association. (2022). *Diagnostic and statistical manual of mental disorders* (5th ed., text rev.). American Psychiatric Publishing.

Anderson, F., Downing, G. M., Hill, J., Casorso, L., & Lerch, N. (1996). Palliative performance scale (PPS): A new tool. *Journal of Palliative Care, 12*(1), 5–11.

Bjelland, I., Dahl, A. A., Haug, T. T., & Neckelmann, D. (2002). The validity of the hospital anxiety and depression scale: An updated literature review. *Journal of Psychosomatic Research, 52*(2), 69–77. https://doi.org/10.1016/S0022-3999(01)00296-3

Byock, I. (2012). *The best care possible: A physician's quest to transform care through the end of life*. Avery.

Doka, K. J., & Martin, T. L. (2010). *Grieving beyond gender: Understanding the ways men and women mourn*. Routledge.

Flückiger, C., Del Re, A. C., Wampold, B. E., & Horvath, A. O. (2018). The alliance in adult psychotherapy: A meta-analytic synthesis. *Psychotherapy (Chicago, Ill.), 55*(4), 316–340. https://doi.org/10.1037/pst0000172

Friedman, M. M., Bowden, V. R., & Jones, E. G. (2003). *Family nursing: Research, theory, and practice* (5th ed.). Prentice Hall.

Hui, D., & Bruera, E. (2017). The Edmonton Symptom Assessment System 25 years later: Past, present, and future developments. *Journal of Pain and Symptom Management, 53*(3), 630–643. https://doi.org/10.1016/j.jpainsymman.2016.10.370

Kroenke, K., Spitzer, R. L., & Williams, J. B. W. (2001). The PHQ-9: Validity of a brief depression severity measure. *Journal of General Internal Medicine, 16*(9), 606–613. https://doi.org/10.1046/j.1525-1497.2001.016009606.x

Kübler-Ross, E. (1969). *On death and dying*. Macmillan.

Larson, D. G. (1993). *The helper's journey: Working with people facing grief, loss, and life-threatening illness*. Research Press.

Parker, S. G., McCue, P., Phelps, K., McCleod, A., Arora, S., Nockels, K., Kennedy, S., Roberts, H., & Conroy, S. (2018). What is comprehensive geriatric assessment (CGA)? An umbrella review. *Age and Aging, 47*(1), 149–155.

Puchalski, C. M., & Romer, A. L. (2000). Taking a spiritual history allows clinicians to understand patients more fully. *Journal of Palliative Medicine, 3*(1), 129–137. https://doi.org/10.1089/jpm.2000.3.129

Rando, T. A. (1993). *Treatment of complicated mourning*. Research Press.

Reisz, H. F. (1992). A dying person is a living person: A pastoral theology for ministry to the dying. *The Journal of Pastoral Care, 46*(2), 184–192.

The Joint Commission. (n.d.). *Standards*. Retrieved from https://www.jointcommission.org/standards/

Van der Kolk, B. A. (2014). *The body keeps the score: Brain, mind, and body in the healing of trauma*. Viking.

Walker, T. (2015). *The inspired caregiver: Finding joy while caring for those you love*. Empowerment Press.

Worden, J. W. (2009). *Grief counseling and grief therapy: A handbook for the mental health practitioner* (4th ed.). Springer.

World Health Organization. (2020). *Integrating palliative care and symptom relief into primary health care: A WHO guide for planners, implementers, and managers*. World Health Organization. Retrieved from https://www.who.int/publications/i/item/integrating-palliative-care-and-symptom-relief-into-primary-health-care

Wright, L. M., & Leahey, M. (2009). *Nurses and families: A guide to family assessment and intervention* (5th ed.). F.A. Davis Company.

Chapter 8
Holistic Psychosocial Care Plans

8.1 Holistic Psychosocial Care (HPC): An Integrative Approach

Holistic Psychosocial Care (HPC) applies the Spiral Model of Grieving and Healing and the 4A4C Framework—awareness, acceptance, affirmation, actualization (4A), and compassion, connection, composure, commitment (4C)—to address grief, loss, and end-of-life challenges. Together, these frameworks provide the foundation for actionable care plans introduced in this chapter.

The Spiral Model of Grieving and Healing emphasizes that grief is a nonlinear and dynamic process with diverse expressions, holding the potential for growth and healing. It advocates for support that aligns with holistic and humanistic principles, addressing psychosocial and spiritual dimensions. Recognizing that grief is embedded within sociocultural contexts, the model highlights the interplay of personal, relational, systemic, and societal factors in shaping the grieving experience. Recognizing humans' innate ability to heal, the model advocates a balanced middle-way approach toward support without over-intervention. Refer to Chap. 1 for detailed discussions.

8.1.1 Overview of the Three HPC Plans

The three systematic care plans presented in this chapter are practical applications of the Spiral Model and the 4A4C Framework, reflecting grief as a dynamic process of reflection, engagement, and growth. These care plans guide professionals and their clients to navigate the spiral-like journey of grieving, allowing them to move fluidly between processing loss and restoring balance in their lives. Additional tools

Y. Z. Ciupak, D. C. Smith, *Death, Dying, and Grief*,
https://doi.org/10.1007/978-3-031-88467-2_8

can be found in Part IV: Addressing Psychosocial Needs and Part V: Addressing Spiritual Needs in End-of-Life and Grieving.

(1) **Systematic Model A: Relationship Peaks and Valleys**

This care plan utilizes visual mapping to explore the complexities of a relationship, helping individuals gain clarity and a more balanced perspective. By addressing confusion or selective memories, this model enables individuals to revisit relational dynamics and integrate nuanced perspectives, as emphasized in the Micro layer of the Spiral Model. It also supports Worden's (2009) tasks of "accepting the reality of the loss" and "processing the pain of grief," while the 4A4C Framework fosters awareness and acceptance throughout the process.

(2) **Systematic Model B: Continuing Treasure**

Focusing on remembrance and forgiveness, this care plan broadens perspectives on relationships beyond linear birth and death timelines. It emphasizes the Social Identity dimension of the Spiral Model, helping individuals navigate relational roles and cultural values associated with loss. By fostering enduring bonds with the deceased, it aligns with Klass et al.'s (2014) work on continuing bonds and Worden's (2009) task of "finding an enduring connection with the deceased." The 4A4C Framework enhances this process by fostering compassion, connection, and actualization.

(3) **Systematic Model C: Acceptance and Carrying-On**

This care plan addresses secondary losses and the relational impacts of grief, focusing on roles previously fulfilled by the deceased. It integrates the Institutional Layer of the Spiral Model, addressing how family, workplace, or community systems are impacted by loss. By guiding individuals to adapt to new realities, it aligns with Worden's (2009) task of adapting to a world without the deceased. The 4A4C Framework encourages acceptance and commitment, helping individuals embrace restorative pathways.

8.1.2 Implementation Guidelines

The care plans introduced in this chapter are compatible with therapeutic modalities such as Cognitive Behavioral Therapy (CBT), Acceptance and Commitment Therapy (ACT), and Grief Therapy as Meaning Reconstruction (GTMR). They are applicable to both bereavement and nonfinite losses, such as breakups or divorce. Actually, some tools were originally developed or refined by one of the authors during research on how college students navigate the challenges of breakups. Additionally, these care plans can be adapted to address anticipatory grief, including the emotional, relational, and existential challenges faced by individuals confronting their mortality. Further research and clinical feedback are encouraged to assess and refine the efficacy and parameters of these models.

To optimize their effectiveness, therapists are advised to implement these care plans gradually, allowing clients sufficient time to engage deeply with each exercise. Reflecting the nonlinear nature of the Spiral Model, clients should be encouraged to develop patience and compassion toward the self, acknowledging setbacks and revisiting steps as needed. This adaptability ensures that the care plans remain responsive to each client's unique grieving process.

Therapists should consider conducting the activities sequentially within therapy sessions rather than providing all the materials at once. This approach ensures that each exercise complements and builds upon the therapeutic process. To maximize the benefits, individuals are encouraged to set aside dedicated, uninterrupted time—a full day or evening—to fully engage with the exercises.

Creating a conducive environment for remembrance can also enhance the effectiveness of the exercises. This could involve setting up a picture of the departed loved one, lighting a candle, and playing soothing music in the background, fostering a serene and reflective atmosphere conducive to healing.

Once clients have shifted their focus from predominantly dwelling on the loss to embracing restoration, as symbolized by the broader, more open loops of the Spiral Model (Fig. 1.1), it may be helpful to guide them in composing "A Letter to Finish the Unfinished" found in Sect. 8.5. This process can be paired with a personalized ritual or a culturally relevant guided visualization centered on delivering the letter to the deceased. Rituals provide a structured and symbolically significant means to honor loss, express grief, create meaning, and find solace (Wojtkowiak et al., 2021). While moments of grief may resurface—as depicted by the Spiral Model's twists and loops—writing the letter and engaging in the ritual represent forward-looking, restorative steps toward integrating loss into life.

Healing unfolds through reflection, emotional processing, and looking forward. To ensure ongoing support, Positive Affirmation Exercises in Sect. 8.6 and Monthly Checkups and Affirmations are integrated following the completion of each care plan. These strategies provide continuity and reinforce progress.

8.1.3 4A4C and Honor the Spiral Journey

In supporting individuals as they navigate grief, it is recommended to apply the 4A4C Competency Framework (discussed in Chap. 6). The **4As**—awareness, acceptance, affirmation, and actualization—focus on self-oriented qualities that the grief counselor nurtures within themselves before extending these attributes to others. In contrast, the **4Cs**—compassion, connection, composure, and commitment—are outward-oriented and strengthen the counselor's ability to build meaningful relationships while maintaining their own well-being. Together, these eight interrelated components create a dynamic and holistic competency structure.

By embodying the **4A4C Framework**, therapists can facilitate a rewarding and empowering experience for clients and themselves, collaboratively navigating the complexities of grief and loss.

Aligned with the Spiral Model, grieving is recognized as a dynamic and fluid process influenced by individual and sociocultural factors. The Spiral and 4A4C guide culturally responsive care. In addition, the Spiral represents the grieving journey as a shift from a tightly focused point on loss toward a sense of spaciousness and openness. This journey involves a continual interplay between loss-oriented and restoration-oriented tasks, gradually leading to reconstruction and reintegration of identity and life. Therefore, the care plans in this chapter are not prescriptive stages or phases of grief but flexible therapeutic roadmaps. They provide tools for therapists to collaborate with individuals in untangling their grief experiences and fostering growth and healing.

8.2 Systematic Care Plan A: Relationship Peaks and Valleys

Systematic Model A: Relationship Peaks and Valleys involves three distinct steps, facilitating the processing of the ABCs (affect, behavior, and cognition) of psychosocial care, unraveling the complexities of relationships, and initiating the recovery process.

Step One, "Processing Grief," engages the client in expressing their emotions, challenging self-critical thoughts, and developing effective coping mechanisms. It facilitates and stretches beyond "processing the pain of grief" in Worden's (2009) Task Model of Mourning. This step integrates classical cognitive behavioral therapy (CBT) with Compassion Inquiry (CI) developed by Gabor Maté, incorporating somatic therapy to identify physical sensations behind emotions, explore alternative explanations, and eventually shift any non-constructive beliefs or narratives related to the self, the loss, and the world.

Step Two introduces the innovative concept of "Relationship Peaks and Valleys," which offers a unique approach to understanding past relationships. By employing a visual mapping technique, therapists help clients unravel the layers within their relationships. This process allows individuals to explore the complexities of their past connections in a tangible and comprehensive manner.

Finally, **Step Three**, "5,4,3,2,1—Recovery Has Begun," guides clients through the journey of forgiveness, gratitude, and closure. Through this step, individuals are encouraged to reflect on their experiences, express gratitude for positive memories, and work toward closure on unresolved issues. The systematic nature of this model ensures that clients receive comprehensive support across all dimensions—emotional, cognitive, behavioral, and relational—as they navigate the grieving and healing process. This exercise fosters "accepting the reality of the loss" as delineated by Worden (2009).

Systematic Care Plan A: Relationship Peaks and Valleys
Step 1: Processing Grief

1. Ground sessions with short mindfulness exercises (e.g., breathing, meditation).
2. Help recognize and process somatic emotions.
3. Facilitate narrative and meaning restructuring.
4. Foster inner strengths and develop affirmations.
5. Explore behavioral coping mechanisms and celebrate progress.

Step 2: Relationship Complexity Mapping

1. Reflect on relationship highs and lows (positive and negative memories).
2. Create a visual mapping to identify and process these memories.

Step 3: 5,4,3,2,1—Recovery Has Begun

1. Guide through forgiveness, apologies, gratitude, wishes, and declarations of love, and gently bidding goodbye.
2. End with a closure exercise (e.g., reading and burning the letter).

8.2.1 Step One: Processing Grief

1. **Ground the Session**

   Begin with grounding exercises such as guided breathing, meditation, or gentle movement. These techniques provide emotional stability during intense moments. For cultural and spiritual sensitivity, consider integrating practices meaningful to both the individual and professional, such as intention-making, mindfulness, or holding a symbolic object like a "healing stone."

2. **Connect to Somatic Presence**

   Encourage the client to recognize how grief manifests in their body (e.g., tightness in the chest, tension in the shoulders). Explore these sensations through somatic awareness exercises, drawing on approaches like Peter Levine's Somatic Experiencing or Bessel van der Kolk's insights from *The Body Keeps the Score* (2015). By bringing attention to the body, clients can interrupt racing thoughts and overwhelming emotions. Inviting them to breathe into these sensations fosters reconnection with the present moment, creating space to shift cognitive patterns and release emotional tension.

   This process not only aids in emotional regulation but also facilitates and expands Worden's (2009) mourning task of "processing the pain of grief" (p. 43), addressing the somatic dimension of pain alongside the emotional experience.

3. **Accompany Emotion Processing**

   Reassure the client that there is no "right" or "wrong" way to grieve. Intense emotions, numbness, or a perceived absence of strong feelings are all normal.

Some individuals, especially men, may feel guilt over not expressing emotions outwardly. Normalize these responses by explaining that grief manifests in different styles, such as **expressive** (emotional release) or **instrumental** (problem-solving and action) (Doka & Martin, 2010). Highlight that both are valid ways of coping.

It might be helpful to print out a simple list of common grieving emotions—sadness, anger, guilt, anxiety, loneliness, relief, and numbness (Worden, 2009)—to help recipients articulate their feelings. If they describe a state like "helplessness," explore the emotions underlying this perception and gently guide them to recognize internal strengths or external resources.

It is essential to offer a safe and non-judgmental environment where the client can explore emotions at their own pace. Silence and an empathetic presence often communicate support more powerfully than words. This fosters safety, enabling authentic emotional expression and paving the way for healing.

4. **Facilitate Cognitive and Narrative Reconstruction**

Grief often brings self-critical thoughts or cognitive distortions, such as "I'll never recover from this" or "no one understands me." These beliefs can intensify emotional distress and hinder healing. Guide the client to identify these patterns and challenge them by exploring alternative, compassionate perspectives. For example,

- Replace *"I'll never recover"* with *"Healing is a process, and I've faced difficult situations before."*
- Reframe *"No one understands me"* as *"Some people may not fully understand, but others have offered support."*
- Encourage the client to counter harsh self-judgments with self-compassionate thoughts. Examples include
- *"It's okay to feel this way. Healing takes time."*
- *"I'm doing my best, even if it doesn't feel perfect."*
- Help the client explore the personal meaning of their loss and integrate it into a larger narrative of growth. Ask reflective questions like
- *"What has this experience taught you about yourself?"*
- *"How have your spiritual or cultural values shaped your understanding of this loss?"*

5. **Identify and Foster Inner Strengths**

In alignment with the Spiral Model's recognition of innate strength and healing potential, guide the client in recognizing and nurturing strengths. Encourage reflection on past experiences where they have demonstrated resilience and determination. Help them identify personal qualities and resources to support them through grieving. Refer to Chap. 7 for strength assessment tools.

6. **Develop Affirmations**

Crafting affirmations tailored to the individual's personal, cultural, and spiritual values can help nurture acceptance and appreciation (4A). These affirmations can reshape internal dialogue and encourage resilience. For inspiration, refer to the Sect. 8.6 of this chapter.

7. **Formulate Behavioral Coping Mechanisms**

   Encourage individuals to identify culturally and spiritually meaningful behavioral-based practices or rituals that align with their values. Examples might include.

   - Practicing progressive muscle relaxation to manage anger.
   - Lighting a candle or saying a prayer during moments of sadness to connect with cultural or spiritual traditions.
   - Visualizing the comforting presence of a loved one while engaging in slow breathing or self-soothing gestures such as self-hugging.

8. **Identify Progress and Celebrate Achievements**

   Progress in grief often follows the swirling, nonlinear path described by the Spiral Model. Celebrating little milestones—whether processing a difficult emotion, engaging in a restorative activity, or gaining new insights—reinforces acceptance and commitment **(4A4C)** to the healing journey.

   Recognizing achievements can be tied to cultural or spiritual practices, such as expressing gratitude in prayer or sharing progress with a supportive community. These celebrations help foster self-compassion and build confidence in navigating grief.

9. **Facilitate Progress after Sessions**

   Between sessions, individuals can reflect on insights gained and integrate exercises into their daily lives. Encourage the use of culturally significant or spiritually meaningful practices, such as meditating, journaling, or following rituals, to reinforce self-compassion and coping strategies.

   Regular follow-up sessions allow care providers to guide individuals in revisiting tasks. Scheduling these reflections ensures ongoing support and fosters connection and commitment (4C) as individuals progress in their journey.

8.2.2 Step Two: Relationship Complexity Mapping

All relationships form unique psychosocial landscapes shaped by emotional highs and lows, social dynamics, and personal connections. Peaks of joy, valleys of sorrow, and stretches of love and frustration reflect the intricate nature of human connections. Exploring these layers can help individuals process the end of a relationship—whether through death, divorce, breakups, or other losses.

The "Relationship Peaks and Valleys" exercise offers a therapeutic tool to visually map this psychosocial landscape. By translating experiences—both positive and negative—into a visual representation, the exercise disentangles cognitive and emotional blockages, clarifies selective memories, and fosters deeper understanding. This process aligns with the Spiral Model of Grieving and Healing, encouraging individuals to revisit, reflect on, and integrate relational experiences in a dynamic, nonlinear way. It provides opportunities for forgiveness, appreciation, and resolution while honoring cultural and spiritual beliefs that shape relationship narratives.

The Relationship Peaks (relationship highs and positive memories) and Valleys (relationship lows and negative memories) drawing can be done in two approaches: combined or separate.

In a combined drawing, arrange the peaks and valleys based on the chronological order of events or memories. This approach allows for a comprehensive visual narrative that captures the entirety of the relationship's highs and lows in a cohesive representation.

The **separate drawing** option creates two distinct visuals—one for peaks and another for valleys. This approach allows for a more detailed independent exploration of the positive and negative aspects. The separate method has been found in clinical practice particularly effective in assisting those coping with breakups and divorces ("being dumped," in their own words) and tend to have selective memory or fixation on the positive moments. The method promotes a more comprehensive and balanced perspective on the relationship's complexities. The following outlines step-by-step instructions for the combined approach:

Relationship Peaks and Valleys

1. **Explore the highs and lows:** Guide the client to reflect on their past relationship and list three to five of the most positive memories and three to five of the most challenging ones.
2. **Draw peaks and valleys:** Instruct the client to draw a horizontal line across a piece of paper, symbolizing the spectrum of experiences in their relationship.
3. **Mark memories:** Instruct the client to place their most positive memory at the peak of the line and the most negative memory at the dip, arranging the memories chronologically if preferred.
4. **Depict intensity:** Help the client sort their memories in order of intensity and draw smaller peaks and valleys to represent positive and negative memories, adding notations and dates to each.
5. **Discuss the landscape:** Guide the client to reflect on both the highs and lows of their relationship. Encourage them to view the relationship as a whole, validating the ambiguity and complexity present in any relationship. Help them explore how these experiences shaped their narrative regarding the relationship with the deceased and address any unresolved emotions that may surface.

An alternative approach is to draw positive and negative memories on separate lines. Positive memories are arranged by intensity, with the highest peak symbolizing the most meaningful moment. Negative memories are drawn separately, with the depth corresponding to their emotional impact.

This method allows for independent reflection on both relationship dimensions, promoting a nuanced and balanced perspective. After completing the drawings, guide the client through a discussion to validate the complexities of the relationship, address unresolved emotions, and reconstruct a supportive narrative.

8.2.3 Step Three: 5,4,3,2,1—Recovery Has Begun

The previous Relationship Peaks and Valleys mapping may have prompted clients to revisit overlooked aspects of their relationship and identify unresolved matters. This step provides a structured approach to reflect on relationships, address lingering emotions, and foster closure.

Drawing on Dr. Ira Byock's (2014) framework for nurturing relationships at the end of life and principles from positive psychology, this exercise guides grieving individuals toward forgiveness, gratitude, and acceptance while creating space for enduring bonds.

The **5,4,3,2,1 Exercise** includes five key reflections: forgiveness, apologies, gratitude, wishes, and declarations of love, in good alignment with the 4A4C. Cultural and spiritual elements can be integrated, tailoring the process to individual or group values and beliefs.

Steps for 5,4,3,2,1

1. **Gratitude**: Identify at least five statements of gratitude to acknowledge positive aspects of the relationship. Examples:
   - *"I am grateful for the way you supported me during tough times."*
   - *"I thank you for teaching me about resilience and love."*
2. **Wishes**: Express four unfulfilled wishes related to the relationship. This step provides an outlet to process missed opportunities or regrets. Examples:
   - *"I wish we had more time together."*
   - *"I wish I had shared my feelings with you sooner."*
3. **Apologies**: Reflect on three statements of apology for things left unsaid or actions taken. This step encourages accountability and healing. Examples:
   - *"I apologize for not calling you more often."*
   - *"I apologize for losing my temper that day."*
4. **Forgiveness**: Write two statements of forgiveness. This step fosters emotional release, helping participants acknowledge unresolved emotions without condoning harmful actions. Examples:
   - *"I forgive you for not being able to attend my graduation."*
   - *"I forgive you for the arguments we had about [specific topic]."*
5. **Declarations of Love**: Write an affirmation of love to honor the emotional bond. Examples:
   - *"I love you for your kindness and the memories we created."*
   - *"I love you for the lessons you've left me with."*

   Farewell Message: Compose a farewell message to symbolize closure while honoring the enduring connection. Example,

"__________, *I ask that you please accept my apologies, expressions of forgiveness, unfulfilled wishes, and my unwavering love. Though you are no longer here, I carry your love and memories. I need to say goodbye to some parts of our life together and keeping others close. Goodbye.*"

Upon completion of the letter, the client may read their reflections aloud privately or in a supportive setting. Encourage the incorporation of culturally or spiritually significant rituals, such as writing on a sky lantern for symbolic release, sending it on a river in a paper boat, or burying it alongside a meaningful item. These rituals can provide significant psychosocial benefits.

8.3 Systematic Care Plan B: Continuing Treasure

Contrary to earlier understandings influenced by Freud's psychodynamic theories, which portrayed grief recovery as requiring the relinquishing of previous ties, the newer "continuing bonds" perspective acknowledges that love and connection endure beyond death (Klass et al., 2014). Instead of viewing grief as a journey toward detachment, this perspective suggests that maintaining a connection with the deceased allows clients to find comfort and relief in a sense of continuity, despite the physical absence of their loved ones. As Attig (2010) states, "We can continue to 'have' what we have 'lost,' that is, a continuing, albeit transformed, love for the deceased" (p. 189).

This new perspective aligns with the Spiral Model, which supports the ongoing, nonlinear journey of grieving and healing, allowing individuals to revisit and integrate their connection with their loved ones into their evolving lives.

However, it is important to be cautious when individuals display an anxious attachment style to hold onto the deceased, as this may potentially lead to prolonged grief (Stroebe et al., 2005). This highlights the need for a balanced, client-centered approach, with the counselor playing a key role in helping clients relocate to a space where they can carry on living effectively. In Worden's (2009) revised work on continuing bonds, he emphasizes the importance of embarking on a new life while maintaining an enduring connection with the deceased.

Systematic Care Plan B: Continuing Treasure
Step 1: Honoring Treasured Moments

- Reflect and write down cherished memories and shared joys with the deceased.

Step 2: Giving Forgiveness

- Reflect on forgiveness (both granting and asking).

Step 3: Continuing Bonds

- Reframe memories across time (past, present, and future).
- Create rituals to reinforce connections with the deceased.

8.3.1 Step One: Honor Treasured Moments

Step One focuses on reflecting on cherished meaningful moments shared with the deceased. This step allows clients to contemplate the profound impact these experiences have had on their lives. By expressing gratitude for these treasured moments, space is created to celebrate the beauty of the relationship and find solace in enduring memories that continue to shape their lives. The following activities guide the client through this process:

1. **Cherished Reminiscence**

   Invite the client to recall five things they greatly treasure that their loved one did or said. Instruct them to write five corresponding statements, addressing the deceased as they would have in life.

   Examples: "Sam, I treasure the time you first told me that you loved me. I remember that special evening." "Mom, I treasure all the times you held me when I came home from school crying. I still feel the warmth of your hugs."
2. **Shared Joy**

   Invite the client to reflect on five experiences they deeply treasure, which were shared with their loved one. They should write five corresponding statements, beginning each with how they would address the deceased.

   Examples: "Sam, I treasure the time we vacationed in San Diego together: the long talks, the walks along the beach, our fish and wine dinners." "Mom, I treasure all our Sunday evening telephone conversations: the tears and laughter we shared."
3. **Create a Legacy of Connection**

   Encourage participants to create a tangible or symbolic representation of their enduring bond with the deceased. Examples include
   - Writing a letter or poem addressed to their loved ones.
   - Crafting a keepsake, such as a memory jar or scrapbook.
   - Planting a tree or dedicating a space in their honor.
   - Donate to a charity in memory of them.

These actions align with the 4A4C model in that they foster connection while nurturing meaning-making and commitment to well-being. They also provide a grounding point for revisiting and celebrating the relationship in the future.

8.3.2 Step Two: Giving Forgiveness

Death serves as a poignant reminder of shared humanity, vulnerability, and imperfection. Acknowledging flaws and extending forgiveness can profoundly facilitate the healing process. The following activities are designed to guide clients through this dual journey of seeking and offering forgiveness:

1. **Granting Forgiveness**

   Invite the client to reflect on instances where they may have felt hurt or wronged by their loved one. Instruct them to write five corresponding statements, addressing the deceased as they would have during life. This exercise encourages the release of lingering resentment and promotes healing and reconciliation.

   Examples: "Sam, I forgive you for refusing to attend my dad's funeral. That hurt me, but I forgive you." "Mom, I forgive you for not speaking to me after my divorce. I wanted to talk to you so much, but I forgive you."
2. **Asking for Forgiveness**

   Encourage the client to ask forgiveness for any actions that may have caused the deceased pain. Have them write five statements, beginning each with how they would address the loved one. This fosters accountability and sincere reconciliation.

   Examples: "Sam, please forgive me for the time I cheated on you. I know I was completely in the wrong." "Mom, please forgive me for not spending more time with you toward the end of your life. None of the excuses I gave were acceptable."
3. **Reflective Review or Ritual**

   Encourage the client to review their declarations several times over the next few weeks. Suggest or guide them to experiment with different review forms, such as visualizing the deceased accepting their apologies or reading the declarations to an object that symbolizes their presence while imagining their loved one sitting there. Encourage the incorporation of culturally or spiritually significant rituals, such as writing on a sky lantern for symbolic release, sending it on a river in a paper boat, or burying it alongside a meaningful item.

8.3.3 Step Three: Continuing Bonds

The following exercises guide clients in exploring continuing bonds with their departed loved ones. By reframing relationships across time and transcending the birth-death dichotomy, clients can come to understand that while death may alter the form and details of their relationships, it does not have to signify the end. Instead, they can carry on the legacy and values of their loved ones, allowing the love and connection to continue enriching and inspiring their lives. Through this process, the departed live on through the client's enhanced being and enduring connection.

1. **Reframing Across Time**

   Guide the client to select six to ten declarations from the previous two activities (Honoring Treasured Moments and Giving Forgiveness). Instruct them to reframe these declarations using three distinctive tenses: one in the past tense, one in the present tense, and one in the future tense. Encourage the client to reflect on these different perspectives to deepen their sense of connection with the deceased.

If the deceased was an older figure, such as a parent or grandparent, the client may also consider incorporating statements inspired by family narratives, imagination, or photographs. These might include reflections on how the loved one eagerly anticipated their birth or lovingly cared for them before their earliest memories formed. This perspective allows clients to perceive love and connection that transcends the boundaries of physical presence and time.

[Examples:

"Mom, I loved you so much when you held me when I came home from school crying. I am thinking of those times right now. Although you are not physically with me, I will always carry those moments in my heart."

"Sam, I was so hurt when you refused to attend my dad's funeral. I forgive you for that and all the other times you hurt me. Despite all those hurtful things, I will go into the future cherishing our many good times together."

"Grandma, You spent so much time making those cute outfits and blankets for me before I was born. You sew in your love and blessings into each thread of the blanket. I love you and miss your warm hugs and delicious pies. I will continue to make the pies using your recipe. Each bite will remind me of your sweetness, which is still with me."]

2. **Reflective Review**

   Instruct the client to engage with their reframed declarations over the next several weeks. They can review these declarations privately, share them with a trusted friend or a counselor, or read them to a photo or other object that symbolizes the presence of the loved one. Encourage them to reflect on how these perspectives—past, present, and future—help reinforce the enduring connection with the deceased.

3. **Continuing Bonds**

   Facilitate the creation of a personalized and culturally relevant healing ritual that acknowledges the ongoing bond with the deceased. Using the statements or guided visualizations from this book, clients can craft a ritual that resonates with their cultural or spiritual values. Whether through reading a letter at a special location, burning the letter, releasing it in a drift bottle, or burying it under a beautiful tree, this ritual allows clients to actively cultivate a sense of connection that transcends the physical realm. These intentional acts of remembrance and reflection provide comfort and solace in the ongoing presence of their loved one.

8.4 Systematic Care Plan C: Acceptance and Carrying On

Acceptance is presented as the final stage of the grieving process in Kübler-Ross's (1969) classical stage theory, following denial, anger, bargaining, and depression. This stage marks a significant transition toward reconciliation (for detailed discussions of its legacy and limitations, see Chap. 4). While more recent perspectives challenge the idea of grieving as a linear process, acceptance remains a crucial aspect of grief work (Worden, 2009).

In the **4A4C Framework**, **acceptance** is a multidimensional construct with self-oriented and relational dimensions:

1. **Acceptance of Reality**: Acknowledging the loss as an unchangeable fact. It signifies coming to terms with the reality that the loved one will not return. It does not mean that pain or sadness disappears, but it acknowledges that these feelings can coexist with a newfound sense of peace and understanding. Acceptance enables individuals to integrate the loss into their lives, carrying on with resilience and hope.
2. **Acceptance of Self**: Embracing one's unique grieving process and manifestations without self-judgment or criticism. Validate emotions and self-worth.
3. **Acceptance of Others**: Recognizing and respecting the diverse ways others experience and express grief, even when they differ from one's own.
4. **Acceptance of the Process**: Allowing grief to unfold naturally and understanding it as a dynamic, nonlinear journey.

Acceptance in this framework extends to professionals supporting those who grieve. For therapists, counselors, and care providers, it involves creating a compassionate space where individuals feel seen, heard, and validated. This requires setting aside assumptions, biases, or expectations about how grief "should" look and fully accepting the person as they are in the moment. It also involves professionals acknowledging their own limitations and recognizing that it is not always possible to help everyone in every situation.

Systematic Care Plan C offers a structured approach to honor the deceased, work through the pain of loss, and address the roles previously filled by the loved one, coming to an acceptance and adaptation to a changed world.

Systematic Care Plan C: Acceptance and Carrying On

Step 1: Accepting the Reality of the Loss

- Identify and reflect on the roles the deceased played.

Step 2: Working Through the Pain

- Acknowledge and develop strategies to address emotional and physical pain.

Step 3: Filling Gaps

- Identify secondary losses and explore ways to fill those roles.

Step 4: Carrying on With Life

- Create rituals for closure and incorporate methods to maintain connections.

8.4.1 Step One: Accepting the Reality of the Loss

1. Guide the client to make a list of four to eight specific roles that were fulfilled by the person they lost. These roles should be unique or almost exclusive to the deceased, such as the person who slept beside them or the one who accompanied them on daily walks.
2. For each role, instruct the client to write a paragraph using the deceased's name, acknowledging both their appreciation for the role and the loss they feel without it.

   Example:

   "Sally, I remember you as the person sitting across from me at the dinner table. I miss seeing you there, listening to you, and having you listen to me. I'm now realizing how much that meant to me. Thank you for being there. It's a big loss not seeing you sitting across the table."
3. Encourage the person to select a meaningful photo, piece of clothing, or object that belonged to their loved one and place it in a quiet, comfortable space. Guide them to read these paragraphs aloud in the presence of this item on three separate occasions over the next few weeks. This practice allows them to express their grief and gratitude, fostering acceptance of the loss. Once they have fully engaged with this activity, they may proceed to the next step.

8.4.2 Step Two: Working Through the Pain

1. **Identify Emotional and Physical Pain**: Ask the client to review the paragraphs from the previous step and identify four to eight emotional, physical, or spiritual pains they are experiencing due to the losses. These might include anger, sadness, headaches, or hopelessness.
2. **Develop Coping Strategies**: For each pain, guide the client to write down two strategies to alleviate it. These can be drawn from discussions with a counselor, resources in this book, or other tools. For example, if their pain is anger, they might write strategies like counting to ten and breathing deeply, or trying yoga.
3. **Visible Reminder**: Instruct the client to post these strategies somewhere visible in their home and read them at least three times during the week.
4. **Implement the Strategies**: Encourage the client to begin implementing at least one strategy for each pain. Remind them that what resists persists; by accepting their pain, they can move forward in the healing process. Only after beginning to work through the pain should they proceed to the next step.

8.4.3 Step Three: Filling Gaps

When individuals experience a **primary loss**—the loss of a significant person—they often face **secondary losses** as well. These may include the roles the deceased fulfilled, the activities they shared, or even aspects of identity and routine. While the loved one is irreplaceable, it is possible to find ways to fill some of these roles and address the gaps left behind. The goal is not to replace the person but to help the client find comfort and healing by addressing these secondary losses.

1. **Identifying Secondary Losses**: Help the client identify —two to three roles that the deceased filled which now represent secondary losses. These might include emotional support or shared routines. Once identified, determine whether these roles can be filled by the client themselves or by someone else.

   Example: If the person used to walk with the client in the evenings, encourage them to explore whether a friend or family member might take on this role.
2. **Addressing Secondary Losses**: Guide the client to explore ways to fill these roles over the next few weeks. While these roles will not be replaced exactly as before, finding new ways to meet these needs can improve daily functioning and comfort.
3. **Recognizing Progress**: Before moving on to the next activity, the client should feel some degree of comfort with how these secondary losses are being addressed. While the primary loss is permanent, working through the secondary losses opens opportunities for healing. As the client begins to improve their daily functioning by addressing these gaps, it enhances their ability to cope and adapt to life without the deceased. Progress in these areas not only helps restore a sense of normalcy but also frees up the necessary emotional energy and time to continue processing the deeper pain of the primary loss. Progress does not need to be complete, but acknowledging even small steps is essential for the overall healing journey.

8.4.4 Step Four: Carrying on with Life

Finally, help the client develop personalized rituals to say goodbye to their loved one. Each ritual should honor how the deceased enriched their life while also providing a clear expression of goodbye, acknowledging that the person is no longer physically present.

For example, the client might write a detailed letter to the deceased, reflecting on cherished memories and concluding with a heartfelt farewell. Another option might involve gathering meaningful objects associated with the loved one, offering a prayer or meditation of gratitude, and then choosing to give away, release, or bury the objects.

Alternatively, the client could create a scrapbook by selecting photos and mementos that hold special meaning. As they reflect on each picture or object, they can curate the scrapbook by adding personal notes, captions, or dates that mark important moments in their relationship. This creative process allows the client to honor the loved one's legacy in a tangible way, crafting a lasting tribute they can revisit whenever they feel the need.

Additionally, the client might choose to carry on a tradition that was meaningful to the loved one. For instance, one student shared how she continues her grandmother's tradition of baking a specific pie for family reunions or holidays, using her grandmother's recipe. In this way, she maintains a connection with her grandmother, honors her memory, and supports her family through this shared tradition. Encourage the client to identify similar traditions or practices that were significant to their loved one and continue them as a way to honor their legacy and foster a sense of connection and continuity for themselves and others.

It is important to remind the client that saying goodbye does not mean their love for the person ends. Rather than viewing it as "moving on," which can be difficult to accept, encourage the client to see it as "carrying on" with life while still upholding their loved one's legacy. The love and inspiration the deceased provided have left a lasting impact, and the client can honor that by allowing the essence of their loved one to guide their actions and being. While death may signify the end of physical presence, it does not end love.

8.5 Finish the Unfinished Business Letter

Writing a letter to a loved one who has passed away can be a powerful way to bring closure to unresolved feelings. However, to ensure the letter supports healing most effectively, it is important to fully process their grief beforehand, ideally with the support of a counselor or trusted friend. This involves untangling emotions, exploring both the positive and negative aspects of the relationship, reconstructing meaning, and addressing the secondary losses for functional adaptation. The systematic models presented in previous sections are designed to assist in this process. It is recommended that the letter be written once the client has reached some level of acceptance and has shifted predominantly into restoration orientation from loss-oriented engagement in the upward Spiral Model of Grieving.[1]

The following steps can guide the client in writing the letter:

1. Invite the client to set aside a couple of hours in a quiet, comfortable space where they will not be disturbed. Encourage them to create a peaceful and personal atmosphere. They might want to set up the loved one's photo, dim the lights, light a candle, or play some gentle background music. These small touches can help them feel more connected and supported.

[1] Refer to Chap. 1 for the graphic illustration of the Spiral Model.

2. Advise them to start the letter by addressing the deceased in a way that feels most natural to their relationship. Examples might include "Dear Mom," "Dear Tommy," "My Dearest Sweetheart," or "To My Best Friend."
3. Follow the greeting with a statement such as, "I have been reflecting on our relationship lately, and there are several things I feel I need to say."
4. Next, the client should write about things they feel they need to **apologize** for—actions or words they regret. Suggest they aim for two to five sentences in this section, offering a heartfelt reflection.
5. After addressing their own apologies, the client should write two to five sentences offering **forgiveness** for any actions or words from the loved one that caused pain or sadness.
6. In the next section, write two to five sentences expressing the **positive feelings** they had toward their loved one—things they might not have said often enough during the loved one's life. These reflections can include what they admired, appreciated, and loved about the person.
7. Conclude the letter by summarizing its contents and offering a heartfelt **goodbye**. Be sure to include the word "goodbye" somewhere in this closing.

Writing this letter can be profoundly therapeutic, allowing the client to express their feelings and begin moving toward closure. The systematic models discussed earlier may already have guided the bereaved individual toward this point, or they may serve as inspiration for creating this letter. If the client has already written a similar letter, they may be encouraged to revisit it, or use the "inhibited writing" method to address any residual emotions.

Once the letter has been written, creating a personalized ritual incorporating the letter can help the client take another step forward in their healing journey. This ritual can be a symbolic gesture of closure, honoring the emotions expressed in the letter and marking a meaningful moment in the grief process.

Here are some suggestions for the client to consider when planning their ritual:

1. **Read the Letter Aloud**: Encourage the client to find a quiet, meaningful location—such as a peaceful spot in nature, a cozy corner of their home, or their loved ones' resting place. Bring an object that symbolizes the presence of the loved one, such as a photo or an object that belonged to them. They can read the letter aloud, fully engaging with the emotions as they do so.
2. **Burn the Letter**: After reading the letter, the client may choose to ceremonially burn it. Watching the flames consume the paper and release their words into the air can symbolize letting go of unresolved feelings and opening the door to a new chapter of healing.
3. **Float the Letter**: Another option is for the client to fold the letter into a small boat, perhaps decorating it with flowers or other meaningful symbols. They can then set the boat adrift on a nearby stream, symbolizing the release of their thoughts and emotions as they watch the letter float away.
4. **Release with a Lantern**: The client could also attach the letter to a biodegradable lantern and release it into the sky. As the lantern rises, they may feel a sense of peace and connection, allowing themselves to let go and move forward.

No matter which ritual the client chooses, it should be seen as a significant milestone in their healing journey. While grief may resurface at times, engaging in this ritual signifies a shift toward hope and acceptance. It is a beautiful way to honor their loved one's memory while also acknowledging their own healing and growth.

8.6 Affirmations

During times of grief, affirmations can serve as powerful tools for guiding individuals toward a more holistic view of life. Research from around the world demonstrates that affirmations help reduce anxiety and depression, foster a more positive mindset, and enhance self-esteem (Cohen & Sherman, 2014). Neuroscience research also supports the role of affirmations in rewiring the brain—a process known as *neuroplasticity*. Through consistent repetition, affirmations help build new neural pathways, gradually shaping the brain to function in alignment with the new intended direction.

When individuals engage with affirmations, they activate brain regions related to self-evaluation and emotional regulation, particularly the ventromedial prefrontal cortex (vmPFC), which plays a key role in how one perceives oneself and manages emotions (Cascio, et al., 2016). Over time, this rewiring process replaces negative thought patterns with healthier, more empowering beliefs. By consciously repeating affirmations, individuals reinforce neural pathways tied to optimism, resilience, and overall well-being.

Pairing affirmations with visualization can further enhance their impact. Visualization engages additional brain areas, strengthening the neural connections associated with personal growth and recovery (Mishra & Gazzaley, 2014). By linking affirmations with corresponding emotions—such as gratitude or confidence—individuals can deepen the effect, reinforcing positive emotional states more effectively.

8.6.1 Tips for Affirmations

Here are some tips for effectively creating and applying affirmations:

1. **Select Affirmations that are Personally Meaningful:** It is important to choose affirmations that truly connect with one's emotions and personal journey. Affirmations should feel meaningful, so clients should either select affirmations that speak directly to their current experiences or modify them to better reflect their unique situation.
2. **Use Concise and Present Tense:** Affirmations are most impactful when framed in the present tense and stated positively. For example, instead of saying "I will be at peace," suggest saying, "I am at peace." Using present-tense language rein-

forces the belief that positive change is happening now, creating a stronger emotional and mental shift.

3. **Repetition is the Key:** Like any habit, affirmations become more powerful with regular use. Encourage individuals to repeat their affirmations daily for at least 3–4 weeks. This repetition strengthens new neural connections and helps integrate the affirmations into their subconscious mind, fostering lasting change.
4. **Believe in the Words and Method:** Affirmations are not just words—they reflect a mindful reconstruction of cognitive narrative. While it is natural to feel some skepticism at first, it is important to approach affirmations with an open mind. Trust in the process and research-based technique. Self-belief amplifies the effectiveness of affirmations in improving well-being.
5. **Connect to the Emotion:** The key to a powerful affirmation is emotional engagement. Encourage clients to feel the emotion behind the words—whether it is peace, confidence, or gratitude. If this is challenging, suggest focusing on physical sensations, such as a calm breath or a relaxed chest, to help evoke the associated feeling. Connecting affirmations with emotion strengthens their impact.
6. **Pair with Visualization:** Visualization can deepen the impact of affirmations by engaging multiple areas of the brain. Encourage individuals to visualize themselves living the affirmation or guide them through imagery. For example, if the affirmation is "I accept the flow of life" or "I am peaceful," they could imagine floating gently down a stream in a flower meadow, feeling the warmth of the sun and the gentle breeze. Whether self-led or guided by a professional, this practice strengthens the neural connections that support positive emotional states and helps embed the affirmation more deeply into their mindset. Remind the client that they could always return to such a space whenever they need it.
7. **Make Affirmations Visible:** Keeping affirmations visible throughout the day serves as a reminder to stay connected to positive intentions. Suggest placing them in high-traffic areas, such as near a mirror, on a desk, or as phone backgrounds, so they are consistently reinforced through repetition and visibility.
8. **Morning and Night Routine:** Incorporate affirmations into morning and night routines. Start and end the day with positive intentions.
9. **Combine with Action:** Affirmations are most powerful when paired with tangible action. While positive thinking is important, aligning thoughts with real-world actions can reinforce beliefs and drive results. For example, if an individual's affirmation is "I am deserving of happiness," suggest they take a step toward self-care, such as enjoying a relaxing warm bath or reaching out to a supportive friend, to reinforce that belief.

8.6.2 Sample Affirmations

The following affirmations are offered to help individuals on their healing journey. Selecting one to three affirmations from the list, or better yet, crafting personalized ones, allows the affirmation to resonate more deeply with each person's unique experience. The true power of affirmations lies in their ability to connect with emotions and aspirations. Inspiration can also be drawn from other sources that hold personal significance.

Affirmations become most effective when they are not just repeated but internalized and embodied. When individuals choose affirmations that truly speak to them, they create a pathway for healing, peace, and resilience.

A. I allow myself to feel my emotions fully and without judgment.
B. Every moment I have a choice. I choose peace.
C. I embrace myself with kindness.
D. Loving myself fills me with limitless love for others.
E. Each day, I find moments of peace and comfort amidst the pain.
F. I accept. I let go.
G. I am not alone in my grief; countless others have walked this path and found solace.
H. Today, I spread positivity and find joy.
I. One day at a time. Focus on the present.
J. I trust my innate power to heal.
K. Each step brings me closer to peace.
L. I release grief and welcome love and joy.
M. The universe cares for me. I surrender my worries.
N. I am guided, protected, and loved.
O. I give myself permission to feel good now.
P. I am surrounded by love and support.
Q. I choose to feel good now, releasing negativity.
R. I connect to compassion and strength within.
S. I invite light, courage, and peace into my life.
T. I embrace healing and choose love.
U. Today is great. I embrace new experiences and peace.
V. I am free, worthy, and deserving of happiness.
W. Everything leads to growth. I welcome positivity.
X. Every day, I grow stronger, wiser, and more peaceful.
Y. I am gentle and kind with myself.
Z. I celebrate each day with kindness, compassion, and hope.

8.7 Monthly Review

The monthly review offers clients a reflective space to document their experiences, serving as both a healing tool and a means to assess progress. Over the first 6–12 months following a significant loss, this practice helps them evaluate past goals, identify emerging challenges, and adjust care plans as they progress through their grief journey. Incorporating models like Worden's Tasks of Mourning (2009) or Swarbrick's Eight Dimensions of Wellness (2006)—including physical, emotional, social, intellectual, environmental, spiritual, occupational, and financial wellness—provides a comprehensive framework for understanding progress. Additionally, the Spiral Model of Grieving and Healing emphasizes the natural movement between loss-oriented and restoration-oriented coping, reminding individuals that setbacks are part of the process and that small victories should be celebrated. By reviewing effective coping mechanisms and setting specific goals for the upcoming month, clients can continue to foster healing and growth.

8.7.1 Step 1. Review and Reflection

1. What positive changes are noticeable in the grieving process compared to the previous month? Identify one to three improvements. What contributed to this progress?
2. Are there areas where new challenges have surfaced? Name at least one aspect where additional support might be needed.
3. Looking ahead, what progress would be most meaningful for the upcoming month? Identify one main area to focus on and set one to three specific, measurable goals.

8.7.2 Step 2: Identify Area of Focus

The following are two different models to help identify areas of progress or new focus:

Model 1. Inspired by Worden's Tasks Model (2009)
In this new month:

- I allow more acceptance of my loss.
- I process and release the pain of grief.
- I am making progress in adjusting to a new world.
- I allow enduring connection with my loved one while embarking on a new life.

Model 2. Swarbrick's "8 Dimensions" of Wellness (2006)
These dimensions—physical, emotional, social, intellectual, environmental, spiritual, occupational, and financial—serve as a holistic guide for identifying areas of progress and setting new goals during the monthly review.

Based on the review and reflection, identify the primary and secondary areas of focus for the new month.

8.7.3 Step 3: Set SMART Goals

At the onset of care, collaborative goal-setting creates a foundation tailored to the client's strengths, challenges, and needs. Revisiting these goals regularly and refining them periodically encourages ongoing commitment and clarity. Models like Worden's tasks or the Eight Dimensions of Wellness can guide this process, helping identify areas for focus and development.

Even beyond formal therapy or counseling, regular reviews of progress and goals foster continued healing. Encouraging clients to anticipate upcoming challenges and set proactive and realistic goals. By integrating goal-setting into daily life, clients can build self-awareness, confidence, and a greater sense of control over their healing process.

A practical tool for setting and maintaining goals is the *SMART Framework* (MacLeod, 2012), which breaks down goals into *Specific, Measurable, Attainable, Relevant,* and *Time-bound* components.

- **Specific**: What is the goal?
  Example: To increase daily water intake to 7 cups a day, at least five days a week.
- **Measurable**: How will progress be tracked?
  Example: Use a phone app or planner to track daily intake. Refill a 32-ounce bottle twice daily.
- **Attainable**: Is this goal realistic, and what resources or obstacles exist?
  Example: Already drinking 5 cups per day, increasing to 7 is achievable. The obstacle is disliking plain water, so strategies like fruit-infused water or herbal tea will be used.
- **Relevant**: Why is this goal important?
  Example: Improving hydration will enhance energy and overall well-being.
- **Time-bound**: When will each step be achieved?
  Example: Set reminders immediately, research and purchase a water bottle by a set date, and reach the 7-cup goal by a specific deadline.

Using this framework, individuals can set their SMART goals for the upcoming month. Refer to Table 8.1 for a template.

Table 8.1 SMART goal template

Primary area of focus	____
SMART criteria	Details
Specific	My goal is:
Measurable	I will track my progress by:
Achievable	This is achievable because:
Relevant	This goal is important because:
Time-bound	I will complete this goal by: (1) Milestone 1 (item and date): (2) Milestone 2 (item and date): (3) Milestone 3(item and date):

8.8 Concluding Reflections

The holistic psychosocial plans outlined in this chapter offer a comprehensive and structured approach for therapists working with individuals experiencing grief, whether from bereavement or nonfinite losses like divorce and breakups. By integrating emotional, cognitive, and behavioral dimensions, these care plans guide both therapists and clients through the complexities of the grieving process. The three models—Relationship Peaks and Valleys**,** Continuing Treasure, and Acceptance and Carrying-On—offer varied pathways for processing grief, honoring memories, and adapting to life after loss.

The care plans presented here are flexible and can be adapted to the unique needs of each client, ensuring a personalized therapeutic experience. Additional tools can be found in Part IV: Addressing Psychosocial Needs and Part V: Addressing Spiritual Needs in End-of-Life and Grieving. The model also emphasizes taking time in the process, allowing clients time to engage fully as the grieving and healing process unfolds.

Therapists are encouraged to maintain a nurturing, non-judgmental environment that emphasizes compassionate companionship and empowers the client to navigate their grief with resilience. By applying these systematic care plans within the framework of the Spiral Model of Grieving and Healing and the *4A4C* competencies of awareness, acceptance, affirmation, actualization, compassion, connection, composure, and commitment, therapists can help clients move toward healing while honoring their unique grief journey.

As with all therapeutic practices, ongoing evaluation and reflection are essential. Therapists should remain open to adjusting care plans as recovery progresses, normalizing setbacks, and celebrating even small steps forward. These tools, combined with therapeutic presence, provide a powerful mechanism for fostering healing, offering hope, and cultivating resilience in clients as they navigate the intricacies of grief and loss.

As Rumi beautifully expressed, *"The garden of Love is green without limit and yields many fruits other than sorrow and joy. Love is beyond either condition:*

without spring, without autumn, it is always fresh" (Rumi, 2016, p. 55). This serves as a reminder that while grief may oscillate between sorrow and joy, both are expressions of love, and the love shared with those lost endures beyond time and space, ever fresh and nourishing, continuing to inspire life beyond loss.

References

Attig, T. (2010). *How we grieve: Relearning the world*. Oxford University Press.

Byock, I. (2014). *The four things that matter most: A book about living*. Simon & Schuster.

Cascio, C. N., O'Donnell, M. B., Tinney, F. J., Lieberman, M. D., Taylor, S. E., Strecher, V. J., & Falk, E. B. (2016). Self-affirmation activates brain systems associated with self-related processing and reward and is reinforced by future orientation. *Social Cognitive and Affective Neuroscience, 11*(4), 621–629. https://doi.org/10.1093/scan/nsv136

Cohen, G. L., & Sherman, D. K. (2014). The psychology of change: Self-affirmation and social psychological intervention. *Annual Review of Psychology, 65*, 333–371. https://doi.org/10.1146/annurev-psych-010213-115137

Doka, K. J., & Martin, T. L. (2010). *Grieving beyond gender: Understanding the ways men and women mourn* (Rev. ed.). Routledge.

Klass, D., Silverman, P. R., & Nickman, S. (2014). *Continuing bonds: New understandings of grief*. Taylor & Francis.

Kübler-Ross, E. (1969). *On death and dying*. Macmillan.

MacLeod, L. (2012). Making SMART goals smarter. *Physician Executive, 38*(2), 68–70, 72. Retrieved from https://www.proquest.com/docview/1284082621

Mishra, J., & Gazzaley, A. (2014). Harnessing the neuroplastic potential of the human brain & the future of cognitive rehabilitation. *Frontiers in Human Neuroscience, 8*, 218. https://doi.org/10.3389/fnhum.2014.00218

Rumi. (2016). *Love is a stranger* (p. 55). Shambhala Publications.

Stroebe, M., Schut, H., & Stroebe, W. (2005). Attachment in coping with bereavement: A theoretical integration. *Review of General Psychology, 9*(1), 48–66. https://doi.org/10.1037/1089-2680.9.1.48

Swarbrick, M. (2006). A wellness approach. *Psychiatric Rehabilitation Journal, 29*(4), 311–314. https://doi.org/10.2975/29.2006.311.314

Wojtkowiak, J., Lind, J., & Smid, G. E. (2021). Ritual in therapy for prolonged grief: A scoping review of ritual elements in evidence-informed grief interventions. *Frontiers in Psychiatry, 11*, 623835. https://doi.org/10.3389/fpsyt.2020.623835

Worden, J. W. (2009). *Grief counseling and grief therapy: A handbook for the mental health practitioner* (4th ed.). Springer.

Part IV
Supporting Psychosocial Needs in End-of-Life and Grieving

Chapter 9
Psychosocial Support for End-of-Life Transition

9.1 Introduction

Navigating terminal illness and the dying process is a complex journey, often accompanied by various challenges for both the dying persons and their loved ones. This section reviews major theoretical models of psychosocial needs, with more in-depth discussions in Chap. 5. This chapter applies the practical tools and strategies to support patients and loved ones through this profound transition.

A particularly helpful framework in end-of-life care is the 5Rs: Remember, Recognize, Respect, Reinforce, and Reminisce (as cited in Corr et al., 2019). These guiding principles provide a compassionate and person-centered approach to interactions.

The tools discussed in this chapter are grouped into key thematic areas: emotional support, legacy building, spiritual exploration, and practical support. These tools are adaptable to the needs of each person and their family, with careful attention to cultural values, practices, and preferences.

9.1.1 Emotions and Tasks in Terminal Illness

Terminal illness and impending death often induce a wide range of intense responses. Psychiatrist Dr. Elisabeth Kübler-Ross (1969) identified a series of common emotions that she observed in terminally ill patients, known as the famous Stage Model. These include denial, anger, bargaining, sadness (referred to as depression), and acceptance.

It is important to note, however, that not everyone goes through this sequence or experiences all the responses. Later research has emphasized that these coping

Y. Z. Ciupak, D. C. Smith, *Death, Dying, and Grief*,
https://doi.org/10.1007/978-3-031-88467-2_9

defense mechanisms can vary greatly between individuals, lasting for different periods, and sometimes occurring simultaneously or cyclically (Corr, 1992).

Denial: Denial often manifests as a refusal to accept the reality of a terminal diagnosis. This response may be characterized by shock, fear, confusion, or avoidance, with representative statements such as "This can't be true," or "This isn't happening."

Anger: Anger may surface as frustration, helplessness, or a sense of injustice, often expressed through questions like, "Why is this happening?" or "How is this fair?" This emotion can sometimes be directed inward or toward others.

Bargaining: Individuals may attempt to negotiate with themselves, a higher power, or reality in an effort to change or mitigate their situation. Common expressions include "If only…" or "Yes, but…"

Sadness/Depression: Sadness often arises as reality settles in. It may be accompanied by regret, loneliness, withdrawal, and changes in sleep or appetite. Some individuals may say, "What's the point?"

Acceptance: Acceptance involves coming to terms with the reality of the situation. This can range from emotional numbness to a more constructive engagement with new opportunities or plans. It may be reflected in statements such as "I can't change this, but I can move forward."

While these coping mechanisms provide a helpful framework for understanding common responses, they are not definitive or prescriptive. The most crucial consideration is to view individuals facing terminal illness as living, dynamic human beings with their unique journey. Care providers should cultivate compassion and a person-centered approach to help individuals find meaning, resilience, and comfort in their final journey. Exploring and recognizing each person's strengths and learning from them helps ensure person-centered care.

9.1.2 Corr's Task-Based Model

The task-based approach developed by Charles Corr provides a structured method for understanding how individuals cope with terminal illness. This model focuses on organizing daily tasks on the basis of their importance to the individual without adhering to a strict timeline. This approach emphasizes the proactive nature of coping, helping individuals manage their situation by prioritizing tasks that matter most to them (Corr, 1992).

Corr's model outlines four primary areas of task work in coping with dying, each addressing different dimensions of a person's experience:

1. **Physical dimension**: Lessening or managing physical pain and distress.
2. **Psychological dimension**: Addressing emotions such as anger, sadness, anxiety, and fear and helping individuals process these emotions to find comfort.

3. **Social dimension**: Connecting with important people and building a social network to provide security and comfort and address concerns about the family's future and unfinished projects.
4. **Spiritual dimension**: Facilitate patients' meaning-making and spiritual exploration as they integrate new experiences and reassess challenged beliefs due to illness, imminent death, and other life disruptions. For detailed guidance and tools, refer to Chaps. 11 and 12.

The task-based model acknowledges that each person copes differently and may shift priorities on a daily or even hourly basis. It encourages continuous engagement with these tasks, allowing them to be revisited and worked through over time (Corr, 1992). Those who assist them can use this model to identify the care receiver's priorities during each interaction, ensuring that the support provided is aligned with the individual's current needs and preferences.

9.2 Five Essential Themes for Supporting Dying Individuals

Caring for and supporting people who are facing the end of life is a rewarding and delicate process that requires empathy, respect, and understanding. The Colorado Collaboration on End-of-Life Care has outlined five essential themes—known as the 'Five Rs' for caring—that guide caregivers and professionals in providing compassionate and effective care (as cited in Corr et al., 2019). These Five Rs offer a practical approach to ensure that those facing death receive care that honors their individuality and dignity.

1. **Remember:** Each person's experience with death and dying is unique. Care providers should approach their role as one of support rather than fixing. It is crucial to recognize that the dying person embodies a multitude of cultural identities, some visible and others not. Be cautious when offering advice or sharing personal perspectives. Insights should be shared only when asked and framed as personal experiences rather than absolute truths.
2. **Recognize:** Recognize the profound, individualized experience of facing death. This theme emphasizes compassionate presence, active listening, and holding a safe space for the dying person to share their thoughts and emotions. Active listening—expressed through attentive body language, eye contact, and responsiveness—fosters trust and connection. Embrace moments of silence, recognizing that attuned presence, without filling the space with words, can be one of the most supportive actions.
3. **Respect:** Respect is foundational to building trust and meaningful connections with the dying person. It requires honoring their values, beliefs, and cultural backgrounds, even when they differ from one's own. Cultural humility is key here: acknowledge personal limitations and remain open to learning from their unique cultural and spiritual perspectives. This approach not only fosters an

environment where the person feels valued and understood but also enriches the care provider's perspective, creating a mutually rewarding experience.

4. **Reinforce:** Reinforce the person's autonomy and decision-making capabilities. This theme encourages care providers to support the dying person in making decisions that align with their values and preferences. Ask clarifying questions that help them articulate their needs and preferences. Advocate for their wishes with other care providers, ensuring that their decisions are respected. Reinforcement also involves validating their feelings and reactions.
5. **Reminisce:** Finally, reminiscing involves encouraging the dying person to reflect on their life and share their memories. This process can be deeply meaningful, helping individuals find comfort, closure, and a sense of continuity. Encourage the person to tell stories about their life, relationships, and experiences. Provide resources that support this reflection, such as poems, songs, readings, rituals, or photographs tailored to the person's cultural and personal preferences. Reminiscing allows people to process and integrate their life experiences, facilitating a peaceful transition.

9.3 Honoring and Facilitating Final Wishes

In the initial stage of the caregiving relationship, the following question can help develop a dying person's care plan. It can also address emotional or psychological concerns in the later stages of the relationship:

> Some say that we are all sentenced to death from the day we are born. Often, when people are given a death sentence, they are granted one last request. What would you want your last request to be?

This question opens the door to meaningful conversations, helping care providers understand the wishes and priorities of the person they are supporting. It allows for a compassionate and candid conversation about what truly matters to them in their final days and what unfinished business they might have. The following real-life cases provide some examples of the last requests.

9.3.1 Case Example: Smelling of a Horse

A dying cowboy's last request to his nurse was not for food or drink, nor was there a person he felt he needed to see or a task he wanted to finish. His request was simple: all he wanted was to smell a horse. He missed that special smell, which he associated with many fond memories from his life as a cowboy.

Two days later, the nurse wheeled the cowboy's bed outside. A horse was brought to the bed, and the cowboy held his face up against the horse's head, smiled, and breathed in that unique smell that evoked all his cherished memories.

9.3.2 Case Example: Werther's Candy and a Beer

Anthony[1] had been in a coma for several weeks. His family had been at his bedside throughout that time, faithfully awaiting his death. Anthony was attached to several machines.

One day, a nurse was in the room checking the machines when Anthony suddenly bolted upright into a sitting position and blurted out, "I want Werther's candy and a beer." The nurse gasped in surprise and immediately ran out of the room in search of the assigned doctor.

One of the family members casually walked out of the room, went down the street to a convenience store, bought Werther's candy and beer, and returned to the room. Before the nurse could get back with the doctor, Anthony had enjoyed one candy, taken two sips of the beer, and peacefully passed away.

9.3.3 Case Example: Just One Little Pill

Leland made an unusual request of his nurse. He said there was only one thing he wanted before he died. "What do you want, Leland?" she asked. He replied, "All I want is one pill, just one pill." The nurse was concerned. She asked, "Are you in pain, Leland?" "Well, not really," he said. "But I suppose you could call it a type of pain. But it can be solved with only one pill. All I want is one. Just one. It's my dying wish: one Viagra. That's all I need, and I will die happy."

Reflection When expressing the intent to honor people's wishes and provide choices and control, care providers must remain mindful of any limitations they may unconsciously impose. Thoughts such as "I don't mind giving people control as long as they follow what I believe is best" may arise, even with the best intentions. Thus, it is essential to examine the underlying assumptions: Am I truly prepared to honor individuals' wishes when they differ from my own? Am I willing to allow choices that might not align with my preferences? Am I ready to support strengths that challenge my own comfort?

Sheldon Kopp emphasized the importance of meeting people where they are and respecting their self-defined well-being and satisfaction without imposing external judgments (Kopp, 1972). True acceptance, in Kopp's view, involves recognizing a patient's sense of what is "okay" or "unsatisfactory" without overlaying one's own criteria. By honoring this perspective, care providers create a therapeutic space rooted in empathy, respect, and autonomy, reaffirming each patient's right to self-determination—including their final stages of life.

[1] All the examples are based on real-life cases. Names in this text except the authors are pseudonyms, and identifying details have been removed to protect the confidentiality of individuals.

9.4 Emotional and Practical Support

An African proverb goes, "If you are never angry, then you are unborn." Anger is a primary human emotion that often emerges alongside other intense feelings such as fear, guilt, sadness, and more. Terminal illness may induce profound emotional turmoil, such as anger, denial, fear, and depression. Supporting patients' coping processes requires care providers to provide appropriate tools for their coping styles and strengths. These tools are especially important for coping styles that might be seen as unacceptable by the general public. Offering support that aligns with the person's values and strengths can help them navigate their unique challenges in a way that feels authentic and empowering. Recognizing that emotions such as anger and denial are valid responses to their situation fosters patience and compassion. Providing practical assistance with daily tasks or facilitating meaningful activities can also alleviate the emotional burden on the person.

9.4.1 A Tool: The Imaginary Sledgehammer

For people experiencing anger, this tool provides a safe and imaginative way to confront and release their frustrations. Begin by gently guiding the person to identify and name what they feel angry or unfair about. These could be recent frustrations or challenges they have encountered throughout their life—anything that has prevented them from achieving their goals or fulfilling their desires. Examples might include interrupted education, family responsibilities, financial hardships, or illness.

Encourage the person to focus on these anger "objects" one at a time and imagine using an imaginary sledgehammer to completely destroy each one in their mind. To enhance the activity, they can physically mimic the motion of swinging the sledgehammer, accompanied by shouting or vocalizing their frustration with each swing.

For a more tangible approach, provide safe objects such as a plush hammer, boxing gloves, a pillow, a stuffed animal, clay, or old newspapers. These items allow the person to channel their anger into a physical and safe outlet. Play dynamic music to energize the activity, and offer verbal encouragement such as, "Squeeze harder—get it all out!" or "Tear it up—let it all out!" In group settings, the facilitator can participate by sharing something they are angry about and demonstrating the activity to engage others.

9.4.2 Case Example: Get Out of My Room

Phyllis was angry, and she made sure everyone knew it. When the nurse entered her room, she snapped, "You know, if you were doing your job, I wouldn't be in this bed. You haven't been doing your job. I don't like you. Get out of my room!" When the social worker came in, Phyllis said, "You've been wasting my time. Go waste someone else's time. I don't like you. Get out of my room!" And when the chaplain visited, she said, "You're living in a world of illusion. You need to grow up. I don't like you. Get out of my room!"

Phyllis felt she had no control over what was happening to her, but she could be angry about it. Her anger might have been her last way of asserting herself, her last way of feeling any strength and control. If her care providers tried to calm her down or take that anger away, they might be doing her a disservice rather than a service.

The social worker working with Phyllis wrote in her care notes: "My role is to be yelled at." It can be emotionally challenging for care providers to work with angry patients. Understanding anger as a coping mechanism and a way to release frustration helps the provider avoid burnout.

9.4.3 Case Example: Susan's Release Room

Susan's remarkable calmness and her easygoing character in the face of her circumstances were puzzling to others. At just 47 years old, her life was taken away by cancer. She lived with constant pain that would likely not subside until her death. Susan certainly had many reasons to be sad and angry, yet she was so serene—almost cheery—with everyone. A visitor to her home once asked her, "What is your secret, Susan? How do you stay so calm with all that is happening to you?"

"Follow me," she replied. "I'll show you my secret." She led the visitor to a spare bedroom and opened the door, revealing her "release room." This was where she would go whenever she felt hurt, angry, or very sad—a space dedicated to releasing her emotions.

The room was simply furnished with a bed, one chair, and two stuffed animals: a bear and a giraffe. When she felt the need to cry, she would lie on the bed, hold the stuffed bear tightly to her, and sob until she felt completely cried out. When angry, she would sit in the chair and yell at the giraffe, which she imagined as her disease or someone who had wronged her. At times, she would wring the giraffe's long neck with all her strength.

9.4.4 Case Example: Martha's Denial and Naughty Words

Cancer had metastasized throughout Martha's 80-year-old body. Her condition was apparent to her family, friends, and medical advisors, but Martha refused to allow the word "cancer" to be spoken in her presence. She also refused to let anyone around her mention the words "dying" or "death." For Martha, those words were all "naughty words." Whenever any of those words were inadvertently mentioned, she turned away from the speaker, faced the nearest wall, and thrashed her arms in agitation.

This was Martha's way of coping. For whatever reason, she felt this was the only way she could manage her situation. By respecting Martha's choice, her care provider enabled a sense of control and a coping mechanism that worked for her.

Reflection Denial is a coping mechanism often discouraged or seen as counterproductive, despite its potential to serve a patient's needs. For those providing end-of-life care, it is essential to examine whether there is a bias against denial because it does not align with their own expectations. Denial has indeed been viewed critically; one limitation of the classical Stage Model of terminal illness (Kübler-Ross, 1969) is that it assumes that all patients should reach acceptance when, in reality, some may not follow each stage or may never arrive at acceptance. This raises several questions: Could denial not serve a positive role for some? Could it provide a sense of control or act as a legitimate coping style?

In practice, many patients use denial as a means to navigate their final journey. Most remain aware of their condition but may simply prefer not to confront or discuss it openly. Some researchers and practitioners argue that the expectation of death with a "positive attitude" can place an additional burden on both patients and caregivers. It can be helpful to honor a patient's choice to use denial if it brings them peace and dignity (Wasow, 1987). Forcing acceptance or open discussion on patients who are not ready can inhibit candid conversations about end-of-life plans, yet respecting their choices affirms their autonomy. By acknowledging any emotions and coping mechanisms including denial as valid responses rather than a failure to cope, care providers can create a compassionate and relaxed space that honors the patient's chosen path.

9.4.5 Case Example: Sam's Defiant Clarity

Sam's family did not think Sam could handle the fact that he was dying. In their initial meeting with the hospice nurse in the hospital's family conference room, they requested that she not inform Sam of his terminal status. They explained that their request came from their love for Sam and their desire to protect him from something they believed he could not handle.

The nurse informed the family that she would honor their request as long as Sam did not bring the topic up himself. She explained that she would not want to hide something from Sam if he really wanted to know it. The family responded by saying that they were convinced that Sam was completely unaware of the seriousness of his illness, and they reiterated their request for the nurse not to initiate any conversation with Sam about his dying.

The nurse left the family in the conference room and then entered Sam's hospital room down the hall. Before she could even introduce herself, Sam greeted her: "Are you the one who's going to work with me while I'm dying?"

The nurse responded affirmatively.

Then, Sam just started talking away. "You know I'm ninety-five," he said. "You don't live that long and not accumulate some wisdom. My family thinks I'm stupid; they treat me like I don't know anything. You don't reach ninety-five without knowing a thing or two. They're the ones that are in the dark. They're such idiots; you'd think they'd never heard of death before."

This situation highlights the complexity of denial and the importance of respecting each individual's and family's unique coping mechanisms. While the family intended to protect Sam, Sam's awareness and acceptance of his situation underscored the need for honest and open communication. By balancing these perspectives with priorities that are in alignment with professional ethics codes and guidelines, care providers can better support both patients and their loved ones.

Reflection Coping with dying involves more than one person. It also involves family, friends, and other social networks around the person. It involves multiple perspectives and motivations. The aim is to honor patients and their loved ones as fully as possible while adhering to professional ethical codes.

Care providers may sometimes underestimate how much the people they support are capable of doing, knowing, and understanding. Many have a deep desire to stay engaged and involved in their care and lives. Recognizing and enabling this capacity is at the heart of compassionate and meaningful care.

9.5 Respecting and Engaging with "Unresponsive" Patients

Even when patients seem unresponsive, it is essential to offer them choices and respect their independence. Those labeled "unresponsive" may simply communicate in ways that are not immediately recognizable, such as through subtle changes in breathing, skin temperature, or expressions. Recognizing and honoring these different forms of communication allows for meaningful, compassionate interactions that respect each person's dignity.

Treating everyone with respect, regardless of their communication style, is key. Care providers can support individuals labeled "unresponsive" with a sense of control by keeping these gentle guidelines in mind:

1. **Greet the person first**: Upon entering, take a moment to acknowledge the person first. Hearing often lasts longer than other senses do, and individuals may listen to every word.
2. **Speak with them, not about them**: When others are present, avoid talking about the person as though they weren't there. A gentle approach reminds everyone in the room that they are still very much part of the conversation.
3. **Respond to all signals**: Any change—whether it is a shift in breathing, an expression, or even a sound—is a form of communication. Respond to these signs as they occur, knowing that they are meaningful.
4. **Offer choices, no matter how small**: Simple choices, such as saying, "I'll move you to your right side now, if that's okay," allow the person a moment to respond in their way, helping them feel involved in their care.
5. **Show gratitude**: Before leaving the room, say a warm "thank you." This gentle acknowledgment shows respect for their space and autonomy.

Additionally, some people may choose to be "unresponsive" as a way to cope. Whether this is a choice, these small steps affirm each person's dignity and autonomy, creating a respectful and supportive environment.

9.5.1 Case Example: Richie's Response to Kind Words

Richie was anesthetized and undergoing his second open-heart surgery and was fading fast. As he was fading, he was receiving frantic care from a doctor and a nurse. The nurse was saying kind and encouraging words to Richie during the surgery. However, the doctor twice blurted out, "The son of a bitch is not going to die on me!"

Three weeks later, as he was being transported out of the hospital in a wheelchair, Richie heard a nurse's voice in the hall. He had the wheelchair attendant stop. Richie addressed the nurse: "You're the one who operated on me. I appreciate your kindness. I appreciated it very much. Would you please tell that doctor that I did not at all appreciate what he was saying about me. Tell him I found him quite offensive… A person like that doesn't deserve to be a doctor."

9.5.2 Case Example: Dottie's Son

Dottie had been unresponsive for five days and death appeared to be imminent. Upon hearing the news, Dottie's son was driving to see her from his home in Toronto. It would take 20 hours to reach his mother's bedside.

Even though Dottie was unresponsive, her nurses periodically informed her about her son's progress. "He'll be here in fifteen hours." "It's only twelve more hours now." "Eight more hours, Dottie. Eight more hours." Even though Dottie did not assure the nurses that she had heard a single word, the nurses continued to inform her of the son's progress. "Four more hours. Now only four hours."

The son arrived. As soon as he entered the room, he said, "Mom, I'm here."

Dottie slowly opened her eyes for the first time in five days. She then spoke with much labor, "My boy. I knew you'd make it. I knew my boy would make it. All along I knew." She smiled at the nurse with the warmth of gratitude.

Dottie died an hour later, holding hands with her son and the nurse.

9.6 Life Review and Legacy Building

Reminiscing is one of the five essential themes in supporting a person nearing the end of life. Individuals often turn to life reviews, reflecting on their experiences and the meaning their life has held. James Hollis (1996) eloquently stated, "Life is not a problem to be solved but an experiment to be lived. It is enough to have suffered through into deeper meaning. Such meaning enriches and is its own reward." Reviewing one's life to find a sense of coherence assists in psychological healing when biological curing is out of reach.

Supporting the meaningful life review process involves inviting them to share stories—either about their own lives or their loved ones' experiences—and listening with compassion and openness. This reinforces their sense of value and the impact they have had on others. Offering meaningful poems, songs, readings, rituals, or prayers that hold personal significance can enrich this remembrance, honoring the life they have lived and the legacy they leave behind.

9.6.1 Tool: A Simple Life Review

When facilitating a life review, two key elements contribute to a positive experience: showing genuine interest and encouraging validating aspects. A review with just two to four thoughtfully chosen questions can offer meaningful insights and foster genuine connection. It's important to demonstrate interest not only through the questions asked but also by actively listening and valuing each response.

A. What event or achievement from your past makes you feel proudest? Can you tell me more about it?
B. When did you first truly understand the meaning of love in your life? What was that moment like?
C. Thinking back on your life, what are some of the most fun or joyful memories you have?
D. Is there a particular event from your past that stands out in your memory? What made it so unforgettable?

E. How would you describe your "good old days"? What made that time special for you?

Life reviews may sometimes lead to difficult memories or unresolved matters. Holding a compassionate presence helps release these unresolved memories to foster a sense of peace. A more systematic counseling process may be needed to examine unconstructive narratives and shift beliefs.

9.6.2 Tool: Photographic Life Review

When entering a room filled with photographs, view each picture as if it has an invisible sign that says, "Ask me." Photographs often carry layers of meaning—both in what they reveal and in what they leave out. For example, if all the photos displayed are from the 70 s and 80 s, a natural question could be, "What made the 70s and 80s so special?" Another gentle question might be, "What about the 60s or 90s? Did they feel different for you?"

These questions invite individuals to share personal memories and reflect on the chapters of life that hold the most meaning, providing a beautiful opening for storytelling and connection.

9.6.3 Tool: Pass It On

Rather than focusing on events that have happened, this "life review" emphasizes lessons that have been learned and can be passed on to others. In this life review, meaning is borrowed from the past to lend significance to the present and future. The person would complete the following sentences:

1. I feel that people need to cherish ______________________________ __________.
2. The best thing people can do with their lives is ____________________ _________.
3. My formula for getting fun out of life is ________________________ _________.
4. I have found that friendships work if people ______________________ _________.
5. I have found that the secret of feeling content is ____________________ _________.
6. The one thing for which I most want to be remembered is ______________________.

This activity could be followed by a discussion on how these lessons might be passed on to relatives, friends, and others:

To involve family and friends, organize a gathering where the person can share their completed life review. This gathering can be in person, virtual, or a combination of both, depending on what is most comfortable and practical for everyone involved.

First, make sure the person feels comfortable and ready to share their insights. Invitations could be sent out to family and friends, allowing them to know the purpose of the gathering and encouraging them to join. When everyone is gathered, start with a brief introduction to set the tone, emphasizing the importance of sharing life lessons and wisdom.

The person can then share their completed sentences. If they need help, the care provider or a participant can assist them in reading aloud. After individuals share their insights, they encourage an open discussion. Invite family and friends to share their own thoughts, feelings, and related memories. Ask them to reflect on how these insights have impacted their lives or how they might incorporate them forward.

To preserve these valuable lessons, consider creating a memory book. Document the person's insights and allow family and friends to add their own reflections and memories. The use of photos and artwork can be transformed into a cherished scrapbook for future generations. Additionally, if the person is comfortable, recording the session on video can provide a lasting record of their wisdom and the heartfelt responses from loved ones.

Finally, discuss practical ways to weave these lessons into everyday life. Talk about revising family traditions or establishing new ones, engaging in community service, or making personal commitments to live by these insights.

This activity not only honors the person's experiences but also strengthens the bonds among all participants. By sharing and acting on these life lessons, the person's wisdom and legacy can continue to inspire and guide those they leave behind.

9.6.4 Tool: Leaving a Message

Recording a message for posterity can be a meaningful way to leave a lasting legacy. Classical methods include writing letters, creating audio recordings, or making videos. Additionally, modern digital platforms offer innovative ways to create and store legacy messages. These services allow individuals to record video, audio, or written messages that can be securely stored and scheduled for future delivery to loved ones.

9.6.5 Tool: A Tribute

People see themselves through the eyes of others. This tribute-style life review is designed for the people receiving care and gathers other people's impressions to reflect back to the person. Some approaches that can be taken are as follows:

1. **Remembrances from the past:** Various people can offer remembrances of special moments they have shared. This can be done in person or through letters, phone calls, audiotapes, or videotapes.
2. **Life history presentation:** Several people can present a short history of key events and accomplishments in a person's life.
3. **Artistic expressions:** Remembrances and recollections can be expressed through poetry, music, or artwork. These artistic tributes offer a unique and imaginative way to honor the person, capturing their essence in a way that words alone might not.
4. **Theatrical performance:** Family and friends can perform a play to portray a person's life.

9.6.6 Case Example: Linda's Healing Journey

As Linda entered the last few months of her life, the physical characteristics of her illness were dramatic reminders of psychological and physical trauma from her past. At the age of 44 years, Linda had cancer of the uterus with metastasis in her spinal cord and subsequent paraplegia from her mid-thoracic region. When the hospice staff met her for an initial interview and assessment, she volunteered that she had been sexually abused by a babysitter. The incident was still of major significance to her after several decades. She revealed this history before she even mentioned other important concerns of the present: the emotional state of her three young children, her own feelings about her debilitation, and worries about her husband's welfare. Linda's childhood nightmare was crying out to be confronted and explored immediately. She needed to discuss it before she could address all the other issues associated with her imminent death.

Addressing that old trauma was frightening for Linda because she had only previously told her husband. However, after sharing all the details with the hospice staff, Linda experienced a sense of great relief. Telling her story was so therapeutic that she decided to tell others, first her children and then her friends. As she told them one at a time, even more relief was experienced. She even invited members of her church prayer group to visit her and hear her story. With each of these meetings, Linda gave her listeners an empathetic charge: do your best to end the horrors of sexual abuse in whatever way you can. That charge was particularly powerful because it came from Linda, only a few weeks away from death. It was her last attempt to release herself from that trauma.

Reflection Reflecting on life can be a deeply personal and transformative experience, especially for those nearing the end of their journey. Engaging in a life review not only honors their past but also helps them find clarity and meaning in their experiences, approaching a sense of coherence in one's life biography. As Dag Hammarskjöld stated, "Do not seek death. Death will find you, but seek the road which makes death a fulfilment … In the last analysis, it is our conception of death which decides our answers to all the questions that life puts to us" (Hammarskjöld, 1982, p. 138), encouraging individuals to embrace their stories and the lessons learned along the way. Meaning-seeking is the underlying force of human actions and resilience, even in the most challenging circumstances (Frankl, 1984). This process often involves reconstructing one's narrative, allowing individuals to weave their experiences into a cohesive story that highlights their resilience and growth. By sharing memories and reflecting on their journeys, they celebrate the lives they have lived and the connections they have forged, fostering a sense of peace and purpose. Ultimately, this journey not only enriches their understanding of their own legacy but also deepens their connection to the lives they have touched and the love they have shared.

9.7 Healing Power of Touch

Many healthcare workers have observed a heightened sense of life and a strong desire for human contact among terminally ill individuals, fostering conversations about purposeful touch as a therapeutic intervention in end-of-life care (Snyder, 1997). Physical touch has significant benefits for both mental and physical health, including reducing stress, lowering blood pressure, and enhancing feelings of safety.

However, it is crucial to assess before offering physical contact. Assessing someone's desire for touch can be simple and intuitive. People's eyes and body language often indicate whether they want you closer or farther away. For example, if you step forward and they step back, that is an assessment. When in doubt, ask them directly.

Care providers can enhance their care by thoughtfully and appropriately incorporating touch into their practice and considering how and when touch is effectively and appropriately utilized.

People use the term "in touch" to indicate being connected to the people and moments that matter most. This suggests not only physical touch but also emotional and psychological connections. Engaging in meaningful conversations and being present in the moment with the person are essential aspects of this connection. Simple gestures of touch, such as a hug, a pat on the back, or holding someone's hand, can foster a sense of connection and support.

9.7.1 Case Example: Candy's Touching Moment

Candy weighed over 400 pounds, and her weight became life-threatening. Although she was only 36 years old, she was living in a nursing home. Each of her days in that nursing home began with four staff members coming into her room to lift her into a sitting position. One morning, one of the staff members, Jan, after helping Candy get up, stayed in the room and talked. Jan asked if she might hold Candy's hand while they talked. After giving Jan her hand, Candy looked down at their hands and started crying. Jan asked, "What's wrong, Candy?" Candy responded, "No one has ever sat down with me and held my hand. The last time I think someone held my hand was when I weighed only sixty-five pounds. I was in second grade. Thank you. Thank you. Thank you."

9.7.2 *Case Example: A Loving Family's Final Touch*

Mabel was a young grandmother. On the day that she died, she was lying in a bed surrounded by her children and grandchildren. Everyone was holding her. One person held one hand, one another. Her feet, shoulders, legs, arms, and head were all held. Then, one at a time, each relative said some words of love they associated with their touch.

The first to speak was a young granddaughter: "Grandma. I remember all the times you would come and visit us, and you would have a surprise behind your back. You would not show us the surprise until we gave you a hug. Grandma, I would have hugged you without the surprise."

Next, a daughter spoke: "Mom. I remember that when I was a little girl, I would often come home from school crying. You would hold me until I stopped. Sometimes, you had to hold me for a long, long time. I remember your love, Mom. I remember your touch, Mom. I'm trying to send that back to you now with my love and my touch."

9.7.3 *Case Example: Role Modeling Touch*

Nelson was lying in a hospital bed, surrounded by his wife, sister, brother, and hospice director, Doug. As Nelson's pain intensified, his wife and sister comforted him, while his brother paced anxiously. Uncertain how to help, Doug decided he would model touch and give permission for his brother to connect with Nelson.

Doug stood up and gently tapped a wet washcloth on Nelson's forehead. Then, he offered the washcloth to the brother. He took the washcloth and touched Nelson briefly and then bent down and hugged him tightly.

9.7.4 *Case Example: The Final Touch*

It was Rosie's first home visit as a hospice nurse in rural South Carolina, where an elderly woman was dying in the presence of her daughter and a deaconess.

The woman periodically gasped loudly, and whenever that happened, her daughter burst into tears while the deaconess spoke in tongues. This process continued for more than one hour.

Finally, Rosie walked to the daughter and suggested that she hold her mother's hand. The daughter went over, took hold of her mother's hand, and said, "Mom." Her mother took a final gasp and died. The daughter turned to Rosie and said with tearful eyes, "I almost missed that, didn't I?"

9.8 Humor and Joy in Care

Many authors have eloquently highlighted the role of humor during times of adversity. Harriet Rochlin wrote, "Laughter can be more satisfying than honor; more precious than money; more heart-cleansing than prayer" (Deger & Gibson, 2024, p. 698). This quote captures the deep relief humor brings, serving as an effective coping mechanism. Likewise, Moshe Waldoks's insight that "A sense of humor can help you overlook the unattractive, tolerate the unpleasant, cope with the unexpected, and smile through the unbearable" (as cited in Mason, 2008, p. 49) reflects the way humor lifts and strengthens us through hardship.

These insights align with research on humor's impact within palliative care settings. Pinna and colleagues conducted a systematic literature review on the use of humor in palliative care (Pinna et al., 2018), examining 34 empirical studies. Their review illustrates that humor serves an unquestionable role in providing comfort, fostering connection, and creating moments of lightness in the terminal phase of life. Thoughtfully applied, humor not only eases emotional strain but also supports resilience, empowering both patients and their families to navigate end-of-life challenges with grace and empathy. This capacity to bring ease, even in the most trying times, is what makes humor such a valuable tool in care.

As with touch, it is essential to assess the appropriateness of humor before it is expressed. It is crucial to ensure that humor is appropriate and welcomed by the people and context involved. When incorporating humor into care, observe the person's reactions and preferences. Some people might appreciate light-hearted jokes or funny stories, while others might find them inappropriate or offensive, especially during serious or painful times. Be sensitive and responsive to each person's unique needs and boundaries.

Care providers can often recognize that patients enjoy humor, as they are frequently the ones who initiate joke-telling. Many patients express feelings about the atmosphere in their rooms, saying things such as "I'm sick and tired of people coming into my room and putting on a mask of seriousness. I can hear people laughing down the hall. Do you know how that makes me feel? It's dehumanizing." This sentiment shows some patients' desire for a more light-hearted environment that respects patients' needs for connection and levity.

9.8.1 Tool: Smiling and Laughing Permitted Here

If patients want to signal to visitors that humor is okay in their rooms, they can pick one or more of the following signs to place in their room, or they can create their own:

A. "This is a frown-free zone."
B. "Danger: Excessive seriousness can prove hazardous to your health."
C. "No business transacted here except for funny business."
D. "I could die laughing if you would be willing to tell me a joke."
E. "I am not afraid of death. I just do not want to be there when it happens."
F. "Everyone allows joy to come to this room: some when they arrive, some when they depart."

9.8.2 Tool: A Funny Life Review

This activity uses the principle of recalling past events and reliving them to bring humor into the present situation. Care providers can ask those they care for to choose three questions from the list below. Rather than answering immediately, suggest that they save their responses for the next visit. This approach not only ensures an enjoyable time during the next visit but also provides moments of levity between visits.

A. What do you remember as a funny thing that happened to you in grade school?
B. What is the funniest thing that ever happened to you during a meal?
C. When did you laugh the hardest in your life, and what was the situation?
D. What is the funniest joke that you have ever heard?
E. What is the funniest prank you have ever played on someone or someone played on you?
F. Describe a time when you could not stop laughing at something that was not supposed to be fun.
G. What is the funniest misunderstanding or miscommunication you have experienced?
H. What was embarrassing when it happened at that time but fun, as you think back?

9.8.3 Tool: Funny Videos

Explore the humorous selection at video stores or take recommendations from patients and friends who enjoy movies. When individuals are ill or have limited mobility, watching these tapes with care providers can be a delightful experience. Sharing popcorn, ice cream, or candy can increase enjoyment. However, it is important to consider their preferences first: "I heard about a funny video recently. It is about this and that … Would you be interested if I brought it next time?"

9.8.4 Willy's Dance

Willy and Clara both lived with dementia. Willy often spent his days in the recreation room, waltzing with an imaginary partner to imaginary music. Clara, on the other hand, would sit in the same room, her head bowed, occasionally glancing up at Willy with a look of disapproval.

One day, Karen, a social worker, decided to join Willy in his dance. The two of them waltzed around the recreation room together. Clara got up from her chair, walked to Karen, and tapped Karen on the shoulder.

"Just wait a minute, Clara," Karen said gently. "I will be done pretty soon, and then I can spend some time with you."

Clara shook her head in frustration, briefly sat down, but quickly got up again to tap Karen on the shoulder.

"Just a minute, Clara. I will be with you soon," Karen repeated. "We are still dancing."

Again, Clara shook her head in disgust, sat down for a moment, and then rose to tap Karen on the shoulder once more.

"Okay, Clara," Karen finally said, turning to her. "How can I help you?"

"There's no music." Clara replied with a hint of irritation.

"Yes, Clara," Karen said softly. "For you, there is no music. However, for Willy, there is."

Reflection Humor can serve as an invaluable coping tool, lightening the weight of the medical and institutional environment. Research highlights that humor provides numerous physiological and psychosocial benefits, from reducing stress and alleviating pain to strengthening social bonds and uplifting the overall mood (Wilkins & Eisenbraun, 2009). Laughter also builds connections and eases tension, making difficult situations more manageable. That said, humor must be sensitive to those present and appropriate to the context, ensuring it is well received and adds to the moment.

9.9 Cognitive and Spiritual Shift

Just as life offers opportunities for reinvention and discovery in midlife, it can also provide avenues for personal growth and fulfillment in later years. When people experience a "mid-life crisis," they often change their career goals, adopt new political causes, return to education, seek new friendships, alter their life philosophies, and even embrace new styles of clothing and hairstyles. These changes can bring about a renewed sense of energy and purpose.

Therefore, why not embrace an "end-life crisis" as well? Is there any reason why individuals in their final years cannot experience a similar period of exploration and growth? What's wrong with someone in their later years enrolling in college courses? What is wrong with them joining a political group such as the National Organization for Women or the Sierra Club? What is wrong with embarking on a spiritual retreat or exploring a new religion? What is wrong in expressing themselves through vibrant clothing choices such as fluorescent orange shirts or bright green pants?

Thoughts and attitudes at the end of life can deeply influence a person's well-being and quality of life. Encouraging constructive thinking while compassionately exploring cognitive errors and harmful beliefs helps the person to find peace and meaning. Gently addressing destructive narratives can help individuals reconnect with their self-worth, reframe their perspectives, and focus on the present while preparing for the future.

9.9.1 Tool: Eliminating Self-Blaming Over Illness

When reflecting on their lives, people sometimes harbor thoughts of self-blame. Much of this self-blame reflects irrational cognitive processes, which can hinder the ability to assert control and make constructive choices. These thoughts often stem from underlying beliefs about themselves or the world. These beliefs can be transformed through mindful practices and cognitive shifts, helping individuals move from irrational personalization to reasonable depersonalization. The following activity is designed to facilitate these cognitive shifts:

1. **Discover self-blaming beliefs**: Write down various self-blaming thoughts that frequently occur in one's mind. Aim to generate a list of at least five self-blaming thoughts. Examples include:
   - "If I had followed a healthier diet when I was younger, I wouldn't be so sick now."
   - "If I only had more positive thoughts, I could overcome this illness."
   - "God is punishing me because of my lack of religiosity."
   - "I am not worthy. I am useless."
2. **Brainstorm alternative causes**: Consider other possible causes or explanations for your situations, reminding yourself that some causes are unknown and that some events occur purely by chance.
3. **Create cause-related statements**: Review each self-blaming belief and write a corresponding statement that shifts the blame away from oneself, using similar vocabulary. Examples include:
   - For "If I had followed a healthier diet when I was younger, I wouldn't be so sick now," write "People can get sick regardless of their diet."

- For "If I only had more positive thoughts, I could overcome this illness," write "If positive thinking could eliminate all illness, optimists would never die, yet they die of the same diseases as everyone else."

4. **Journaling:** Journal events and your thought process to raise awareness and aid cognitive exploration.
5. **Post reminders**: Place statements and affirmations around your living space to remind yourself to be compassionate toward the self.

Reflection Everyone has dirt in their lives. Some people grow roses in the dirt, and some people grow weeds.

9.9.2 Tool: The Grass Could Have Been Browner

People nearing death often feel cheated, questioning why their life is ending and longing for more time. This can lead to fantasies of a better existence. To examine this, follow these steps:

1. Close your eyes and envision the fantasies coming true forever.
2. Write down elements of the fantasy world, such as "no aches and pains," "live forever," or "freedom to eat anything."
3. Create a detailed picture of this life, considering both positives and negatives. For instance, think about how pain can be protective or how constant access to food might reduce enjoyment. Similarly, living forever may entail enduring the pain of all loved ones dying or Earth's resources running out without mortality.
4. Shift focus to the current life, identifying its pleasures and advantages. Reflect on meaningful relationships and recent joys that might have been missed without the experiences of the present life.

9.9.3 A Tool: Positive Affirmations

Affirmations can also be used with patients and loved ones. One to three of the following affirmations could be chosen by a terminally ill person to be their personal affirmation(s). Or, even better, a person could create their own affirmation(s). Each affirmation used would be posted on a place visited every day (on a mirror or a refrigerator). Each time the person sees the affirmation, the affirmation is internally (or verbally) repeated three times.

A. Every day, in every way, I am getting more at peace with myself, my family, and my environment.
B. I am a powerful person because I am filled with love.
C. I accept and love myself just as I am.
D. I have already done what I needed to do with my life.

E. My life has truly been full of joy.
F. I am letting go in peace and joy.
G. My body might be leaving this world, but my influence/love will surely remain.
H. I am going into my future with gratitude and courage.
I. I am grateful for the love and support that surrounds me during this journey.
J. Each breath is a gift. Each moment is a blessing.
K. I am at peace with the life I have lived and the legacy I leave behind.
L. I embrace this moment and look forward to merging with infinity/divinity.

9.9.4 Tool: Empowerment by Care

A German proverb goes, "The hand that gives, gathers." Giving implies abundance; helping fosters a sense of empowerment. Those who receive care can experience joy and purpose when given opportunities to care for others.

The loss of jobs and family responsibilities in their final years often leaves people feeling a lack of self-worth, meaning, and purpose. The following activities require minimal time or physical energy; however, they can bring immense satisfaction to everyone involved, fostering a cycle of simultaneous giving and receiving.

A. Bake cookies, make lemonade, and set up a table outside your home with a sign saying: "FREE LEMONADE AND COOKIES."
B. Visit a nursing home or home for individuals with disabilities and spend at least half an hour with someone who rarely receives visitors.
C. Visit a neighborhood playground or shopping mall and give out free balloons to children.
D. Go to a shopping mall and distribute flowers with a tag saying "Have a good day. Please give this flower to someone else." Enjoy watching people walk by with their flowers.
E. Randomly send one- or five-dollar bills to people chosen from a telephone book, imagining how the money might brighten their day.
F. Sit outside a beauty parlor and compliment everyone who exits.
G. Write and send handwritten letters or cards of appreciation to friends, family, or acquaintances.
H. Offer to teach a skill or hobby you enjoy to others, such as cooking, painting, or gardening.
I. Knit infant hats, make baby blankets, or create other handmade items, and donate them to birth centers or hospitals.

9.9.5 Guided Visualization/Imagery: Dialog with Death

The following guided imagery can be read with pauses between sentences to allow them to verbalize the images, thoughts, and responses that come to mind. This dialog can be adapted for different occasions, such as a "Dialog with Pain" or a "Dialog with Stress." Participants may imagine Death in any form—masculine, feminine, genderless, abstract, or symbolic—whatever feels most resonant or meaningful to them. For clarity and consistency, the script uses "it" or "Death" when referring to this figure.

Since these visualizations can be intense, it is essential to assess and customize the script to align with the person's cultural and personal context before introducing more intense visualization. It is often helpful to first create a safe and protective environment. Additionally, a check-in and reflection at the end are important. During the process, be attentive to the reactions to the prompt to provide the needed support.

(1) **Preparation**

Close your eyes and take a deep breath, allowing your chest and abdomen to expand. Hold the breath for a moment, then slowly exhale, letting go of any tension. This deep breathing is repeated a few times until you feel a sense of calm wash over you.

Now, imagine a warm, protective light coming into your crown and surrounding your body. This light can be any color that makes you feel safe and secure. Visualize it to form a protective and loving barrier around you, shielding you from negative energy or thoughts. Know that within this light, you are completely safe and protected. When you feel ready and fully embraced by this protective light, we begin visualization.

(2) **Visualization**

Imagine yourself sitting across from an empty chair. Now, picture Death sitting in that chair as a person. What does it look like? ... How does its face appear? ... What kind of clothes is it wearing? ... What do its hands look like? ...

Think about what you want to say to Death. Speak in the present tense, as if it is truly sitting in front of you...Say everything you want to say and want to do to death...

Now, imagine yourself in Death's chair, looking at yourself. What would it say to you? Speak as if you are Death, responding to the things you said earlier... How would Death reply to your message? ...

Although you cannot make Death disappear, you have some control over how you relate to it. Go back to your original chair and tell Death what you want Death to do. Give Death some instructions. Tell Death how you want it to act from now on... Describe how you want it to look and wear for the next visit...

Now, focus on yourself. Focus on the ideal state of mind and being you want at this moment. Every moment, you have the choice of what state of mind you want to be in. Is it peace? Courage? Clarity, awareness, or love? What is your chosen state of mind? Breathe in, and go to that state of mind.

Now, tell Death to stand up and leave the room… As you watch it leave, tell Death that you know you will see it again, but you expect Death to wait for your invitation before returning and the way you expect it to look. In addition, you will be in your chosen state of mind for the visit…

For now, say goodbye to Death, slowly open your eyes, and rest in your chosen state of mind and being.

(3) **Reflection and Sharing**

Please take a moment to reflect on your experience. How are you feeling? What insights or emotions surfaced during the exercise?

This activity might seem silly to some, but it explores a profound truth. For many, the personification of death can change. Death can transform from an intruder to a welcome guest, from something ugly to something that might even be beautiful, from an enemy to a friend. This activity helps people realize that our relationship with death can change; death can change. Even though it can be intense for the first time, when it is performed multiple times, this exercise may eventually help ease death anxiety when the transitional moment actually arrives. The exercise also opens up conversations to examine attitudes, beliefs, and emotions related to death.

9.9.6 Guided Imagery: My Funeral

(Use the preparation and apply the same caution discussed in the previous exercise before starting the visualization.)

Lying down on the floor, close your eyes, and try to make your body as quiet as you possibly can… Relax deeply… Relax until you feel as though your body and the floor are one… Your life has left you. Only your body remains on the floor…

Your body no longer moves. Your body is dead. Your physical being is gone … Only your consciousness survives, and your consciousness realizes that it is the day of your funeral … Your funeral is about to begin …

You see your body lying in a casket at the end of a funeral parlor. Picture the lid open on your casket and see your dead body lying inside… Notice how you appear … Notice how you have been preserved. Notice what you are wearing …

See the people who have come to your funeral. Look around at who has come. Recognize the individuals. Look into their faces … Notice their expressions … Notice their emotions … Notice those who are mingling with others … Notice those who are silent and reserved …

Imagine people coming up to the casket one at a time. Who is the first person to come up to your casket? … How does this person react to seeing your body? … What would you like to say to this person? Remember you are dead and cannot say anything … Notice the second person who comes up to your casket. What reactions does this person have? … What do you want to say to this person? How do you feel being unable to say those words? … Who is the next person to look at your body? How does this person react? … What thoughts do you have about this person? …

Looking around, is there someone missing that you hoped would be there? … Who is the missing person? … What has caused this person to be absent? … What would you like to say to that person? …

Notice your emotions as you picture your funeral… Focus on those feelings… Experience your feelings. What do you feel?…

Notice the music that is playing at your funeral… Listen to the music as it is being played… Is the music what you wanted to hear?…

Notice the flowers… Are there many? Are there few?… Visualize and smell the flowers at your funeral… How do you feel about these flowers?…

Notice who is getting up to give your eulogy… Listen to what this person says… How do you feel as you listen?…

The funeral is now ending, and the people are leaving… Notice how people look as they are leaving the service… Prepare yourself to leave the service and return to your body…

Now take your attention back to your present physical body, the living body, the body that is lying on the floor at this very moment… Feel the weight of your head… Feel the weight of your pelvis… Feel your heels… Feel your upper body… Feel your upper body move as you take in each breath… Feel the life-giving air enter your body, allowing its life-giving energy to swirl throughout your entire body… You are alive!… Your life is not over yet!… You have more time. What do you want to do with this time?… What did you learn from imagining your funeral? What do you need to do? Who do you need to talk to?…

Slowly open your eyes…

Reflections and Sharing Follow this guided imagery with reflections and discussions:

1. What negative experiences or images did you encounter during the guided imagery? What aspects did you dislike?
2. How can you reduce the likelihood of those negative experiences and images becoming a reality?
3. What positive experiences or images did you have during the guided imagery? What aspects did you enjoy?
4. How can you increase the chances of those positive experiences and images becoming a reality?
5. I noticed that you displayed (a specific body movement or facial expression) when I mentioned (certain words). Would you like to share what you were feeling at that moment?

9.9.7 Case Example: Amanda's Breakthrough

During one of the initial interviews with Amanda, she said, "I feel angry, and I feel cheated." It was easy to assume she felt this way because of her illness and the sense that her future had been taken from her. However, when asked to explain more, Amanda revealed something unexpected.

She shared that she had discovered her husband had been having an affair for seven years with a close friend. Amanda, not feeling assertive, chose not to confront him and continued living with him for three more years, knowing the affair continued, until he eventually left. She felt angry and cheated—not because her future was taken, but because her past felt stolen. She even said, "How can I talk about my future? I didn't have a past."

The hospice director suggested that Amanda might be "stuck" in those years and asked how she planned to get "unstuck" and move beyond them. She said she needed to confront him, though she admitted to not being very assertive. She asked if she could do it over the phone and if someone could be there with her. The agreement was made to do it that way.

Once Amanda got on the phone, she did not need any help. She said everything she needed to say, and she said it with strength. After that visit, she became known as "Amanda the Hun."

9.10 Autonomy and Control at End-of-Life

Respecting the patient's autonomy is a fundamental principle in end-of-life care emphasized by many professions, such as the American Medical Association (AMA, n.d.). This respect involves honoring individuals' wishes and autonomy, ensuring that their preferences guide medical decisions. Empowering patients to actively participate in their care—such as setting personal goals, making informed treatment choices, and advocating for their preferences—enhances their sense of control and dignity. Offering options in daily routines, including meals, activities, and scheduling, further supports this autonomy.

The AMA also recognizes the importance of advance care planning, encouraging physicians to help patients identify what matters most to them when cure is no longer possible and to negotiate difficult decisions about what trade-off to accept between quality and quantity of life.

9.10.1 *Jonathan's Pain Management*

Jonathan was a 36-year-old man with AIDS, total blindness, an esophageal ulcer, and HIV cardiomyopathy. He was receiving a great deal of pain medication, including durable patches, nitroglycerine tablets, propoxyphene napsylate tablets, morphine sulfate liquid, and lidocaine viscous liquid.

As his ailments progressed and medications increased, Jonathan decided to reduce his intake. He sought an acupuncturist to treat the pain associated with his peripheral neuropathy, which caused an intense burning sensation. Nevertheless, he chose acupuncture and discontinued the use of duragesic patches and some medicines.

Even though acupuncture was less convenient and provided about the same level of pain relief as the patches, Jonathan chose to stay with acupuncture because, he explained, it was something he decided for himself, which gave him a sense of empowerment.

9.10.2 *Case Example: Elmer's Empowerment in Pain Relief*

Elmer was living with lung cancer and celiac disease, struggling with constant pain. However, Elmer was resistant to the use of morphine, which to her was a sign of "giving in" to the illness. The couple decided to try reflexology. Each evening, Elmer's wife performed therapeutic foot massages for Elmer. The practice helped ease Elmer's pain and even reduced the need for morphine. More than anything, it gave Elmer a renewed sense of control and connection.

9.10.3 *Case Example: Conflicting Wishes*

Tricia, a young nurse, cared for a woman in her seventies who expressed not wanting artificial feeding. The patient frequently reassured Tricia that she was ready to die and that there was no need to fear death. When Tricia had difficulty eating and became weak, her oldest son insisted that she be fed through a tube and pressured the healthcare team to do so.

For a few weeks, the woman refused to communicate with anyone. When the tube was finally removed, the woman broke her silence during a sponge bath, quietly saying to Tricia, "Thank you, deary. You've been very kind to me. Not everyone has been kind." Days later, she passed away peacefully, never speaking another word to her son or doctor.

Reflection Honoring a patient's choices at the end of life is a principle agreed upon by most but is complicated in reality. This may involve ethical dilemmas, conflicting opinions, and compounded by the family and medical system. All of these factors can obstruct the fulfillment of a patient's end-of-life wishes. The stories above are stark reminders of the need for clear communication, ethical responsibility, and establishing support systems, such as ethics committees and collective advocacy, to navigate these complex situations. Ultimately, it is about ensuring that those at the end of their lives can pass away peacefully with dignity.

9.11 Love and Connection

In today's world, the concept of the family goes beyond traditional definitions. An increasing number of families are composed of diverse and nontraditional structures. So, what exactly defines a family? At its core, a family is characterized by connectedness, interdependence, and intimacy. It is defined by the emotional bonds and mutual support shared among its members, rather than its structural composition. Whether it consists of biological relatives, close friends, or a chosen family, the strength of a family lies in its ability to provide love, respect, and support to one another.

9.11.1 Tool: Activities and Games for End-of-Life Conversations

For those who are terminally ill, knowing that their family members are prepared for their passing can be incredibly reassuring. Various engaging methods designed to facilitate these sensitive discussions in a nonthreatening manner can be incorporated. Here are some ideas:

1. **Reflection and Writing Exercise**
   Each family member spends time alone reflecting on their thoughts and feelings about death and life. Family members write their thoughts in a stream-of-consciousness style, addressing prompts such as the following:
   - What causes people to die?
   - What is the best death you can imagine?
   - Your opinions about an afterlife.
   - Feelings about your own death.
   - The most important aspects of a worthwhile life.
     Family members share their writings in a judgment-free environment, respecting all their opinions as being equally valid.
2. **Hello Game:** The **Hello Game** is designed to start conversations about end-of-life values in a comfortable and engaging way. It involves question booklets and thank-you chips to facilitate discussions on what matters most to the participants through life and death. https://commonpractice.com/products/hello-game.

3. **Heart-to-Heart Cards: Heart-to-Heart Cards** help family members understand each other's wishes for end-of-life care. Originally designed for the Chinese-speaking community, these cards can be used by anyone to discuss various end-of-life scenarios and preferences.
4. **The Death Deck: The Death Deck** is a party game that prompts players to answer thought-provoking questions about death in a group setting. It's a way to explore personal preferences and beliefs about dying in a light-hearted yet meaningful manner.
5. **Go Wish: Go Wish** cards help individuals articulate what is most important to them if their life is shortened by illness. This game encourages participants to prioritize their wishes and discuss them with family members https://gowish.com/
6. **Now and Then Board Game:** "Now and Then" board game guides players through their past, present, and future, prompting discussions on significant life decisions and end-of-life preparations through a mix of fun and deep challenges.

These activities facilitate open communication surrounding end-of-life by incorporating elements of play and reflection. These activities are also beneficial for community workshops and events. For further details and resources, you can visit the Conversation Project https://theconversationproject.org/.

9.11.2 Tool: Coupons

To enhance a sense of care and love, family members might offer personalized coupons that are redeemable at their discretion. Here are some examples:

A. "This coupon is good for a 10-minute back massage."
B. "This coupon is good for one ice cream cone. You choose the flavor."
C. "This coupon entitles you to have me as your slave for a whole afternoon."
D. "This coupon means that I will read to you for an hour from a book of your choice."
E. "This coupon is good for a manicure."
F. "This coupon means that I will be the guardian of your peace and quiet for a whole day."
G. "This coupon entitles you to a three-hour outing of your choice."

9.11.3 Tool: Sharing Dreams

Research shows that people facing death often dream about it, and their family members may experience similar dreams before or after their loved one's passing. Dr. Christopher Kerr's work on dreams related to death and bereavement describes how patients frequently have vivid dreams involving deceased loved ones, providing comfort and reassurance as they approach the end of life (Kerr et al., 2014). Additionally, researchers at the Center for Hospice and Palliative Care in New York reported that nearly all hospice patients in their final weeks experience dreams and visions involving deceased and living friends and relatives, typically offering comfort and appearing highly realistic (Wright et al., 2014). Family members who are terminally ill also report dreaming about death, which can help open discussions about dying within the family, fostering a sense of connectedness and emotional preparedness (Rosen, 2013). Furthermore, these dreams can ease bereavement and strengthen continuing bonds after death occurs (Hewson et al., 2023).

It could be a fun and profound experience to share and discuss dreams. As a group or family activity, each participant could describe one dream they had during the past week, followed by a discussion of feelings and thoughts about that dream. This practice can deepen bonds and provide mutual support during challenging times.

9.11.4 A Tool: Giveaway Ceremony/Party

Giving away a person's possessions can be meaningful when done in a group setting. This ceremony can be conducted by the dying person before they pass away or by an executor (or other designated person) after their death.

1. Send invitations to all those who will receive a gift. Choose music and other elements that reflect the dying person's personality and preferences.
2. During the ceremony, share special memories about each item and explain why it is being given to a particular recipient.
3. Ask each recipient to give a verbal response after receiving their gift.

9.11.5 Tool: Family Litany as Death Is Near

When the dying person is ready to let go, the family might want to gather and recite the following litany, inserting the dying person's name or family title in the blank spaces.

1. **Family spokesperson:** "__________, in knowing that you have led a good and complete life,"
   Family: "We release you."
2. **Family spokesperson:** "__________, in knowing that we are not at all angry with you,"
   Family: "We release you."
3. **Family spokesperson:** "__________, in knowing that you have all our love,"
   Family: "We release you."

4. **Family spokesperson:** "__________, in knowing that we have heard and received your love,"
   Family: "We release you."
5. **Family spokesperson:** "__________, in knowing that there is no more that we can do for you,"
   Family: "We release you."
6. **Family spokesperson:** "__________, in knowing that your suffering will soon be relieved,"
   Family: "We release you."

In presenting this litany to a family, the care provider should explain that only the family will know the right time and place to use it. The care provider can mention that other families have found it helpful but stress that the decision is up to them. The family can also decide whether to recite the litany in the presence of the dying person or in another room. The wording can be customized to reflect love, forgiveness, and gratitude.

9.11.6 Case Example: Priscilla's Birthday Party

Priscilla knew she would be alive for her eightieth birthday, but it would almost certainly be her last. She often reminisced about her relatives, clearly missing them. A couple of weeks before the event, her daughter decided to organize a special surprise. She called about thirty of Priscilla's relatives to see if they could be available to call Priscilla on her birthday. A schedule was formed, staggering the telephone calls throughout the day. As each call came in, her daughter held the phone up to Priscilla's ear. Priscilla received calls from relatives in twelve different states that day, each one filled with greetings and fond memories.

9.11.7 Case Example: Carlo's Wedding Anniversary

Carlos was dying of emphysema. Although he was told that he had only a couple of months to live, he set his heart on making it to his fiftieth wedding anniversary, which was nine months away. His three daughters decided to honor his wish in a unique way. They designed a different fiftieth wedding anniversary celebration each month that he remained alive, with each celebration having a different theme. One month later, they had a tacky gift party. Another month, they organized a remarriage service. Another, they hired an accordion player to serenade the couple. They even had a thirty-one-flavor ice cream party for one month. Carlos and his wife had a ball at each celebration. Carlos managed to celebrate his real fiftieth wedding anniversary and enjoyed eight more wonderful parties before he passed away a couple of weeks later.

9.11.8 Case Example: Christopher's Last Bath

Christopher, in his mid-thirties and nearing the end of his life, spent his final days in a hospice, where he had lost over fifty pounds. Each morning, a nursing assistant would bathe him. One day, Christopher asked to have his father give him the bath instead, and he passed away the next day.

His father honored the request and later reflected, "As I held him in the tub, his whole life rushed back to me. I remembered washing him as a baby, treating his scraped elbow, seeing him on his first day of school, and the moment he told me he was dying. I'm so glad I was able to do that for him; it meant a lot to both of us."

9.12 Concluding Reflection

In the delicate dance of life and death, living and dying, people give, receive, serve, and love. The concepts, stories, and tools shared in this chapter are intended to empower care providers, enabling them to offer holistic, person-centered care that acknowledges and honors the unique journey of each person.

As renowned physician Dr. Elisabeth Kübler-Ross reminds us, the focus should be on seeing the patient as a living human, recognizing their ongoing need for meaning, closure, and dignity. This perspective shifts the focus from merely addressing symptoms to nurturing the whole person, moving from an emphasis on impending death to a fulfilling life. With this approach, care providers are better positioned to offer care that resonates deeply with the emotional, cognitive, and spiritual needs of each person.

The conceptual frameworks, tools, and real-life stories provided in this chapter also aim to enrich the caregiving experience, making it more fulfilling and meaningful for care providers—professionals or family alike.

In the face of human vulnerability and mortality, the bonds created through caregiving stand as a testament to shared humanity. Each act of care, moment of empathy, and gesture of support weaves a strong fabric of love, connection, and mutual healing. Through these interactions and sincere intentions, care providers honor the enduring spirit of those they serve, celebrating their lives and the profound impact they have on each other's growth and healing. While the outcomes of care may not be fully within control, there is reassurance and peace in knowing that these efforts and good intentions contribute to a degree of "heartwarming." The world does not need any more global warming, but any degree of "heartwarming" will bring more peace and healing to the world.

References

American Medical Association. (n.d.). *Caring for patients at the end of life*. AMA Code of Medical Ethics. Retrieved November 24, 2024, from https://code-medical-ethics.ama-assn.org/chapters/caring-patients-end-life

Corr, C. A. (1992). A task-based approach to coping with dying. *Omega: Journal of Death and Dying, 24*(2), 81–94.

Corr, C. A., Corr, D. M., & Doka, K. J. (2019). *Death & dying, life & living* (8th ed.). Cengage Learning.

Deger, S., & Gibson, L. A. (2024). *The book of positive quotations* (p. 698). Globe Pequot.

Frankl, V. E. (1984). *Man's search for meaning: An introduction to logotherapy* (Rev. ed.). Beacon Press.

Hammarskjöld, D. (1982). *Markings* (J. M. Stewart, Trans.). Knopf.

Hewson, H., Galbraith, N., Jones, C., & Heath, G. (2023). The impact of continuing bonds following bereavement: A systematic review. *Death Studies, 48*, 1001. https://doi.org/10.1080/07481187.2023.2223593

Hollis, J. (1996). *Swamplands of the soul: New life in dismal places*. Gotham Books. Retrieved from https://jameshollis.net/hollisBooks/swamplands.htm

Kerr, C. W., Donnelly, J. P., Wright, S. T., Kuszczak, S. M., Banas, A., Grant, P. C., & Luczkiewicz, D. L. (2014). End-of-life dreams and visions: A longitudinal study of hospice patients' experiences. *American Journal of Hospice and Palliative Medicine, 32*(3), 269–274. https://doi.org/10.1177/1049909113517291

Kopp, S. B. (1972). *If you meet the Buddha on the road, kill him! The pilgrimage of psychotherapy patients*. Bantam Books.

Kübler-Ross, E. (1969). *On death and dying*. Macmillan.

Mason, J. (2008). *You can do it--even if others say you can't*. Baker Publishing Group.

Pinna, I., Mahtani-Chugani, V., Cruz-Oliver, D. M., Bonati, P., Ercolani, G., Marchini, F., & Palma, S. (2018). The use of humor in palliative care: A systematic literature review. *American Journal of Hospice and Palliative Medicine, 35*(10), 1344–1352. https://doi.org/10.1177/1049909118764414

Rosen, D. (2013). The dreams of the dying. *Psychology Today*. Retrieved from https://www.psychologytoday.com/us/blog/sleeping-angels/201310/the-dreams-the-dying

Snyder, J. R. (1997). Therapeutic touch and the terminally ill: Healing power through the hands: Krieger/Kunz Method. *American Journal of Hospice and Palliative Medicine, 14*(2), 83–87.

Wasow, M. (1987). The burden of dying with a positive attitude. *Health & Social Work, 12*(3), 239–247.

Wilkins, J., & Eisenbraun, A. J. (2009). Humor theories and the physiological benefits of laughter. *Holistic Nursing Practice, 23*(6), 349–354. https://doi.org/10.1097/HNP.0b013e3181bf37ad

Wright, S. T., Kerr, C. W., Doroszczuk, N. M., Kuszczak, S. M., Hang, P. C., & Luczkiewicz, D. L. (2014). The impact of dreams of the deceased on bereavement: A survey of hospice care provider s. *American Journal of Hospice and Palliative Medicine, 31*(2), 132–138. https://doi.org/10.1177/1049909113479201

Chapter 10
Psychosocial Support for Grieving

10.1 Introduction: Navigating the Complexities of Grief

Consider the following true story: A dedicated student began struggling in class about 6 months after his father died from kidney failure. Prior to that, he had made plans to donate a kidney to his father. He wanted to move forward immediately when testing confirmed his match. However, his father, worried about disrupting his education, insisted on waiting until spring break. The doctor had assured them of his stable condition.

Tragically, a week before the surgery was scheduled, his father's condition worsened, and he passed away unexpectedly. Upon hearing the news, the student tried to rush home but was involved in a car accident and missed the chance to say goodbye. Afterward, he kept himself busy, stepping into the role of "man of the house" to support his mother and younger siblings. Though he believed he was handling the loss, the weight of his grief became overwhelming 6 months later.

He found himself struggling to focus and feeling both physically and emotionally drained. Juggling multiple jobs to support his family financially while wrestling with guilt for not acting sooner, his grief was overwhelming.

This story highlights how grief is more than an emotional response; it is a holistic experience that may manifest in physiological, cognitive, behavioral, social, and spiritual dimensions. Responses to loss are shaped not by the events alone but by the meanings assigned to them and the resources available, influenced by social positioning and cultural expectations around gender, ethnicity, and more.

Earlier theories, such as Kübler-Ross's (1969) Stage Model, depicted grief as a linear, emotion-based process. Contemporary understandings, including the Spiral Model of Grieving and Healing (Ciupak, 2025), present grief as a multifaceted, nonlinear journey shaped by sociocultural dimensions. For example, modern capitalist societies often emphasize productivity, discouraging emotional vulnerability

Y. Z. Ciupak, D. C. Smith, *Death, Dying, and Grief*,
https://doi.org/10.1007/978-3-031-88467-2_10

(Granek, 2014). In individualistic cultures, grief may become privatized and even pathologized, contributing to shame and disconnection (Harris, 2010).

The student's experience exemplifies these dynamics. Pressured by societal ideals of masculinity, he prioritized financial obligations over emotional needs. This internalized conflict deepened his guilt, shame, and sadness. Cultural expectations of productivity left little space for healthy grieving, while his gender identity as a strong and mature man prohibited him from seeking help.

Holistic psychosocial care addresses these complexities by integrating socioculturally embedded affective, cognitive, and behavioral strategies. These approaches explore cognitive constructions, process emotions, and foster constructive behaviors to honor the multidimensional nature of grief. The following section examines how grief intersects with disease, guilt, and depression, providing a foundation for practical tools to support those navigating loss.

10.2 Relationship to Disease

Grief is not an abnormality or a disease but a natural reaction to loss, rooted in human evolution and attachment. It is a "dis-ease," a disturbance of equilibrium triggered by life-altering stressors. While most grief responses are healthy and normal, grief can manifest through physiological symptoms due to its psychobiological connections. Similar to depression, it can impact the immune system, disrupt bodily functions, and elevate stress hormones like epinephrine, norepinephrine, and glucocorticoids, which may increase the risk of inflammation, illness, and cognitive impairment. Although grief is not a direct cause of disease, evidence supports a correlation between physical ailments and mortality (Fagundes & Wu, 2020).

The physiological effects of grief vary based on coping abilities and mechanisms. Healthy methods to manage grief-related stress include exercise, meditation, journaling, and cognitive-behavioral therapy. While normal grief often causes emotional distress, prolonged or complicated grief may lead to heightened symptoms. Non-health-related issues such as poor diet, sleep disturbances, and financial stress during grief can also negatively affect overall health.

10.3 Relationship to Depression

Grief and depression are distinct yet connected experiences, sharing signs such as low energy and sadness. While grief arises from a specific loss, depression may develop independently and often requires clinical intervention. Individuals with a history of depression are more vulnerable to depressive episodes during grief, which can complicate or prolong the grieving process. Unprocessed grief may develop into depression, and a lack of social support increases the risk, often resulting in social withdrawal and isolation.

Distinguishing between common grief, maladaptive grief, and depression can be complex for clinicians and support professionals. The Diagnostic and Statistical Manual of Mental Disorders (DSM-5), published by the American Psychiatric Association, recently included prolonged grief disorder (PGD), a condition characterized by persistent and intense grief lasting more than a year that disrupts daily functioning. Symptoms of PGD include a strong longing for the deceased, difficulty accepting the loss, and a preoccupation with the deceased that hinders adaptation to life without them. Based on the DSM-5 descriptions, key differences between grief and depression include the following: grief develops following a loss and is directly tied to it, whereas depression may develop at any time and encompasses pervasive feelings of despair and worthlessness. Grief symptoms typically improve over time, while depression often requires ongoing treatment (American Psychiatric Association, 2021).

Clinicians may use self-reports or self-assessments to establish symptomatology before treatment. It is advised not to misdiagnose major depressive disorder in the context of bereavement, as symptoms may overlap. Chapter 3 contains a detailed discussion about PGD, which also summarizes the boundary between clinical depressive disorders and PGD.

For most people, acute grief manifestations diminish within a year—a timeline adopted by the DSM-5 (Moreira et al., 2022). However, this trajectory varies depending on factors such as cultural norms, developmental stages, and the circumstances of the loss. Traumatic or unexpected losses, such as those involving violence, are closely linked to prolonged grief and depressive disorders (Fagundes & Wu, 2020). Lenferink et al. (2019) describe traumatic grief as an overlap of persistent complex bereavement disorder (PCBD), depression, and post-traumatic stress disorder (PTSD), which may deepen emotional distress and impede recovery. Meanwhile, unresolved guilt can also intensify depression (Li et al., 2019).

Depression related to grief is not confined to any age group. Older adults, despite their familiarity with loss, face heightened risks of loneliness and depression as social connections diminish over time (Schladitz et al., 2021). At the other end of the spectrum, younger adults also report significant challenges; for instance, 34% experience mild to severe depression following a loss (Moreira et al., 2022).

Socioeconomic factors also shape grief experiences. Limited access to counseling or other resources is often linked with lower education levels and increases vulnerability to depression, PCBD, and PTSD (Lenferink et al., 2019). Financial difficulties can increase feelings of guilt and sadness, while access to resources and supportive systems can help alleviate these effects.

10.4 Relationship to Guilt

Guilt is a deeply interpersonal emotion, arising from one's perception of failing to meet social or personal expectations in relation to others (Bushman & Baumeister, 2025). Mild guilt is a common part of the grieving process, often reflecting the natural tension between what was done and what could have been. Bereavement guilt, as defined by Li et al. (2019), is a remorseful emotional reaction stemming from perceived failures regarding the deceased. It encompasses a range of feelings, including guilt for not preventing the death, for not doing enough, or even for moments of joy after the loss. This complexity often reflects an interplay between helplessness and self-recrimination.

Research indicates strong correlations between guilt, depression, and complicated grief. Li et al. (2019) found that guilt not only coincides with elevated levels of complicated grief and depression but also predicts persistent symptoms a year post-loss. Persistent guilt can overwhelm the grieving process, inducing stress and hindering meaning reconstruction, which ultimately obstructs healing.

If unaddressed, guilt may escalate into shame, a deeper form of self-consciousness involving feelings of inferiority and inadequacy (Gilbert, 2019; Matos & Steindl, 2022). Unlike guilt, which focuses on actions, shame often involves negative perceptions of self-worth, impairing social interactions and creating additional barriers to healing.

Self-compassion offers a powerful pathway for addressing guilt and shame, fostering a kinder and more understanding relationship with oneself. By encouraging individuals to acknowledge their imperfections without judgment, self-compassion helps reframe self-blame and create space for healing (Gilbert, 2019). Developing self-compassion not only alleviates emotional distress but also supports resilience and the ability to move forward meaningfully. The Social-Emotional Tools section contains many tools to foster self-forgiveness.

10.5 Forgiveness

Forgiveness is a complex cognitive-emotional process involving the release of emotions, such as anger, sadness, and guilt. It also involves cognitively reframing the experience in a way that promotes understanding and empathy. Behavioral changes may occur too, such as reconciling with the person who caused harm or adopting rituals to signify emotional release and healing. Alexander Pope, the Enlightenment poet, famously wrote, "To err is human, to forgive, divine" (1888). This reminds us that while making mistakes is a natural part of life, the act of forgiveness transcends our human flaws. Forgiveness is a powerful and transformative process that has been examined by philosophers, social scientists, theologians, and alike. It is more than just a personal emotional release—it serves as a moral and social practice that fosters individual and collective well-being.

From a sociological view, forgiveness functions as an essential tool for maintaining social harmony and cohesion. Sociologists emphasize that forgiveness is not just about individuals—it plays a crucial role in communities and societies by helping to resolve conflicts and reduce cycles of retaliation. In post-conflict societies or fractured communities, forgiveness can serve as a bridge toward reconciliation and peace. This perspective extends the philosophical view of forgiveness as a moral act

(Griswold, 2007), highlighting its capacity to repair not just individual relationships but the broader social fabric. Communities that embrace forgiveness often see it as essential for collective healing, whether in small groups or larger societal contexts.

Psychologists such as McCullough (2001) support this perspective by showing how forgiveness helps individuals contribute to well-being and form pro-social behaviors. His research suggests that those who are more agreeable and emotionally stable are more likely to forgive, fostering healthier, more resilient relationships. At the same time, some studies shift the focus to the transgressor. These found that factors, such as the severity of the transgression, relational closeness, and guilt all play critical roles in motivating offenders to seek forgiveness. Guilt, in particular, was a major driver in prompting transgressors to make amends, which highlights the relational and social importance of forgiveness (Riek, 2010). When offenders actively seek forgiveness, it allows not only for personal reconciliation but also for the restoration of social bonds that might otherwise be damaged.

From a spiritual perspective, forgiving others often serves as a pathway to forgiving oneself. Mother Teresa's insight that "it is by forgiving that one is forgiven" (Kolodiejchuk, 2009, p. 238) reminds the reciprocal nature of forgiveness. When individuals extend forgiveness, they not only release the burden of resentment but also create space for healing within themselves. This journey of forgiveness nurtures personal growth and deeper connections, emphasizing that to truly heal, one must often start by offering forgiveness to others.

Taken together, these insights reveal that forgiveness operates on both personal and societal levels, affecting the relationships with others and oneself. It is not an easy task, but through consistent practice, individuals can cultivate their ability to forgive. As noted by various thinkers, the journey of forgiveness requires effort and dedication; it is often said that "forgiveness is not an occasional act; it is a permanent attitude" (King Jr., 1964). Like any skill, it can be developed over time, reinforcing the idea that continual practice is essential for mastering the art of forgiveness.

It is also necessary to remember that sometimes forgiveness cannot be given, and care providers must accept this reality. It is important not to force the person into a process not ready for. Instead, the care provider's role may simply involve being present, validating the emotions, and meeting people where they are.

10.6 Social-Emotional Tools

10.6.1 Forgiving the Deceased

Forgiving someone who has passed away can become particularly challenging in the context of ambiguous attachment, where emotional bonds are unclear or unresolved. Such ambiguous relationships can leave individuals grappling with emotional turmoil, compounded by the physical absence of the deceased. Finding meaning and acceptance can help dismantle these complexities and foster reconciliation. The following exercise offers an opportunity for such a practice.

Steps

1. Gather three colored papers: yellow, red, and green. On the yellow paper, write things that caused sadness; on the red paper, note what caused anger; and on the green paper, list other hurts from the deceased.
2. Place your hands on the papers and say aloud:

   _________, I forgive you for all the times you made me sad.
   _________, I forgive you for all the times you made me angry.
   _________, I forgive you for all the times you hurt me.
   _________, I, too, have been less than perfect. I may have caused you sadness, anger, and hurt. I love you and cherish the good and love you showed me. Life has its challenges, and I must learn and grow from them. I forgive you. I love you. I must go on learning and growing.

3. Turn the papers over and cut them into flower shapes: a circle for the center from the yellow paper, petals from the red paper, and a stem with leaves from the green paper.
4. Paste these pieces on a large sheet of white paper, with the written sides facing down.
5. Place the completed forgiveness flower on a refrigerator door or another visible spot as a daily reminder of your forgiveness and acceptance of the deceased.

10.6.2 From Guilt to Self-Forgiveness

Guilt often arises from the stories individuals construct about their actions in relation to others, making it a relational and cognitive-mediated emotion. Approaches like Byron Katie's four-question inquiry (Katie & Mitchell, 2017) and Gabor Maté's Compassionate Inquiry (Compassionate Inquiry, n.d.) offer effective tools for reframing these narratives and releasing emotions.

The Work employs structured self-inquiry to challenge guilt-inducing thoughts, repeatedly questioning one's narratives: *Is that true? Are you absolutely sure it's true?* This process uncovers alternative perspectives and fosters cognitive reframing (Katie & Mitchell, 2017).

In contrast, *Compassionate Inquiry* emphasizes the connection between body and mind, encouraging individuals to observe how emotions manifest somatically—through physical sensations—while gently questioning the beliefs sustaining it. This process of somatic awareness and connection creates a space to release emotions, question cognitive narratives, and thereby shift beliefs (Compassionate Inquiry, n.d.). This focus on somatic awareness aligns well with Schachter and Singer's (1962) two-factor theory of emotion, which recognizes that emotions are shaped by both physiological responses and the meaning assigned to them. The exercises below draw on these approaches, providing practical tools that professionals can use to guide individuals to work through guilt.

Step 1: Connect to guilt somatically:

- Where does the guilt show up in the body? If comfortable, close the eyes and allow a little time to connect to the sensation.
- Feel and describe it—does it have a shape or color?
- Breathe deeply and slowly into the area, noticing any shifts.
- If it has a voice, what would it want to say?

Step 2: Ask: Is that true?

- Ask*: Is that (belief/narrative) true?*
- Ask: Can you *absolutely* know your assessment of yourself is justified, given the circumstances at the time?

Step 3: Alternatives:

- Could there be alternative explanations or possibilities?
- How do you react when you believe that thought?
- What does that make you?
- If your friend judges themselves like this, what would you say to them?

Step 4: Forward-Looking:

- What can you now say clearly and sincerely?
- What can you do now for yourself or someone else?
- What can you redo or improve for someone else?
- What actions can you take now to address your deepest regrets?

Step 5: Commit to specific actions that address these reflections.

Step 6: Express gratitude to the deceased for the lessons learned and growth gained through the guilt experienced with them.

10.6.3 Ritual of Self-Forgiveness

1. Prepare three pieces of colored paper: yellow, red, and green. On one side of the yellow paper, write all the things you did or said that might have caused sadness for the departed person. On the red paper, jot down actions or words that might have caused anger. On the green paper, list other ways you may have unintentionally hurt the loved one.
2. Place your hands on the three pieces of paper and recite an affirmation statement like the following:

   > I am just human, and I have made mistakes—we all do. I have hurt people and been hurt. Yet, I choose to focus on the good I've done and not let past mistakes trouble me excessively. I forgive myself for my mistakes. I forgive myself. I forgive myself. I forgive myself. I forgive myself. I have intended well. I've done many good things. Moving forward, I embrace the present with compassion. I am committed to ongoing growth and making positive contributions.

3. Turn the three pieces of paper over and cut them into flower shapes: a yellow circle for the center, red petals, and a green stem with leaves.
4. Paste these paper pieces onto a large sheet of white paper with the written sides facing down.
5. Finally, mount the completed forgiveness flower on a refrigerator door or another prominent place as a daily reminder of self-forgiveness and acceptance.

10.6.4 Forgiving Those Who Hurt Us

When considering forgiveness, it is essential to clarify that forgiving someone who has caused deep hurt or abuse does not condone or validate their actions. Instead, forgiveness allows individuals to release stored pain and reclaim their power. Research supports the idea that forgiveness can reduce psychological distress, depression, and anxiety while fostering emotional well-being and post-traumatic growth (PTG) (Martinčeková & Klatt, 2017; Toussaint et al., 2015). It enables individuals to move beyond the pain of past harms, creating space for healing and growth, irrespective of whether forgiveness of the person is possible or desired.

Forgiveness is often vital for post-traumatic growth, the positive transformation that can arise from adversity (Tedeschi & Calhoun, 2004). Self-forgiveness and forgiving others can play a key role in this process, as they help facilitate emotional release, enhance coping strategies, and reduce feelings of shame. Studies have shown that individuals who integrate forgiveness into their healing journey often experience greater resilience and improved relationships with themselves and others. For example, forgiveness writing therapy has been shown to significantly enhance post-traumatic growth by helping individuals reframe their trauma and find meaning through their pain (Ha et al., 2019).

Furthermore, forgiveness can foster post-traumatic growth by involving spiritual or religious dimensions. Schultz et al. (2010) found that the positive relationship between forgiveness and PTG was mediated by the importance of religion and spirituality, suggesting that these factors can influence how individuals process forgiveness after experiencing interpersonal transgressions.

However, forgiveness should not be seen as a required outcome in all cases. In situations of severe abuse or trauma, healing may not necessarily involve forgiveness, and this is a valid path. Research suggests that other approaches, such as trauma-informed therapy, focusing on self-compassion and consideration of justice in forgiveness, can offer alternative routes to recovery when forgiveness is neither possible nor desired (Winders et al., 2020).

Case Example: Darcey[1]

Darcey's experience highlights the complexities of forgiveness in abusive relationships. As she cared for her dying partner, who had abused her physically and

[1]All stories are based on real-life cases. However, all names in this text except the authors are pseudonyms, and identifying details have been removed to protect the confidentiality of individuals.

emotionally, she faced overwhelming feelings of resentment and guilt. "I had to be his caregiver as he was dying … begging me to forgive him … I couldn't. How could I? I hated myself for even what I was doing." Darcey's story underscores the emotional toll of caregiving in such contexts and how the expectation of forgiveness may feel unattainable or even unjust.

Research indicates that, in cases like Darcey's, the immediate focus may need to be on self-compassion rather than forgiveness. Acknowledging her own strength in surviving and caring for someone who caused her harm is a crucial step toward her healing. Forgiveness may not be the goal, but creating emotional space for self-compassion and setting boundaries can support her in processing the trauma.

Case Example: Treena

Treena's case reveals another dimension of forgiveness after trauma. After her abusive stepfather died, she found that her anger toward him intensified, rather than dissipating. Her anger, that rage, had been complicated by the fact that the object of her anger was no longer present to receive it. In this case, the absence of her abuser complicated her ability to resolve her feelings, leaving her trapped in unresolved emotional turmoil.

In situations where direct forgiveness feels out of reach, individuals like Treena can still experience post-traumatic growth. Reframing the situation and working through anger with therapeutic support can allow for healing, even without reconciling with the person who caused harm. Studies indicate that emotional processing, rather than forgiveness, can foster growth and recovery in such cases (Tedeschi & Calhoun, 2004).

10.6.5 Grieving Diary

A grief diary helps process emotions and preserve memories. Choose a blank book with a meaningful and appealing design. Use it to record thoughts, feelings, and memories, both positive and challenging, without restrictions. Do drawings, add stickers or pictures.

10.6.6 Memory Book

A memory book honors and remembers a loved one by collecting meaningful items.

1. The book's cover can be made from a special material, such as a favorite pattern or a former article of clothing of the deceased.
2. The book could hold items such as

- Birth certificate
- Various photographs

- Diplomas
- Wedding announcement
- Menus from favorite restaurants
- Reminders of vacations taken
- Person's favorite passages from literature or scripture
- Newspaper announcements (birth, school events, marriage, retirement, etc.)
- Letters sent and received
- Funeral service program
- Sympathy cards

3. If multiple family members are participating in the project, each member can take responsibility for gathering materials related to a specific time in the deceased person's life or a particular role they had, such as father, husband, businessman, golfer, or community activist.
4. Leave blank pages for future additions, like new memories or reflections
5. Place the book in a special place to revisit and share over time.

10.6.7 Memory Collage

Gather old magazines, beautiful pictures, a large poster board, scissors, and glue to create a meaningful and personalized collage. Then, cut out pictures and words from the magazines that remind them of the person who has passed away and make a beautiful collage. This collage can be shared with family and friends to remember and honor their loved ones. This activity is also an excellent fit for grief support groups.

10.6.8 Memorial Quilt

The project is to create a quilt where each square represents a special time or different role in the life of a departed person. Some suggestions for creating this quilt are as follows:

- Use fabric paint, embroidery, or special items/mementos to stitch onto the cloth squares.
- This project can be done by a single participant, a couple of bereaved individuals, an entire bereaved family, or several friends and family members.
- After completing the quilt, consider organizing a party to invite family members and friends to come and admire the quilt and share stories about the person being memorialized.

10.6.9 Memory Jar

A memory jar can support grieving by creating a space to collect and reflect on memories. This activity is particularly meaningful for families with children and can be customized with creative touches like drawings, painted notes, or origami. A jar, glass bottle, or box can be used.

Steps to create a memory jar:

1. Choose a large container and place it in an accessible spot. It can hold personal significance, such as belonging to the deceased, but this is not required.
2. Write down memories or thoughts about the loved one whenever they come to mind, and place the notes inside the container.
3. At regular intervals, such as the first day of each month, the person/family can take some time to sit down with the jar and read through the memories that have been added since the last review. This can help them to remember and honor the person they've lost.

Case Example
The Memorial Sculpture

Brad was a popular teen. When Brad got sick, he had many visitors who would come to his room during visiting hours. Typically, there were at least four or five people in the room at any given time. They would talk, reminisce, tell jokes, and act silly.

One day, a couple of weeks before he died, Brad's mother entered his room just before visiting hours and found him crying. "What's wrong, dear?" she asked.

He replied, "Mom, I know I have a lot of friends, and everyone comes and visits me, and everyone seems to have a good time when they're here. But have you noticed that no one ever touches me anymore? They don't touch me. People used to give me hugs all the time. They'd put their arms around my shoulders. Sometimes a handshake. But now, no one touches me, no one hugs me. No handshakes. It's tearing me up inside. It's tearing me up. No one, no one anywhere, should have to die without being touched and held."

Brad's mother later shared Brad's remarks with some of his friends. His friends were moved to show more physical expressions of their love; there was plenty of touching in Brad's room after that.

Brad's friends also decided to make a memorial to Brad after he died. Twenty-seven of his friends gathered one day to put their hand prints in a mold. A wall sculpture was made for the hospital. The sculpture had 27 pairs of hands appearing to reach out from the wall. At the bottom of that sculpture was the Brad's conversation with his mother:

No one, no one anywhere, should have to die without being touched and held.

10.6.10 Service of Remembrance

The funeral service typically takes place within a week of the person's passing when most mourners are still in shock and confusion while handling many logistic matters. A remembrance service held 3–12 months after passing can provide time for planning and allow attendees to process their grief and strengthen connections.

Steps to organize a service:

1. Select a location: Options include a church, a meaningful place frequented by the deceased (e.g., a park or restaurant), or a home.
2. Choose an officiant: This could be a minister, a family member, or a close friend.
3. Determine attendees: Decide whether to include family, friends, or community members.
4. Plan the format: Include elements such as readings, speeches, music, or refreshments.
5. Send invitations: Clearly outline the purpose and structure of the event.

Case Example: Creating Remembrance
A "Dead Denny Party"

When Denny was alive, he used to relax and entertain himself by wearing an old sweatshirt and jeans, taking a stereo to his backyard, listening to Grateful Dead music while enjoying Chianti, and smoking a big cigar. That was his favorite form of relaxation. After Denny's death, his friends started holding an annual "Dead Denny Party" on his birthday. They would gather in someone's backyard, wear sweatshirts and jeans, listen to Grateful Dead music, drink Chianti, and smoke big cigars to honor Denny's memory.

10.6.11 Litany of Remembrance

The following litany can be repeated periodically by someone grieving. A good time for this to be said is when feeling sad or guilty. Just insert the departed person's name in the blank. Feel free to modify or customize it as needed.

"For the good times we spent together, for all those fond memories, for all those special moments we shared: __________, I give you thanks. Thank you for all of those special moments."

"For all the times I said or did something that hurt you, for all the times I caused you any pain or suffering: __________, I ask your forgiveness. Please know that I loved you and did not want to cause you any hurt."

"For all the times you said or did something that hurt me, for all the times you caused me any pain or suffering: __________, I forgive you. I believe you loved me and did not want to cause me any hurt."

"For the early days in our relationship: __________, I will always remember. How could I ever forget?"

"For the easy times in our relationship, when the two of us experienced oneness with each other in thought and heart: __________, I will always remember."

"For the rough times in our relationship, when the two of us had separate ideas and actions: __________, I remember them too. But I will always remember the bigger picture, the greater context."

"For our last good moments together: __________, I will always remember. How could I ever forget?"

"For our future together: knowing that you are no longer with me physically, but you are still a very great part of me nonetheless—a very great part. Thank you."

"__________, I give thanks to you for sharing your life with me. I am so thankful we were able to share our lives together. You have meant so much to me; you mean so much to me now. Thank you. Thank you. Thank you."

Case Example
The Best Sermon

A clergyman had been a minister at a large congregation for a couple of years when his best friend Ray passed away. Ray was a member of the congregation. Although this minister wanted to deliver the eulogy, he asked one of his assistants to do the funeral service.

When it came time for the eulogy, the minister mounted the pulpit. However, before he could even say a single word of his prepared eulogy, he started crying and couldn't stop. Eventually, he simply left the pulpit, unable to say anything.

At the end of the service, three of the minister's parishioners approached him and said, "That was the best sermon I had ever seen."

Reflection: It is okay to allow ourselves to be authentic and vulnerable. This forms the basis for genuine relationships and healing.

10.6.12 Guided Visualization: Dialogue with the Lost One

(Opening) Please make yourself comfortable. Take in a nice, big, and deep breath. As you exhale, allow yourself to let go of any tension you may be experiencing. If you feel comfortable, please close your eyes. Take in another deep breath, feeling the muscles in your body relaxing and softening. As you exhale, release all anxiety or other emotions. Now, take in one more deep breath, feel the body begin to let go, noticing how good it feels just to relax. Then, gently exhale once again. Begin to allow yourself to let go fully. Notice the rhythm of your breathing. Relax as my words flow in and out of your awareness.

(Visualization) Remember your loved one at a time when the two of you were at your best together... Remember your loved one's appearance at that time... Now imagine your loved one sitting in a chair across from you... Imagine the two of you breathing together. You and your loved one breathe in together, ... and out together, ... and in together, ... and out together... Look at your loved one's total appearance... Look at your loved one's face... Look into your loved one's eyes...

You are now going to have a dialogue with your loved one. You are going to be imagining yourself asking some questions and making some statements. You will imagine your loved one responding to your questions and statements... Looking into the eyes of your loved one, imagine yourself giving thanks for all your times together. Imagine yourself thanking this person... What does your loved one say in response to what you have just said?... Looking into the eyes of your loved one, imagine yourself asking forgiveness for all the times you caused your loved one to hurt... What does your loved one say in response?

Looking into the eyes of your loved one, imagine yourself giving forgiveness for all the times your loved one hurt you... What does your loved one say in response?... Looking into the eyes of your loved one, imagine yourself verbalizing some of your greatest fond memories in your relationship... What does your loved one say in response?... Once again, thank this person for your times together...

Once again, imagine yourself breathing in unison with this person. Breathing in together, ... and out together, ... and in together, ... and out together...

You are now about to say goodbye to this person... You will say goodbye, but you can always revisit this person whenever you close your eyes. You will say goodbye, but you will always know that this person is as close to you as your very lungs, breathing in, ... and breathing out, ... and breathing in, ... and breathing out. Slowly say goodbye to this person, watching their image slowly disappear, knowing that your loved one is as close to you as your very lungs, ... breathing in, ... and breathing out, ... and breathing in, ... and breathing out...

(Closing) Return your attention to your body now. Notice where your body connects to the surface you are sitting/lying on. Wiggle your fingers and toes, then bring your arms above your head and have a good stretch. When you're ready, open your eyes.

10.6.13 Guided Visualization: Experiencing Unity

The following could be read to someone or placed on a tape recording for periodic use. It is designed to awaken the senses to refresh the spirit. It can take away tension. It can eliminate preoccupation with personal problems.

(Opening) Please make yourself comfortable. Take in a nice, big, and deep breath. As you exhale, allow yourself to let go of any tension you may be experiencing. If you feel comfortable, please close your eyes. Take in another deep breath, feeling the muscles in your body relaxing and softening. As you exhale, release all anxiety or other emotions. Now, take in one more deep breath, feel the body begin to let go, noticing how good it feels just to relax. Then, gently exhale once again. Begin to allow yourself to let go fully. Notice the rhythm of your breathing. Relax as my words flow in and out of your awareness.

(Visualization) You are walking along a beach. You are breathing in the fresh ocean air… Feel the summer air fill your lungs with gentle warmth… You feel the air's warmth enter your lungs… Warm, fresh, ocean air… It is about five o'clock in the afternoon. The sun is just resting above the horizon, about to go to sleep for the night… The sun is brilliant, glowing orange. The sky is a hazy blue. The sand beneath your feet is a warm, soothing beige… As you walk along the beach, you can feel the massaging warmth of the sand through your toes…

Your lips are brushed with a thin coating of salt. You lick your lips and taste the salt… You hear the refreshing splashes of the waves coming in and going out, … coming in and going out with the same rhythm as your breathing, the breathing of the warm, fresh, ocean air. Coming in and going out… Coming in and going out… A distant seagull, flying toward the setting sun, cries out. Its cries become more and more distant. More and more distant…

As you are walking along the beach, you see in front of you a sand dune, bending and bulging on the horizon. The sand dune is covered with flowers, splashes of yellow, blue, orange, pink… You reach the sand dune and sit down, … stretch your arms to the sky, … and gaze in wonder out to the sea… The ocean shimmers in silver, reflecting the last rays of the setting sun… As the sun slowly dips into the water, you become more and more relaxed. The lower the sun, the deeper your relaxation… The warmth of the ocean air enters your lungs and relaxes you even more, … and more, … and more… All of your being begins to be absorbed into everything that surrounds you… You are the radiant sun… You are the shimmering sea… You are the massaging warmth of the sand… You are the flowers splashed with color… You are the ocean air swirling in your lungs… You are the distant gull crying in joy to the horizon… You are the world at peace, … at rest, … comfortable, … relaxed….

(Closing) Return your attention to your body now. Notice where your body connects to the surface you are sitting/lying on. Wiggle your fingers and toes, then bring your arms above your head and have a good stretch. When you're ready, open your eyes.

Case Example
Tom Was a Gruff Man

Tom was a gruff man. Tom never spoke to people; he always shouted at them. One day, I (Doug Smith) was in Tom's living room along with his wife and sister when suddenly he shouted, "I want the women out of the room! I want them out now!"

After the women left, Tom turned to me and shouted, "Doug, I have a problem!"

(continued)

(continued)

"What's your problem, Tom?" I calmly responded.

"I can't cry, dammit! I can't cry!" shouted Tom.

"You sound angry," I calmly responded.

"I am angry! I can't cry, dammit!"

"People are usually sad when they want to cry. Are you sad, Tom?"

There was this pause. Then Tom shouted, "Yeah, I'm sad, dammit! I'm sad!"

I calmly said, "Tom, I want you to come over here and give me a hug."

"What?!" He shouted.

"I want you to come over here and hug me."

"No! I'm not going to give you a hug!"

"Tom, just come over here."

He took a step forward and gave me this look as if he were trying to determine my sexual preferences.

"Tom, just come over here," I repeated.

Tom slowly walked over, still giving me that look.

"Now, wrap your arms around me." He wrapped what felt like two baseball bats around my shoulders.

"Relax, Tom," I said… He tightened up even more.

"Relax, Tom. It's okay to relax." … He loosened up a little.

"It's okay, Tom. It's okay to relax." … He loosened up some more.

"Relax, Tom… If you would like to cry, it's alright… It's alright… Tom, I want you to know that it's alright." I heard two swallows, a gulp, some quivering, some shaking, and then, all at once, tears started gushing out, going down the back of my shirt.

Tom cried for at least five minutes. Afterward, I felt his hands on my back as he wiped away his tears before standing up.

Tom stood back and exuded a peacefulness I had never seen. He softly said, "You know, Doug, that felt real good." He paused. Then he shouted, "That felt real good, dammit! That felt real good!"

Reflection: Tears can often be the most therapeutic approach and offering a hug can be the warmest language when providing emotional support.

10.7 Cognitive Tools

10.7.1 Relationship Life Review

Reflecting on and sharing memories of a loved one can bring comfort. The following questions can guide the process:

- When did you first meet? Where were you, and what happened?
- What is your fondest memory from the early part of your relationship?

- What was the most challenging time in your relationship? What happened, and how did you overcome it?
- What is your most cherished memory from the later stages of your relationship?
- What will you miss the most and the least about this person?
- How were your last few days together? Were they similar to other days, or were they different?
- If your story were a book, what would the title be?

10.7.2 The Fun(ny) Times

Reflecting on humorous and joyful memories can bring lightness during grief. Consider these questions:

- What is the funniest memory you shared with this person?
- What is the funniest thing they ever said or did?
- What is the funniest movie, show, or event you experienced together?
- What did they enjoy most for fun?
- What could you do or say to make them smile?

10.7.3 Intentions

When grieving, it can feel as though time is standing still. This activity can help in making progress on the healing journey.

1. Write about your intentions to improve physical well-being.
2. Write about your intentions to improve intellectual well-being.
3. Write about your intentions to improve emotional well-being.
4. Write about your intentions to improve social well-being.
5. Write about your intentions to improve spiritual well-being.
6. Conclude with a paragraph to motivate yourself. Celebrate small progress daily, even hour by hour.

10.7.4 Opening Up to Wonder

Routines and habits often dominate one's life. People wake up every morning and go to the same workplace, using the same car and route. The job can be monotonous, involving the same tasks, methods, and colleagues every day. Grieving persons may feel that life has become repetitive, meaningless, and dull.

Here are three ways to break the cycle:

1. Before leaving your house, take a moment to observe your surroundings. Try to notice something that you haven't seen in a while.
2. While driving to work, pay attention to your route. Look for something new or interesting that you haven't noticed before.
3. When interacting with someone familiar, look closely at their appearance, personality, and communication style. Try to identify something that you haven't noticed before.

10.7.5 Life-Giving Energy

This activity focuses on connecting with the life-giving energy within and around:

1. Take a moment to imagine yourself as a young child, full of life-giving energy. Consider the life-giving energy that exists within all children.
2. Now, imagine the life-giving energy that existed between you and your mother during your birth. This energy is present during all childbirths.
3. Think back to the love that your parents shared, which gave birth to you. Imagine the life-giving energy that exists within all love shared by couples.
4. Take your imagination way back to the beginning of time, when the first life-giving energy brought this world into being. Imagine the same energy that brought all worlds into existence.
5. Bring forth into your present consciousness, into your present state of being, the life-giving energy of creation that was expressed through this world and all other worlds that came into being. All of that life-giving energy. All of that is in you.
6. Bring forth into your present consciousness, into your present state of being, the life-giving energy of love that was expressed in your parents and all other lovers of all time. All that life-giving energy. All of that is in you.
7. Bring forth into your present consciousness, into your present state of being, the life-giving energy of your youth, the life-giving energy that is in all children. All of that life-giving energy. All of that is in you.

10.8 Social-Behavioral Approaches

10.8.1 Creating a Buddy System

A buddy system can connect individuals experiencing similar losses (e.g., spouse, child, or suicide-related losses). Groups of two to five grievers provide mutual support by checking in with one another. When a member is struggling, they can reach out to another for a visit or a phone conversation, fostering connection and comfort during difficult times.

10.8.2 Being My Own Best Caregiver

When feeling overwhelmed, practicing self-care can help nurture well-being. Consider these acts of kindness:

- Visualize yourself as healthy, grounded, and at peace.
- Engage in physical activity such as uninhibited dance or simple workouts to stimulate the body and lift the mood.
- Observe and journal little beauty or wonders in the surroundings.
- Spend time with supportive and nurturing people.
- Practice body-mind connection exercises, such as yoga, Taichi, meditation, and more.
- Eat nutritious foods and drinks.
- Take a nap.
- Take a hot bath or walk in nature.
- Breathe deeply, noticing the long and calming exhales.
- Take a massage or warm water foot bath with aromatic herbs.
- Listen to relaxing music or motivational/inspirational talks.

10.8.3 Becoming Proactive with the Reactive

Many responses to grief are natural and normal. However, some repetitive responses may negatively impact health. This activity helps redirect those responses toward positive and constructive possibilities.

1. **Identify responses**: Choose four intense grief responses from this list:
   - Numbness
   - Confusion
   - Exhaustion
   - Denial
   - Anger
   - Hate
   - Cynicism
   - Guilt
   - Sadness
   - Hopelessness
2. **Describe the response**: Share or write a sentence describing how each chosen response manifests.
   - Example: *"Anger: I often feel angry at people, myself, and everything around me since the loss."*
   - Example: *"Guilt: I feel guilty for not spending more time with my loved one."*

3. **Plan an alternative**: For each response, outline a constructive alternative action or mindset.
   - Example: *"Anger: I will manage my anger by reading a book on anger management and applying its strategies."*
   - Example: *"Guilt: I will focus on spending more time with family to honor their memory."*
4. **Keep sentences accessible**: Place these sentences somewhere easy to find. Revisit them when the feelings arise to remind yourself of your goals and how to move forward.

10.8.4 Commitment to Myself

After processing the pain and releasing tears, a firm commitment to healing and growth can be transformative. As the Chinese proverb says, "You cannot prevent the birds of sorrow from flying overhead, but you can prevent them from making nests in your hair." Writing down intentions can turn them into measurable, actionable steps toward healing.

I, ____________________, make the following commitments to myself and those I love. I make these commitments as my personal contribution to my healing process, realizing that I must help myself if I am ever going to heal. I agree to do the following, commencing on the dates stated.

1. Physical Revitalization

   I will enhance my physical well-being by engaging in the following activities:
   Activity (a): ____________________________ Date: __________
   Activity (b): ____________________________ Date: __________
   Activity (c): ____________________________ Date: __________
   Activity (d): ____________________________ Date: __________
2. Mental Revitalization

   I will nurture my mental well-being by engaging in the following activities:
   Activity (a): ____________________________ Date: __________
   Activity (b): ____________________________ Date: __________
   Activity (c): ____________________________ Date: __________
   Activity (d): ____________________________ Date: __________
3. Social Revitalization

   I will enrich my social connections through the following activities:
   Activity (a): ____________________________ Date: __________
   Activity (b): ____________________________ Date: __________
   Activity (c): ____________________________ Date: __________
   Activity (d): ____________________________ Date: __________
   Signature: ______________________________ Date: __________
   Witnesses (Who will hold me accountable?):
   ____

10.9 Concluding Reflection

Grieving is a nonlinear process that ebbs and flows. This chapter adopts a holistic approach to grief support, using holistic psychosocial tools structured around cognitive, social-emotional, and social-behavioral dimensions of human experience. While each tool may emphasize a specific aspect of grieving, all are interwoven to foster emotional expression, reflection, and actionable coping strategies. Activities such as creating memory books, practicing forgiveness, or engaging in guided visualizations help individuals explore their feelings while nurturing connections and self-compassion. These tools embrace the dynamic and evolving nature of grief, empowering individuals and their supporters to navigate the complexities of loss with understanding and grace. The real-life stories featured in this chapter inspire customized rituals and exercises. As Vicki Harrison eloquently noted, "Grief is like the ocean; it comes in waves, ebbing and flowing. Sometimes the water is calm, and sometimes it is overwhelming. All we can do is learn to swim" (as cited in Newmark 2022, p. 140). These tools hopefully serve as a helpful hand, offering strength to navigate the waves and regain balance.

References

American Psychiatric Association. (2021, September 22). *APA offers tips for understanding prolonged grief disorder*. [News Release]. Retrieved from https://www.psychiatry.org/newsroom/news-releases/apa-offers-tips-for-understanding-prolonged-grief-disorder

Bushman, B. J., & Baumeister, R. F. (2025). *Social psychology and human nature* (6th ed.). Cengage Learning.

Ciupak, Y. (2025). *Spiral model of grief and healing: An integrative sociological, psychological, and cultural framework [Unpublished manuscript]*. Northern Michigan University.

Compassionate Inquiry. (n.d.). *The approach*. Retrieved November 27, 2024, from https://compassionateinquiry.com/the-approach/

Exline, J. J., Worthington, E. L., Hill, P., & McCullough, M. E. (2003). Forgiveness and justice: A research agenda for social and personality psychology. *Personality and Social Psychology Review, 7*(4), 337–348. https://doi.org/10.1207/S15327957PSPR0704_06

Fagundes, C. P., & Wu, E. L. (2020). Matters of the heart: Grief, morbidity, and mortality. *Current Directions in Psychological Science, 29*(3), 235–241. https://doi.org/10.1177/0963721420917698

Gilbert, P. (2019). Distinguishing shame, humiliation and guilt: An evolutionary functional analysis and compassion focused interventions. In *The bright side of shame: Transforming and growing through practical applications in cultural contexts* (pp. 413–431). Springer.

Granek, L. (2014). Mourning sickness: The politicizations of grief. *Review of General Psychology, 18*(2), 61–68.

Griswold, C. (2007). *Forgiveness: A philosophical exploration*. Cambridge University Press.

Ha, N., Bae, S. M., & Hyun, M. H. (2019). The effect of forgiveness writing therapy on post-traumatic growth in survivors of sexual abuse. *Sexual and Relationship Therapy, 34*(1), 10–22.

Harris, D. L. (2010). Healing the narcissistic injury of death in the context of Western society. In J. Kauffman (Ed.), *The shame of death, grief, and trauma* (pp. 75–86). Routledge.

Katie, B., & Mitchell, S. (2017). *A mind at home with itself*. HarperOne.

King, M. L. Jr. (1964). *Nobel Peace Prize acceptance speech*. Biography. Retrieved from https://www.biography.com/activists/martin-luther-king-jr

Kolodiejchuk, B. (2009). *Mother Teresa: Come be my light*. Doubleday.

Kübler-Ross, E. (1969). *On death and dying*. Macmillan.

Lenferink, L. I., Nickerson, A., de Keijser, J., Smid, G. E., & Boelen, P. A. (2019). Reciprocal associations among symptom levels of disturbed grief, posttraumatic stress, and depression following traumatic loss: A four-wave cross-lagged study. *Clinical Psychological Science, 7*(6), 1330–1339.

Li, J., Tendeiro, J. N., & Stroebe, M. S. (2019). Guilt in bereavement: Its relationship with complicated grief and depression. *International Journal of Psychology, 54*(4), 454–461. https://doi.org/10.1002/ijop.12483

Martinčeková, L., & Klatt, J. (2017). Mothers' grief, forgiveness, and posttraumatic growth after the loss of a child. *OMEGA—Journal of Death and Dying, 75*(3), 248–265.

Matos, M., & Steindl, S. (2022). Shame in the context of grief. In *Compassion-based approaches in loss and grief* (pp. 157–166). Routledge.

McCullough, M. E. (2001). Forgiveness: Who does it and how do they do it? *Current Directions in Psychological Science, 10*(6), 194–197. https://doi.org/10.1111/1467-8721.00147

Moreira, D., Azeredo, A., Moreira, D., Favero, M., & Sousa-Gomes, V. (2022). Why does grief hurt?: A systematic review of grief and depression in adults. *European Psychologist, 28*, e490. https://doi.org/10.1027/1016-9040/a000490

Newmark, A. (2022). *Chicken soup for the soul: Grieving, loss and healing: 101 stories of comfort and moving forward*. Chicken Soup for the Soul.

Pope, A. (1888). *Selected poems: The essay on criticism; The moral essays; The Dunciad*. Google Books.

Riek, B. M. (2010). Transgressions, guilt, and forgiveness: A model of seeking forgiveness. *Journal of Psychology and Theology, 38*(4), 246–254. https://doi.org/10.1177/009164711003800402

Schachter, S., & Singer, J. (1962). Cognitive, social, and physiological determinants of emotional state. *Psychological Review, 69*(5), 379–399. https://doi.org/10.1037/h0046234

Schladitz, K., Löbner, M., Stein, J., Weyerer, S., Werle, J., Wagner, M., Heser, K., Scherer, M., Stark, A., Kaduszkiewicz, H., Wiese, B., Oey, A., König, H.-H., Hajek, A., & Riedel-Heller, S. G. (2021). Grief and loss in old age: Exploration of the association between grief and depression. *Journal of Affective Disorders, 283*, 285–292.

Schultz, J. M., Tallman, B. A., & Altmaier, E. M. (2010). Pathways to posttraumatic growth: The contributions of forgiveness and importance of religion and spirituality. *Psychology of Religion and Spirituality, 2*(2), 104–115.

Tedeschi, R. G., & Calhoun, L. G. (2004). Posttraumatic growth: conceptual foundations and empirical evidence. *Psychological inquiry, 15*(1), 1–18.

Toussaint, L. L., Worthington, E. L., & Williams, D. R. (2015). *Forgiveness and health: Scientific evidence and theories relating forgiveness to better health*. Springer Netherlands.

Part V
Supporting Spiritual Needs in End-of-Life and Grieving

Chapter 11
Spiritual Support for End-of-Life and Grieving

11.1 Introduction: Human's Search for Meaning

Significant losses and encounters with death often evoke existential anxiety, prompting individuals to seek meaning and order in their experiences. Humans are inherently driven by a need for meaning. People strive to create order, make sense of their daily encounters, and attach significance to their experiences. Viktor Frankl (2006) considers that meaning underlines all human motivation and is essential for mental health. Sociologist Peter Berger (1969) identifies two forms of order that provide structure: *nomos,* which brings coherence to daily life, and *cosmos*, which situates individual lives within a greater sacred whole. These frameworks help people understand both the mundane and profound aspects of human existence, particularly when confronting mortality. Anthropologist Morton Klass (2018) describes how diverse cultures construct "ordered universes" to address life's ultimate questions, such as "Why is this happening?" or "What will happen after death?"

The search for meaning and the existential quest are not solely personal endeavors; they are deeply influenced by cultural traditions, communal practices, and societal narratives. Collective spiritual experiences connect individuals to a broader social identity, fostering a sense of purpose and resilience during crises (James et al., 2003). While spirituality is often deeply personal, it is embedded within social and cultural contexts. For professionals supporting individuals at the end of life or in grief, understanding these broader contexts is crucial.

Y. Z. Ciupak, D. C. Smith, *Death, Dying, and Grief*,
https://doi.org/10.1007/978-3-031-88467-2_11

11.1.1 Spirituality and Religiosity

The concepts of spirituality and religiosity are distinct yet interconnected. Perspectives in scholarship and clinical practice present a spectrum: some equate spirituality with religion, while others view them as separate, exemplified by the growing "Spiritual but Not Religious" (SBNR) movement. This book adopts a holistic perspective, defining *spirituality* as the human pursuit of meaning, connectedness, and transcendence (Willemse et al., 2020), with religious practice as one of its potential expressions.

Spirituality encompasses more than beliefs; it includes practices, symbols, customs, emotions, and relationships (Roberts & Yamane, 2020). Within Maslow's hierarchy of motivation in human nature, spirituality fulfills belonging needs—by fostering connection and community—and self-actualization needs. At its highest level, spirituality facilitates transcendence, enabling individuals to pursue meaning and connect with something greater than themselves (Maslow, 1971).

11.1.2 Spiritual Diversity

Spiritual and religious expressions are becoming increasingly diverse in today's interconnected world. Religious pluralism has expanded, with many individuals blending traditional practices with personalized beliefs. This diversity underscores the importance of understanding how spirituality is influenced by culture, community, and personal identity. A systematic review of religious beliefs regarding major end-of-life issues across the five major world religions reveals significant heterogeneity within these religions, influenced by factors such as the country of origin, level of education, and degree of intrinsic religiosity (Chakraborty et al., 2017).

At the same time, a growing number of people identify as "Nones" or describe themselves as "Spiritual but Not Religious" (SBNR). Despite increased recognition of these groups, gaps persist in understanding their existential challenges and spiritual needs, particularly during times of loss. Professionals working with these populations must remain open and adaptable, recognizing that meaning-making and spiritual exploration take many forms.

Cultural diversity in spiritual practices necessitates cultural humility. Unlike the fixed goal of "cultural competency," cultural humility involves an ongoing commitment to learning and recognizing the diversity within communities. This approach fosters a deeper appreciation of how spirituality intersects with cultural identity and grief. (Refer to Chap. 2: Culture in End-of-Life and Grief Support)

11.1.3 Spiritual Support in End-of-Life and Grieving

Spiritual support is essential in end-of-life care and grief, addressing existential and emotional needs during these profound experiences. Controlled trials with advanced cancer patients demonstrate that meaning-centered psychotherapy significantly improves spiritual well-being, fosters a sense of meaning, and reduces anxiety. These findings highlight the intersection of spiritual and psychological dimensions in enhancing well-being (Breitbart et al., 2010).

However, as discussed earlier, spiritual support extends beyond individual therapy sessions. Individual or communal rituals and practices enhance resilience and a sense of connection.

The integration of spiritual care into healthcare and social work practice has gained increasing recognition. Research highlights the positive impact of spirituality on mental and physical health outcomes, with spiritual needs now recognized as essential components of holistic care in palliative settings (Puchalski et al., 2009). For example, the World Health Organization (WHO, n.d.) identifies a holistic framework for palliative care that addresses spiritual needs alongside physical, emotional, and social dimensions of care.

In 2009, experts from various disciplines gathered to establish guidelines for improving spiritual care, which resulted in the development of the influential Consensus Report on spiritual care in palliative settings (Puchalski et al., 2009). Participants identified literature-based categories of spiritual care and outlined approaches for implementing these concepts. These recommendations became foundational guidelines, emphasizing the integral role of spiritual care in quality palliative care, in alignment with the National Consensus Project and the National Quality Forum.

The Consensus Report on spiritual care in palliative settings outlines various interventions to support spiritual well-being. These approaches can be grouped into three main categories: therapeutic communication techniques, therapy-based interventions, and self-care and social support practices.

Therapeutic Communication focuses on being present with compassion and deep listening. This approach allows for mirroring and validation, asking about key life events, and helping individuals identify the spiritual strengths that sustain them. Open-ended questions and active listening can invite engagement and offer a safe space to explore deep emotions, personal beliefs, and values. Life reviews and storytelling create meaningful moments, reflections, and reconciliations. Ongoing support reinforces a trusting therapeutic alliance.

Therapeutic Modalities are diverse. Techniques like guided visualization can help transform experiences of "meaningless pain," and work on healing from the subconscious level. Practices such as progressive relaxation, mindful breathing, and contemplation help reduce stress and bring emotional and spiritual balance. Therapies focused on meaning and dignity offer ways to explore life's purpose, maintain a sense of worth, and reconstruct the narrative surrounding the self, loss, and life. If deeper spiritual care is needed, connecting with chaplains, spiritual care providers, and other referrals may offer additional culturally responsive support.

Self-care and Social Support are essential in building spiritual resilience. Practices such as meditation, reading sacred texts, and engaging in rituals are shown to be effective in promoting peace and healing. Mindfulness-based activities such as yoga, and tai chi help strengthen the mind-body connection. Creative outlets such as music, art, dance, and journaling offer powerful ways to process emotions. Seeking reconciliation with oneself or others, along with participating in spiritual support groups and communities, can further cultivate inner peace and connection.

This chapter presents tools grounded in these recommendations, ranging from spiritual assessments to mindfulness exercises and culturally sensitive rituals. Professionals are encouraged to adopt a holistic approach that tailors these tools to individual and cultural contexts.

As Henri Nouwen poignantly stated, "…a shared pain is no longer paralyzing, but mobilizing when it is understood to be a way to liberation. When we become aware that we do not have to escape our pains but can mobilize them into a common search for life, those very pains are transformed from expressions of despair into signs of hope" (Nouwen, 2014, p. 102). The exercises provided in this chapter aim to guide individuals and support providers in transforming emotional wounds into catalysts for growth and healing.

11.2 Spiritual Assessments

Spiritual assessments help understand and utilize people's strengths during end-of-life and grief. They facilitate an exploration of the spiritual vocabulary and needs.

11.2.1 Consensus Report

The Consensus Conference Report on Enhancing the Quality of Spiritual Care within Palliative Care (Puchalski et al., 2009, p. 894; commonly referred to as the Consensus Report) highlights typical spiritual concerns that may arise during this process. These include existential questions, a sense of abandonment by God or others, conflicting belief systems, and feelings of despair. The report suggests that spiritual concerns warrant diagnosis when they meet the following criteria:

1. The spiritual issue results in distress or suffering, such as a lack of meaning, conflicted religious beliefs, or an inability to forgive.
2. The spiritual issue is the root cause of a psychological or physical diagnosis, leading to conditions like depression, anxiety, or acute or chronic pain. For example, severe feelings of meaninglessness may lead to depression or thoughts of suicide, while unresolved guilt may manifest as persistent physical pain.

3. The spiritual issue acts as a secondary cause or influences the psychological or physical diagnosis. For instance, difficulties controlling hypertension may occur when a person refuses medication due to religious beliefs.

The Consensus Report also emphasizes the importance of addressing these concerns through interventions that incorporate therapeutic communication, spiritual therapy, and self-care techniques. These spiritual health interventions serve as a critical component of the care plan, aiming to alleviate suffering and improve the overall quality of life.

To facilitate the integration of spiritual care into palliative care settings, the Consensus Report outlines three key stages of communication and assessment:

1. Initial screening for potential spiritual concerns.
2. A spiritual history conducted by trained support providers, and
3. A comprehensive spiritual assessment carried out by a board-certified chaplain.

This multi-step process ensures that spiritual care is considered a routine part of individual evaluations. Various professionals, such as physicians, nurses, social workers, and spiritual counselors, can conduct spiritual histories, though a formal spiritual assessment often requires specialized training. Board-certified chaplains are typically responsible for documenting these findings and collaborating with other support providers to inform care plans.

11.2.2 Spiritual History Tools

Several spiritual history tools, including the FICA, HOPE, and Domains of Spirituality assessments, are widely endorsed. These tools capture both objective data (such as religious affiliation and spiritual practices) and subjective areas (like the significance of beliefs and sources of hope). Each tool offers a framework for understanding the individual's spiritual landscape and how it intersects with their healthcare and support needs.

Unlike the structured nature of spiritual history-taking, primary spiritual assessments are not limited to fixed questions. Instead, they serve as interpretive frameworks that emerge from listening to and engaging with the patient's unfolding narrative and lived experiences. Due to the complex nature of these assessments and the specialized clinical training required, the Consensus Report recommends that only board-certified chaplains or equivalently trained spiritual care providers undertake this form of assessment.

This section introduces various tools that can facilitate different types of spiritual communication and assessment:

(1) *HOPE Questions:*

- *H*—Sources of Hope, Strength, Comfort, and Peace: What gives you hope, strength, comfort, and peace?

- *O*—Organized Religion: Do you identify with any organized religion or spiritual community?
- *P*—Personal Spirituality and Practice: What role does your spirituality play in your life? Do you engage in any spiritual practices?
- *E*—Effects on Medical Care and End-of-Life Issues: How does your spirituality influence your approach to medical care and end-of-life decisions?

Source: Anandarajah, G., & Hight, E. (2001). Spirituality and medical practice: Using the HOPE questions as a practical tool for spiritual assessment. *American Family Physician, 63*(1), 81–89.

HOPE is a commonly used spiritual assessment too, but the emphasis on organized religion may not be inclusive for the diverse "spiritual but not religious" population. The FICA tool emphasizes the significance of faith and its influence on healthcare decisions.

(2) *FICA Spiritual History Tool:*

- *Faith/beliefs*: What is your faith or belief?
- *Importance/influence*: How important is your faith or belief in influencing your life?
- *Community*: Are you part of a spiritual or religious community?
- *Address in care*: How would you like your healthcare provider to address these spiritual issues in your care?

Source: Puchalski, C., & Romer, A. L. (2000). Taking a spiritual history allows clinicians to understand patients more fully. *Journal of Palliative Medicine, 3*(2), 129–137.

The *SPIRITual History tool* takes a broader approach, considering personal and communal spiritual beliefs and their implications for medical care.

(3) *SPIRITual History Dimensions:*

- *S*: Spiritual Belief System
- *P*: Personal Spirituality
- *I*: Integration and Involvement in a Spiritual Community
- *R*: Ritualized Practices and Restrictions
- *I*: Implications for Medical Care
- *T*: Terminal Event Planning (Advanced Directives)

Source: Maugans, T. A. (1996). The SPIRITual history. *Family Medicine, 28*(1), 11–16.

(4) *JAREL Spiritual Well-Being Scale Dimensions:*

- *Relationship with God*: Exploring the person's relationship with a higher power or God.
- *Purpose and Meaning in Life*: Assessing the individual's sense of purpose and meaning.
- *Connectedness with Others*: Examining the person's sense of connectedness with others.

Source: Hungelmann, J., Kenkel-Rossi, E., Klassen, L., & Stollenwerk, R. (1996). Focus on spiritual well-being: Harmonious interconnectedness of mind-body-spirit—Use of the JAREL spiritual well-being scale. *Geriatric Nursing, 17*(6), 262–266.

11.2.3 Word Association

When assessing spirituality, it is crucial to approach the process with an open mind. Spiritual language can be highly individualized, with interpretations varying even among people from the same tradition. As Sri Ramakrishna beautifully said, "Many are the names of God and infinite the forms that lead us to know Him. In whatsoever name or form you call on Him, in that very name and form you will see Him" (Ramakrishna, 1942/1999, p. 154). This reflects the diversity of spiritual perspectives and the importance of respecting each person's unique spiritual journey. Embracing this diversity requires openness and respect for each individual's spiritual perspectives and experiences.

To perform this assessment, encourage the client to share the first word that comes to mind when they hear specific spiritual terms. Then, invite them to elaborate on their responses. This process should unfold without interruption, allowing space for the individual's spiritual narrative to emerge.

Alternatively, provide a list of quotes and see which one(s) the client resonates with the most. This method can open up a deeper dialogue about their personal connection to spiritual concepts. Some examples regarding "God" include

- *"It is good if man can bring about that God sings within him."*—Rabbi Elimelekh of Lizhensk (Elimelekh, as cited in Buxbaum, 1999, p. 187)
- *"I searched for God and found only myself. I searched for myself and found only God."*—Rumi (Barks, 2004)
- *"The LORD is compassionate and gracious, slow to anger, abounding in love."*—The Bible (Psalm 103:8, New International Version)
- *"If you wish to be free, know you are the Self, the witness of all these, the heart of awareness."*—Ashtavakra Gita (Nityaswarupananda, 1932/2001, p. 10)
- *"Many are the names of God and infinite the forms that lead us to know Him. In whatsoever name or form you call on Him, in that very name and form you will see Him."*—Sri Ramakrishna (Ramakrishna, 1942/1999, p. 154)

These quotes highlight the variety of ways people interpret the concept of "God." Allowing the client to select the quote that resonates with them most can provide meaningful insights into their spiritual worldview.

Suggested terms to explore include

- God
- Suffering
- Prayer

- Life
- Afterlife
- Love
- Consciousness

11.2.4 Spiritual Life Map

A spiritual life map is a tool or visual representation to explore and understand their spiritual journey, beliefs, experiences, and more. It serves as a reflective guide to one's spiritual path. Creating a spiritual life map often involves mapping out key events, milestones, influences, and insights that have shaped an individual's spiritual growth and understanding. Identifying successful tactics that clients have employed in the past often suggests options for addressing current difficulties. Research and clinical findings establish the spiritual life map as an effective client and culture centered tool, respecting the client's autonomy and fostering a strong personal connection (Hodge, 2005; Bushfield, 2010). The spiritual life map brings many strengths to the assessment and therapeutic process.

Prepare a sizable piece of paper, such as 24″ × 36″. Have a variety of drawing tools with different sizes and colors on hand. Additionally, gathering various types and colors of construction paper, along with magazines and scrapbooking materials, can be beneficial. To facilitate the process, include scissors, glue sticks, and rulers. These items will allow the client to cut and paste elements onto their life map, making the activity more interactive and tailored to their preferences.

Guide the client in sketching a chronological path or roadway that depicts their spiritual journey from birth to the present and potentially extending beyond into the afterlife. Encourage the use of hand-drawn symbols, cut-out pieces, and other representations to mark key events along this journey. Since many spiritual traditions view material existence as an extension of sacred reality, the client may want to incorporate significant life events such as marriages, the birth of a child, or the death of a loved one on the map.

To optimize the instrument's potential, invite clients to integrate life crises they've faced into their maps, along with the inner and external resources they utilized to overcome those challenges. Symbols like hills, bumps, rain, clouds, lightning, and the sun, can be employed to illustrate various life situations and sentiments. By delineating successful strategies clients have employed in the past, you can uncover options for overcoming present struggles.

While providing clients with general guidelines may be necessary, actively encourage creativity and self-expression in the life map creation process.

11.2.5 Exploratory Questions

In this spiritual assessment, ask the client to write down or verbalize his or her answers to some or all of the following questions:

A. How would you describe your basic philosophy or belief system? In other words, what is the "glue" that holds your world together?

B. How would you describe your purpose in living? In other words, what do you believe is the best use of your life?

C. Do you believe that there is a force or a being responsible for creating and sustaining of our existence? If so, why? If not, why not?

D. What are your views on the causes of pain and suffering that exist in this world?

E. How would you describe who or what you were before you were born?

F. How would you describe who or what you will be after you die?

G. Is there a symbol(s) that is significant to you?

11.2.6 Imagined Roles

Gauging someone's spiritual beliefs can sometimes be challenging, especially when there's a risk of causing discomfort or offense. One way to gently explore a person's values and beliefs is through imaginative exercises. These hypothetical scenarios allow individuals to express their core principles in a creative and non-confrontational way. The following method offers insights into their spiritual and ethical worldview, helping you better understand and support them.

Exercise 1: The President of the Board of Directors
"Imagine that you are the president of the board of directors of the largest building in your community. You have complete control over how the building is used and what the staff does."

- **A**. How would this building be used to promote your values? What activities or services would take place regularly to reflect what is most important to you?
- **B**. What responsibilities and behaviors would you expect from the staff in order to uphold the mission of the building?

This exercise provides a unique window into the person's value system by allowing them to reflect on how they would manage resources and people to align with their spiritual and ethical beliefs.

Exercise 2: The Dean of a Seminary
"Now, imagine you are the dean of a seminary. You have the authority to determine the core curriculum for all seminarians. You are tasked with selecting four required courses that every seminarian must take, regardless of their spiritual background or denomination."

- What would those four courses be? Why are they essential to the spiritual formation and development of future leaders?

This scenario encourages the individual to think about the fundamental aspects of spiritual education they consider most valuable. Their choices of courses can reveal key insights into their personal beliefs and priorities regarding spiritual growth and moral development.

11.2.7 Case Example: Spiritual Language (Narrated by Doug Smith)

During my first visit to Jim's house, his wife, Barbara,[1] greeted me at the door, asking me to keep it brief because Jim had a rough night. Yet, when I entered, there was Jim at the kitchen table in a sharp three-piece suit, a stark contrast to Barbara's request. I compromised, shortening the usual 40-min visit to 20. In my haste to leave, I accidentally left my overcoat behind.

Back at the office, Jim called, reminding me about my coat and insisting I come by at 5 o'clock sharp. His mysterious tone piqued my curiosity.

At 5, I arrived to find Jim dressed casually in blue jeans, his wig from earlier set aside. He greeted me at the door, saying, "It's okay, Doug. Barbara's in the basement under a hair dryer. We've got twenty minutes. Come on in."

As we settled in, Jim handed me a beer and turned the conversation to something he missed—Stormy's Bar.

Jim: "You know what I miss the most?"
Me: "No, Jim. What do you miss?"
Jim: "I miss Stormy's Bar."
Me: "Why do you miss Stormy's Bar?"
Jim: "That bar was run the way a church ought to be run."

Surprised, I asked him to elaborate, and he revealed his values:

Jim: "At Stormy's, I could wear anything—blue jeans or a suit—and no one would judge me. But at church? If I wore jeans, people would stare. I like church, but I want to feel comfortable being myself."

[1]All stories are based on real-life cases. However, all names in this text except the authors are pseudonyms, and identifying details have been removed to protect the confidentiality of individuals.

He continued, "At Stormy's, I could sit next to someone, and we'd talk—or argue—and by the end, we'd know something about each other. At church, everyone says the same thing in unison. How will I ever learn about the person next to me?"

Then he added, "Stormy's has a few simple rules. If you break them, you're out. But at church, there are so many rules, and no one follows all of them. Everyone pretends, and no one gets kicked out. What kind of rules are those?"

In those 20 min, Jim had just given me his spiritual assessment clearly and simply. He was saying, "Look, Doug, if you want to talk religion with me, you need to understand that I'm a down-to-earth guy. I'll shoot straight with you, and I expect the same in return. It's okay if we argue, but let's cut to the chase—no messing around."

11.2.8 Conclusion

Ultimately, spiritual assessments serve not only as a clinical tool but as a means of creating a more meaningful connection with the client. By acknowledging their spiritual and cultural backgrounds, professionals can provide more compassionate and comprehensive care, addressing both psychological and spiritual needs during the end-of-life journey.

11.3 Dynamic and Diverse Spiritual Exploration Tools

11.3.1 Supporting Spiritual Exploration

The spiritual journey during dying or grieving is inherently dynamic, reflecting the profound emotional, existential, and spiritual transformations individuals undergo as they confront mortality and grapple with the complexities of meaning-making. It is crucial for support systems to remain open, adaptable, and ready to embrace the evolving and sometimes fluctuating spiritual needs of individuals during this challenging time.

1. *Fluidity of Beliefs*

   Spiritual beliefs are not static; they ebb and flow, often shaped by the emotional and existential challenges of the journey. As clients face the realities of illness or loss, they may move through a spectrum of beliefs—ranging from deeply held convictions to moments of doubt and uncertainty. This fluidity requires professionals and support systems to remain sensitive to changes in spiritual perspectives without making assumptions based on past beliefs or religious affiliations.

2. *Questioning and Reflecting*

   The process of dying or grieving frequently prompts intense questioning and introspection. Individuals may begin to reflect deeply on the purpose of life, the meaning of suffering, and the nature of the divine. Swami Paramananda (1923) captures this journey by noting that life offers innumerable opportunities. The lesson we must learn how to shift focus from relentlessly seeking better opportunities to how to make the best use of those we have. This reflection often leads to shifts in perspective as the individual re-evaluates their spiritual frameworks in light of their current experiences. Offer a non-judgmental space for such explorations, understanding that spiritual questioning can be a critical aspect of growth and acceptance.
3. *Exploration of Diverse Practices*

   Individuals may explore various spiritual practices and rituals, drawing from different traditions or personal philosophies. This eclectic approach can be a manifestation of the need for comfort and connection, transcending rigid religious boundaries. Support this exploration with cultural humility, recognizing that diverse practices may offer new avenues for healing and understanding.
4. *Acceptance of Mystery*

   Some individuals may find peace in embracing the mystery and uncertainty of life and death. This acceptance does not necessarily align with specific religious doctrines but reflects a deeper acknowledgment of the limitations of human understanding. As Pema Chödrön (2018) explains, "our life's work is to use what we've been given to wake up… It doesn't matter whether it's wealth or poverty, beauty or ugliness, mental stability or instability, life in a madhouse or a peaceful desert" (p. 32). Valuable support can be provided by respecting the individual's journey toward acceptance without pushing for definitive answers or religious conformity.
5. *Emotional Impact on Beliefs*

   Psychology literature shows that human beings sometimes "think with feelings." Emotional states play a significant role in evaluating spiritual beliefs. While navigating grief, fear, or acceptance, their spiritual perspectives may shift in response to the emotional landscape of the journey.
6. *Individualized Paths*

   Each individual's spiritual path is unique. Some may find strength in reaffirming their existing beliefs, while others may chart entirely new territories. Acknowledging and respecting these diverse paths is essential for a supportive caregiving environment.

In summary, individuals' beliefs often evolve in profound and personal ways during the journey of dying or grieving. Professionals and support systems are essential in creating and holding a space of non-judgmental "unconditional positive regard" (Rogers, 1995), helping individuals seek and make meaning. This process may involve spiritual quest, but it is ultimately about supporting individuals as they navigate their own unique paths toward understanding and healing. Being adaptable and showing deep respect for each person's journey are key to offering meaningful support, ensuring they feel validated and understood, both emotionally and spiritually.

11.3.2 Cases Examples of Spiritual Exploration

The journey through dying and grieving often leads individuals to confront deep, existential questions regarding life, purpose, and suffering. These experiences frequently involve grappling with spiritual questions, meaning-making, and the search for personal truth. For some, these experiences lead to a deepening of faith—a newfound connection to spiritual practices that bring comfort and clarity. For others, the pain of loss can shatter long-held beliefs, leaving them questioning or even renouncing their faith. Each person's journey is unique, shaped by their individual experiences and the meaning they seek. The following cases show just how diverse these journeys can be. Some find their faith blossoming in the face of loss, while others wrestle with anger and disbelief, struggling to reconcile their pain with their previous spiritual beliefs. These stories illustrate the varied ways individuals come to terms with grief, faith, and the desire to make sense in the midst of life's most difficult moments.

(1) *A Withering Faith*

Bernie was angry with God. In his eyes, God had betrayed him. He granted him the woman of his dreams, permitting their marriage, only to snatch her away before they could even celebrate their first anniversary. For Bernie, such a God was too cruel to ever pray to, too cruel ever to worship.

(2) *A God in Pain*

An entry from B.J.'s journal:

"I went to my last counseling session with Pastor Hanson today. He quoted a passage of scripture to me: *'All things work together for good for those who love God.'* How dare he use that against me! How dare he belittle my pain! How dare he belittle my faith!"

"I need someone to acknowledge my pain and to legitimize my suffering. Things do not always work together for good; there are some pains that never go away. The God I believe in is not just a God of peace and happiness. My God has to also be with me when I'm angry, when I'm scared, when I'm depressed, and when I just don't give a damn."

"I do not live in a fairy tale world! And God doesn't either!"

(3) *A Blossoming Faith*

For Ginny, her faith blossomed after the death of her husband, reaching a level of maturity it had never achieved before. She shared with me, "Before, I would only mouth the words. I participated in the worship service simply because everyone else was doing it, with no other reason. But now I understand what the words mean. Now I know that God is truly with us wherever we are, wherever we go—the heights and the depths."

Reflection

The stories of Bernie, B.J., and Ginny reveal the deeply personal and varied spiritual responses to grief. For Bernie, grief shattered his long-held faith. The death of his wife felt like a betrayal by God, leaving him angry and disillusioned. This is not uncommon, as grief often forces individuals to confront profound questions about suffering, which can destabilize even the strongest beliefs (Stroebe & Schut, 1999; Attig, 2011).

In contrast, B.J. found a way to hold onto her faith, but only by reshaping it to fit the lived reality of her suffering. She rejected the simplistic explanations offered by her pastor, feeling they minimized her pain. Instead, B.J. found solace in a belief system that embraced suffering as part of the human experience. Many spiritual teachings suggest that suffering can bring one closer to the divine, but only if it is acknowledged and honored rather than dismissed (Talmud Bavli, Berakhot 5a, n.d.).

In Ginny's case, the loss of her husband became a catalyst for growth, turning her once superficial religious practice into an authentic spiritual strength. Her faith flourished amid adversity, showcasing the concept of post-traumatic growth (Calhoun & Tedeschi, 2014). Ginny's journey exemplifies these research findings about how adversity can lead to increased spiritual awareness, deeper relationships, and other growth (Linley & Joseph, 2004).

These case examples illustrate the wide spectrum of spiritual responses to grief and adversity. Whether a crisis of faith, a redefinition of beliefs, or a deepening of spirituality, each person's journey is unique. Supporting this process means honoring the diversity and fluidity of their responses and providing a non-judgmental space for their spiritual exploration.

11.4 The Wounded Healer: Reflection and Reconstruction Exercises

Rumi famously said, "The wound is the place where the Light enters you" (Barks, 2004). This simple yet profound statement speaks to the transformative potential of suffering. In the face of loss and transitions, it is equally important to validate the experience while fostering healing and transformation.

Through self-reflection and guidance, individuals can learn to see their suffering as a catalyst for profound growth. This process involves adapting to new realities, finding meaning, and building connections. The light that Rumi refers to is the enlightenment, resilience, and self-discovery that can emerge from these difficult experiences.

As Swami Paramananda wisely observed, "If we do not have all that we desire, let us make the best use of what we have" (Paramananda, 1923, p. 29). This section includes exercises designed to engage individuals in personal introspection and meaning reconstruction, empowering them to reconsider pain and transform their wounds into sources of light.

11.4.1 The Wounded Healer Resume

This exercise guides the construction of a resume based on past and present experiences with challenges, including problems, pain and suffering, disabilities, imperfections, and shortcomings. Recognizing these wounds can often lead to personal growth and improvement. The aim is to illustrate how such experiences contribute to growth.

1. Begin by listing major past and present wounds, such as problems, suffering, disabilities, imperfections, etc.
2. After each item, reflect on how it has shaped personal growth and strength. Consider the following questions:
   A. How does this experience equip me to handle future challenges?
   B. In what ways does it deepen my understanding of and empathy for others' struggles?
   C. How does it strengthen qualities like resilience, courage, endurance, faithfulness, and hope within me?
   D. What unexpected qualities has this experience revealed about myself?
3. Finally, organize reflections into a formal resume or cover letter format, similar to a standard resume presentation or cover letter.

11.4.2 Reconstruct the Shattered Assumptive World

The term "Assumptive World" denotes a deeply ingrained framework of conceptual systems underlying one's perceptions of the world and oneself. Evolved and maintained gradually over time, this framework establishes expectations that individuals rely on to interpret, plan, act, and engage with the social milieu (Janoff-Bulman, 1992). These fundamental beliefs form the bedrock of daily emotions, cognition, and behaviors. Losses, especially traumatic events, can shatter our assumptive worlds. Some basic Assumptive World systems that are often found beneficial for mental health include:

- The world is benevolent;
- The world is meaningful;
- The self is worthy.

Janoff-Bulman (1992) emphasizes that, ultimately, the core coping task for post-traumatic growth involves rebuilding trust and reconstructing a viable, non-threatening assumptive world, transitioning from victimhood to survivorship (p. 69). Reflect on the following:

> ...recognize the possibility of tragedy,
> but do not allow it to pervade their self and worldviews.

> The world is benevolent but not absolutely;
> events that happen make sense, but not always;
> The self can be counted on to be decent and competent,
> but helplessness is, at times, a reality...
> There is disillusionment, yet it is generally not the disillusionment of despair.
> Rather, it is disillusionment tempered by hope...
> [In the end, this view] involves an acknowledgment of real possibilities, both bad and good---
> of disaster in spite of human efforts,
> or triumph in spite of human limitations.

Source: Janoff-Bulman (1992), *Shattered Assumptions: Towards a New Psychology of Trauma*. Pp. 174–175

Exercise: Reconstructing Your Assumptive World
This exercise invites individuals to engage in personal reflection, with the option for support providers to guide the process.

1. Reflect on the core beliefs that define one's worldview and how they have changed due to recent losses. Consider: What beliefs have been hardest to maintain after these experiences?
2. Think about the challenges to these beliefs and how an understanding of life has shifted. Validate any feelings associated with disillusionment.
3. Reflect on Janoff-Bulman's quote and the following ideas, and explore new possibilities.

   - Tragedy exists but does not have to dominate one's perspective.
   - The world can be kind but is not always.
   - Sometimes things make sense; sometimes they do not.
   - Competence exists alongside feelings of helplessness.

   Additionally, ask:

   - What good and bad possibilities exist in life?
   - What steps can be taken to rebuild trust in oneself and others?

4. Write down thoughts on how to balance feelings of disillusionment with hope. Consider: How can hope be cultivated despite challenges?
5. Journal reflections and insights on how to reconstruct one's worldview.
6. If comfortable, discuss with a support provider or group.

11.4.3 How Can I Use This

In times of emotional turmoil, validating pain while finding ways to navigate through it with resilience and compassion is essential. As Karen Kissel Wegela notes, "All the juicy, smelly, negative thoughts and feelings we have are the rich compost that lets our hearts mature" (Wegela, 2010, p. 72). The following questions are designed to guide individuals in this introspective process, addressing various emotions such as sadness, pain, anger, and depression, and transforming them into opportunities for personal growth and contributions to the well-being of others:

- What is currently causing the most sadness?
  - In what ways can this sadness be channeled to foster personal growth?
  - How can this experience be utilized to contribute to the well-being of others?
- What is causing the most pain at this moment?
  - How can this pain be transformed into a catalyst for personal development?
  - In what ways can this experience assist others in improving their well-being?
- What is presently causing the most anger?
  - In what ways can this anger be harnessed to foster personal evolution?
  - How can this emotional experience positively impact the well-being of others?

Albert Kreinheder's insight resonates here: "The greatest treasure comes out of the most despised and secret places … This place of greatest vulnerability is also a holy place, a place of healing" (Kreinheder, 1991, p.88). Recognizing that emotional turmoil can lead to profound insights and growth can be transformative for both individuals and those they support.

11.4.4 Refining Personal Philosophy

Beliefs shape thoughts, emotions, and behaviors. Therefore, it is essential to uncover and examine these beliefs to understand their influence and identify steps toward constructive change. As Dean Ornish noted, "During the times that we feel most vulnerable, that which is invulnerable within us becomes uncovered, becomes more apparent" (Ornish, 2006, p. xxix). The following exercise employs a simple cognitive-behavioral approach to navigate these beliefs.

1. *Identify distressing beliefs*: Identify and track philosophical beliefs contributing to distress. Common concerns among individuals in later years might include:
   - "I am old and therefore I am useless."
   - "All the personnel in the nursing home do not care about me."
   - "God must not love me if I'm allowed to become old and infirm."
2. *Facilitate open dialogue*: Creating a safe and compassionate environment to encourage open dialogue. Question whether the belief is fact or just an opinion.
3. *Craft an alternative philosophy*: Question the narratives, identify cognitive errors, and explore alternative explanations. Collaboration can lead to the development of a more empowering philosophy that minimizes distress. This new perspective should be logically sound, practical, and adaptable. For example, a shift from the limiting belief "I am old, and therefore I am useless" to a more

empowering outlook like "My age doesn't determine my worth; I possess choices and have contributions to make." A helpful technique is to ask what the person would say to a friend who would have the same critical self-judgment.

4. *Putting into practice*: Assistance in exploring ways to put this new philosophical position into practice can be invaluable. This can involve documenting thoughts in a journal or engaging in conversations. Consider the following areas:
   - Fostering relationships with partners or spouses
   - Improving interactions with children
   - Strengthening connections with friends
   - Enhancing physical well-being
   - Fostering openness to change
   - Nurturing religious or spiritual growth
   - Developing resilience in handling criticism and rejection
   - Facilitating coping strategies for physical decline
   - Encouraging a constructive approach to embracing mortality.
5. *Integrate the new philosophy*: Simply exploring new ideas is insufficient; these concepts must be lived out. In cognitive-behavioral therapy (CBT), cognitive reflection initiates the process, but true transformation occurs through behavioral practices again and again. Collaborating on specific steps to implement the more constructive philosophy.

Each individual constructs a unique world in their mind, responding to experiences through the lens of such perceptions. Symbolic interactionism indicates that not merely the events themselves that shape one's reality but how individuals interpret and react to those events. This perspective highlights the significance of examining and refining personal philosophies and beliefs, as the beliefs underpin perceptions, shaping emotional responses and behaviors.

11.5 Self-Care Practices

11.5.1 Flexing Spiritual Muscle

Flexing one's spiritual muscle involves tapping into the psychosomatic connection between the body and mind to transform challenging experiences into opportunities for growth.

To practice this exercise, select a muscle group to strengthen, such as the stomach, buttocks, or legs. When encountering a person or situation that triggers negative feelings, pause and take a moment to view the experience as an opportunity for growth and express gratitude for it.

Tighten and relax the chosen muscle group while observing the sensations in the body. Continue this cycle, directing emotions toward this constructive outlet and intentionally releasing any tension.

As the negative energy fades, express gratitude again, acknowledging the lessons learned. Consider future challenges as opportunities to build resilience and deepen spiritual growth.

11.5.2 Giving Thanks

Research consistently shows that practicing gratitude has numerous benefits for mental and physical well-being. It can reduce feelings of depression and anxiety while promoting better sleep and higher energy levels. Additionally, gratitude strengthens relationships by fostering connections and encouraging positive social interactions. By incorporating gratitude into daily life, individuals can cultivate a greater sense of well-being and resilience. While gratitude can be expressed and practiced at any time, it is helpful to dedicate a few quiet moments and space for this practice.

To engage in a gratitude meditation, follow these steps:

1. Find a quiet, comfortable space and focus on breathing for a few minutes, noticing the softening of muscles around the navel and the rise and fall of the chest.
2. Silently express gratitude for the lungs and their role in sustaining life.
3. Acknowledge and thank the heart for its tireless work.
4. Appreciate the senses—sight, hearing, taste, touch, and thought—and the experiences they bring.
5. Extend gratitude to those who have provided support, including family, farmers, and artisans, recognizing their contributions.
6. Thank the universe for the earth, plants, animals, water, sunshine, and the cycles of day and night.
7. Stand, smiling with hands together in gratitude for the present and past, looking around with appreciation.
8. Return to a comfortable position and carry this sense of gratitude throughout the day.

Gratitude shifts focus from lack to fulfillment. Even in difficult times, cultivating gratitude for the little things can reveal hidden opportunities for joy and satisfaction.

11.5.3 Joy and Concerns Altar

The sayings "Every cloud has a silver lining," and the Taoist principle of *Yin* and *Yang* remind the positive aspects even admitting adverse experiences. This activity is designed to help recognize the balance between these opposites.

Start by designating a special place in the home—a coffee table, end table, or dresser top—as a Joys and Concerns Altar. Place two candles on the altar: one for concerns and one for joys. At regular intervals, such as every evening or each Sunday evening, light the candles with intention and dedicate time to prayer or meditation.

Begin by lighting the "candle for concerns." Dedicate this candle to a specific worry, pain, or trouble experienced during the day or week. Spend 3–5 min in quiet reflection, allowing the flame to represent the burning away of these concerns, transforming them into smoke that disappears into the universe.

Next, light the "candle for joys." Dedicate it to a moment of peace, happiness, or pleasure from the same time period. Spend another 3–5 min reflecting on this positive experience, offering your gratitude or joy through the flame.

As Rumi says, "God turns you from one feeling to another and teaches by means of opposites so that you will have two wings to fly, not one" (Barks, 2004). This practice encourages a balance between joy and sorrow, helping to recognize the lessons and beauty in both.

11.5.4 Ritual of Radiant Living

Each sunrise is a reminder of emerging from the darkness to embrace new life. This ritual provides a pathway toward rising from darkness into the light of sacred living, embodying renewal and spiritual alignment through simple yet profound practices.

Begin by selecting a quiet, secluded spot, bringing a candle, a bowl of water, and some incense. To infuse the water with symbolic or spiritual significance, herbs or essential oils such as sage, lavender, or rosemary may be added.

With the candle and incense lit, take 10 min to settle into stillness. Allow the breath to deepen, absorbing the light of the candle and the fragrance of the incense, anchoring presence in the moment.

Next, dipping fingers into the water, touch the forehead, and affirm, "I bless my mind and understanding. May my thoughts focus on all that is good and pure in this life."

The same gesture can be repeated for the ears, saying, "I bless my ears and hearing. May I strive to hear all that is good and pure in this life."

As the water touches the eyes, offer, "I bless my eyes and seeing. May I strive to see all that is good and pure in this life."

Bless the throat with the words, "I bless my throat and speaking. May I strive to say only what is good and pure, benefiting others."

Finally, wash the hands in the water, stating, "I bless my hands and doing. May I strive to do only what is good and pure, benefiting others."

The ritual is completed by sprinkling the water onto the hair, expressing affirmations or intentions related to purity, blessings, and spiritual alignment.

Conclude by sitting in quiet reflection for 10 min, allowing the spoken words to take root, deepening the connection to living a sacred and intentional life.

11.5.5 Reward Yourself

Recognizing and celebrating progress fosters motivation and resilience. Rewarding efforts, both large and small, can reinforce positive behaviors and strengthen a sense of achievement.

1. *Reflect on progress and achievements:* Take a moment to recognize present circumstances, acknowledging every little progress and good efforts.
2. *Choose a meaningful reward:* Celebrate and reward coping efforts and progress. The following list offers some ideas for meaningful rewards:
    - A massage.
    - A new outfit or pair of shoes.
    - Attending an uplifting play, musical, or concert.
    - A retreat out of town.
    - Enrolling in a course at a local community college, YMCA, or YWCA.
    - A sweet treat.
    - Reading a mindful book.
    - Receiving or giving a flower bouquet.

Rumi reflects, "You were born with wings; why prefer to crawl through life?" (Barks, 2004) Celebrating small progresses and milestones helps spread the wounded wings and embrace the growth made, facilitating an unfolding journey toward healing.

11.6 Mindfulness and Contemplative Exercises

11.6.1 Mindfulness, Health, Spirituality

Mindfulness is defined as the act of paying attention, on purpose, to the present moment, non-judgmentally (Kabat-Zinn, 2013). It involves an open and accepting awareness that helps individuals observe their experiences without becoming overwhelmed. This practice creates a space between perception and reaction, fostering clarity, calmness, and resilience in times of emotional turmoil. Mindfulness-based practices, such as meditation, have gained significant attention for their ability to reduce stress, anxiety, and depression while enhancing overall well-being (Creswell, 2017).

Meditation, a foundational practice in many mindfulness traditions, intentionally engages the mind, transforming it from a source of distress into a tool for well-being. By fostering heightened awareness, meditation interrupts habitual identification with thoughts and emotions, offering a pause that prevents reactive behaviors. Rooted in ancient Buddhist and Hindu practices, modern adaptations of meditation, including Mindfulness-Based Stress Reduction (MBSR) and Mindfulness-Based

Cognitive Therapy (MBCT), are widely used in secular settings, including hospitals. Randomized controlled trials of various mindfulness or meditation practices consistently demonstrate their effectiveness in managing chronic pain, preventing depression relapse, and supporting addiction recovery (Davidson et al., 2003; Creswell, 2017).

Beyond its psychological benefits, mindfulness supports physical health. Studies show that regular practice improves cardiovascular health, lowers blood pressure, enhances heart rate variability, and strengthens immune function (Creswell, 2017). For example, Davidson et al. (2003) found that an 8-week mindfulness meditation program increased brain activity associated with positive emotions and improved immune responses. This evidence highlights the holistic value of mindfulness in promoting resilience in both mental and physical domains.

Spiritual Dimensions of Meditation

Meditation also fosters spiritual growth by encouraging a deep inward exploration of the mind and self. Many traditions, such as Yogic and Zen practices, describe this journey as a path toward "Self-realization" with a capitalized *S*—the discovery of a peaceful and luminous oneness that transcends individual identity (Palmo, 2022). Tibetan Buddhist teachings view this awareness as the primordial nature of the mind, often accessed more readily during the dying process when physical and mental distractions fade. This perspective views death as an exciting opportunity for enlightenment. It emphasizes regular meditative practice to prepare for the transition. Such perspectives and practices are detailed in influential texts such as *the Tibetan Book of Living and Dying* (Sogyal, 1994) and *Mind Beyond Death* (Ponlop, 2006).

Research supports the unique benefits of integrating spirituality into meditation. Wachholtz and Pargament (2005) found that spiritual meditation practices, compared to secular techniques, yielded greater reductions in anxiety and enhanced positive mood. Participants engaging in spiritual meditation also reported more profound spiritual experiences and demonstrated a higher tolerance for physical discomfort. These findings suggest that the spiritual component of meditation deepens its psychological and physical benefits, offering a sense of meaning and connection that supports individuals navigating end-of-life challenges.

Whether practiced in secular or spiritual ways, meditation shares a focus on cultivating equanimity and presence. While exploring different techniques can provide initial insights, consistent practice with one method allows deeper benefits to unfold over time—much like digging deeply in one spot to find water.

Incorporating mindfulness and meditation into spiritual care offers a holistic way to address pain management and psychological and spiritual needs. It is highly recommended by the Consensus Report (2009). Whether through structured programs or simple daily practices, these tools bridge inner peace and outward challenges, empowering individuals to navigate their journey with greater clarity, resilience, and acceptance.

11.6.2 Dr. C's ABC Meditation

This meditation, developed and often used by one of the authors, Dr. Yan Ciupak, is one of the favorites among participants to begin grief-related workshops. It helps participants stay grounded and offers practical tools for handling emotional triggers during the workshop and beyond. This exercise combines three key elements: open awareness, *Box Breathing* to promote relaxation and manage stress, and the ABC framework from social psychology—Affect (emotions), Behavior (actions), and Cognition (thoughts). By cultivating self-compassion and guiding participants through handling the various aspects of the psyche, the exercise exemplifies holistic psychosocial care. Drawing on the two-factor theory of emotion by Stanley Schachter and Jerome Singer, emotions are seen as having two parts: the feeling itself and the physical sensations that come with it. By tuning into the body, emotions can begin to shift and release. Thoughts, on the other hand, are recognized without the need to engage or follow them, encouraging a more detached, observational approach.

Instructions

As we get started, I suggest you remove your eyeglasses if you wear them. Sit comfortably in your chair. You can cross your legs or keep your feet flat on the floor, feeling grounded… Keep your spine and neck straight—some people find it easier to sit a little forward on the chair rather than all the way back… Inhale and gently lift your shoulders up toward your ears, then exhale and let them relax… If it feels right, softly close your eyes or keep a soft gaze on the floor ahead.

Now, bring your awareness to your feet. Feel the solid support they have from the ground. Notice how the earth beneath you holds you… Shift your awareness to where your body meets the chair, feeling that same solid support from gravity. There's nothing to do, nothing to control—just allow yourself to feel safe and supported by Mother Earth.

I'd like to invite you to move your attention to your belly. Inhale slowly, noticing how it rises and the muscles soften. As you exhale, feel your belly gently fall. With each inhale, expand and refresh. With each exhale, let go and relax.

Now, bring your awareness to your chest. Stay curious—what sensations are there? Does your chest feel open or maybe a bit tight? Take a full breath in, feeling your chest expand. Exhale, releasing any heaviness or tightness. Breathe out through your nose or mouth—whichever feels most natural. Take a few more breaths at your own pace.

Next, bring your awareness to your nostrils, noticing the breath as it moves in and out. Is the air the same temperature, or does it feel slightly cooler or warmer on the inhalation or exhalation? Do the inhalation and exhalation last the same amount of time, or are they different? There's no right or wrong answer—just stay curious and open, simply observing what's happening as you take a few more breaths.

We're now going to practice *Box Breathing*, a relaxation technique rooted in ancient yogic pranayama practices and used by U.S. Navy SEALs to manage stress and boost focus. Inhale through your nose for a count of four: 1, 2, 3, 4. Pause briefly at the top… Exhale slowly through your mouth for a count of eight: 1, 2, 3, 4, 5, 6, 7, 8. Repeat this cycle a few times at your own rhythm.

As you continue, notice any thoughts that may pop up. Let them float by like clouds drifting across the sky. You don't need to follow or engage with them—just watch them pass. You have a choice.

If any emotions arise, simply notice them. You can label them if that feels helpful, but there's no need to do anything more than observe. Every emotion has its own space and validity. As you continue, notice any sensations in your body—if there's tension, acknowledge it as a call for attention. Breathe into that space. Wrap it with compassion, as if gently cradling a sweet, sleeping baby. Stay soft and aware, and see how the tension might shift or soften.

To close, gently rub your palms together, feeling the warmth and sensation between your hands. Lift your palms and place them over your eyes, feeling the warmth spread. When you're ready, slowly open your eyes behind your palms, then lower your hands and take your time coming back to the room, carrying this sense of calm with you.

Thank you.

11.6.3 Mindful Senses

Mindfulness offers a gentle way to slow down and reconnect with the beauty of everyday moments. Through simple sensory exercises, it's possible to ease into a state of calm presence, where even the smallest details can bring a sense of peace and relaxation. These practices invite an opportunity to pause, breathe, and savor life's quiet wonders.

Mindful breathing Take a few minutes to simply observe the natural flow of the breath. No need to change or manipulate anything—just be open and curious, noticing the gentle rise and fall of each inhale and exhale. Feel the air as it moves in and out, perhaps sensing differences in temperature or rhythm. Is there a soft pause between breaths, or does the breath flow continuously? Let awareness rest on the sensations around the nostrils or the gentle movement in the belly or chest. If thoughts drift away, kindly guide attention back to the breath, allowing it to ground the mind in a state of ease and presence.

Mindful listening Settle into a quiet space and let the ears open and be curious to the sounds around. Whether they are near or far, soft or sharp, let each sound come and go without judgment, simply enjoying the variety. Notice the tones, the pauses, and the spaces between. Gradually, the quieter sounds of the body—perhaps the heartbeat or the soft rhythm of breath—can become part of the experience. This relaxed listening practice creates a calming connection to the present moment.

Sensory bloom Take a slow, deliberate moment to appreciate the delicate beauty of a flower. Let the eyes wander over its colors and shapes, tracing the softness of each petal. Touch the flower gently, feeling its texture. Breathe in deeply, allowing the subtle fragrance to fill the senses and relax the mind. This gentle engagement with nature helps bring a sense of peaceful awareness to the present.

Zestful harmony Enjoy the pleasure of mindful eating by focusing on the simple act of savoring a piece of fruit, like an orange. Begin by noticing the vibrant color and the texture of the peel. Inhale the citrusy aroma as the fruit is peeled, letting the scent awaken the senses. Slowly taste each segment, feeling the juice, the texture, and the layers of flavor as they unfold. With each bite, notice the sensations and allow the experience to become a quiet celebration of the senses.

Coffee/Tea Ceremony Transform the preparation and enjoyment of a cup of coffee or tea into a peaceful, mindful ritual. As the water boils and the utensils softly clink, let the sounds and movements create a soothing atmosphere. Inhale the rich aroma, and feel the warmth of the cup in hand. With each sip, savor the layers of flavors, letting them unfold slowly on the palate. Feel the warmth as it travels down the throat, spreading a gentle heat throughout the body, bringing a sense of comfort and relaxation.

In Zen tradition, the legendary 140-year-old Zen master Zhaozhou Monk would often say, "Zhǐ guǎn chī chá qù," which means, "Just go have a cup of tea." This phrase is a reminder to embrace the present moment and cultivate a sense of contentment, aligning with the Zen concept of the "ordinary mind" as the path to enlightenment (Guo, 1252/2024). The practice invites an opportunity to let go of distractions and complexity, embracing the simplicity and beauty of life.

11.6.4 Mindful Tasting for Non-attachment

Mindful eating is an invitation to fully experience food in a way that opens the senses and quiets the mind. By exploring a variety of tastes and textures while blindfolded, this exercise creates an opportunity to release judgments and expectations, encouraging a deeper appreciation of the present moment. This exercise works great in group settings too.

1. *Prepare the space*: Find a calm, quiet area, free from distractions. Sitting comfortably with eyes closed or a soft blindfold helps to gently turn focus away from sight, allowing the other senses to take the lead.
2. *Choose a variety of foods*: Gather several different types of food within easy reach—something smooth, something crunchy, something soft. Including a range of flavors, from sweet and savory to bitter and salty, creates a rich sensory experience.

3. *Centering breaths*: Begin with a few deep breaths, inhaling through the nose and exhaling slowly through the mouth. These breaths serve as a way to center, bringing focus into the present and setting the tone for mindful awareness.
4. *Introduce the foods*: Before tasting, take a moment to explore each food item by touch. Notice the textures, shapes, and sizes without seeing them. The hands can offer a new way of connecting with food that's often overlooked.
5. *Smell the aromas*: Bringing each food close to the nose, inhale deeply and appreciate the scent. Every aroma has a unique story to tell, and letting it fill the senses can offer insight into the experience ahead.
6. *Tasting*: Take a small bite and allow the flavors to unfold naturally, without rushing or expectations. Chewing slowly, about 35–40 times, reveals layers of taste that might otherwise be missed.
7. *Non-attachment*: With each bite, practice letting go of any preconceived notions about how the food should taste. Simply experience the flavor as it is, in this moment, without holding on to likes or dislikes.
8. *Explore texture*: Tune into the texture of the food in the mouth. Is it crunchy, smooth, chewy, or soft? Let the sensations be noticed without forming any particular judgment or preference.
9. *Non-aversion*: Moving on to a food that might not normally be favored, approach it with openness and curiosity. Even tastes or textures that aren't typically enjoyed can become part of the mindful experience when met without resistance.
10. *Mindful chewing*: Pay attention to the act of chewing, noticing the movement of the jaw and how each bite feels. This rhythmic, deliberate process is an opportunity to fully immerse in the simple act of eating.
11. *Repeat with different foods*: Continue the process with various foods, staying mindful of the shifting tastes and textures. Non-attachment and non-aversion become a guiding principle for each new experience.
12. *Reflect on equanimity*: After tasting a variety of foods, pause for a moment to reflect on any changes in perception or emotional response. Has there been a shift in the relationship with certain tastes or textures? Notice how staying open and balanced brings a sense of ease.
13. *Conclude mindfully*: Gently remove the blindfold and take a few moments with eyes closed, reconnecting with the present space. A few deep breaths can ease the transition back to the visual world. Expressing gratitude for this practice can deepen the sense of peace and mindfulness cultivated throughout the experience.

This mindful eating practice creates a space to embrace food with openness and curiosity, without attachment or aversion. It offers an opportunity to connect more deeply with each sensation, finding a balance between presence and equanimity in the simple act of nourishing the body.

11.6.5 A Mindful Mirror Journey

The mirror reflects more than just a physical appearance—it can offer a window into how emotions are held in the face, and how subtle changes in expression can affect mood and mindset. This mindful mirror exercise is a gentle invitation to explore how expressions shape inner feelings while encouraging awareness and compassion.

1. *Set the scene*: Choose a quiet, well-lit space where it's comfortable to sit or stand in front of a mirror.
2. *Mindful breathing*: Start with a few slow breaths, in through the nose and out through the mouth. Let the breath bring focus to the present, easing the body and calming the mind.
3. *Observation*: Look into the mirror. Notice what is reflected back—expressions, posture, and any thoughts or emotions that come up. There's no need to judge or analyze, just observe with a gentle curiosity.
4. *Frown*: For the first minute, gently frown and observe how the face changes. Notice the lines that form, and be mindful of any emotions that come with this expression. Let the feelings rise and fall naturally, without clinging to them.
5. *Neutral expression*: Let the face return to a neutral expression. Observe the reflection without expectation—just notice how it feels to sit with this softer, relaxed expression. Any thoughts or emotions that come up can be noted, but no effort is needed to change them.
6. *Smile*: Slowly, allow a warm smile to spread across the face. Notice how this shift changes not only the expression but also the internal mood. Let the smile reach the eyes and notice how it feels to hold that gentle warmth. Notice any physical sensations rising.
7. *Positive affirmation*: With the smile still present, quietly affirm something positive—a message of self-love, gratitude, or strength. Let the affirmation settle, allowing it to create a small ripple of positivity.
8. *Express gratitude*: End the practice by acknowledging the time spent in this mindful reflection. A simple moment of gratitude for the opportunity to connect with oneself can gently close the exercise.

One of the "side benefits" of this practice is becoming more aware of how facial expressions might influence interactions with others. Just as the mirror offers insight, so do others in daily life reflect back what is expressed outwardly. This way, this exercise can also foster more intentional and meaningful connections with others.

11.6.6 Free-Expression Dance

Free-expression dance is a practice that combines movement with awareness and focus, enabling spontaneous and uninhibited self-expression. This practice is not about performance; rather, it emphasizes a deep connection with the body and emotions, allowing for the release of tension and fostering a state of full presence.

Studies show that dance can improve psychological health, enhance emotional expression, and contribute to physical health benefits, particularly in aging populations and in cancer prevention (Pessoa et al., 2019). Furthermore, dance therapy has been shown to promote healing through emotional release and body awareness, drawing from established anthropological and therapeutic traditions (Dunphy et al., 2021).

While free-expression dance works wonderfully as an individual practice, group settings often offer additional motivation and shared energy, helping participants feel more connected and engaged. Whether practiced alone or in a group, free-expression dance offers a chance to connect with the body and expression/release emotions.

1. *Prepare the space:* Choose a quiet, comfortable area where movement can happen freely. Clear any obstacles to create a safe and open space for dance. Choosing aroma and lighting to create a sacred environment for expression.
2. *Choose the music:* Select music that resonates with the emotions or intentions of the moment. It might be calming, uplifting, or energizing, depending on the desired experience. The music will guide the rhythm of movement.
3. *Set an intention:* Before beginning, take a moment to set an intention for the dance. This might be about releasing stress, embracing joy, or simply being present in the body. Let this intention guide each movement, no matter how small or large.
4. *Begin with mindful breathing:* Start by closing the eyes and taking a few mindful breaths. Focus on the sensation of the breath moving in and out, helping to center the mind and bring awareness to the body.
5. *Connect with the body:* Tune into the body, noticing any areas of tension or tightness. Begin to move slowly and naturally in response to the music. These movements might be small or large, gentle or energetic—let the body decide.
6. *Connect with emotion:* Take a moment to check in with the emotions present. Whether it's joy, sadness, calm, or excitement, let these feelings be expressed through movement. The body becomes a vessel for the emotions, moving as a response to what's being felt.
7. *Release inhibition:* This is a space free from judgment. Let go of any concerns about how the movements might look, and embrace the freedom to move in an authentic, uninhibited way. The focus is not on appearance but on the experience of letting the body move naturally.
8. *Engage the senses:* Fully engage in the sensory experience of the dance. Feel the texture of the floor beneath the feet, the air against the skin, and the music filling the space. Allow the senses to enhance the depth of connection to the moment.
9. *Embrace flow:* As the body begins to move more freely, allow the movements to flow without effort. Trust the body's natural rhythm and wisdom, letting the dance take shape in its own unique way.
10. *Stay present:* Keep attention grounded in the present, letting go of any thoughts about the past or future. Being fully immersed in the dance creates a powerful sense of presence and mindfulness.

11. *Conclude mindfully:* As the dance draws to a close, gradually slow down the movements. Stand still for a moment, allowing the body to feel the effects of the practice. Notice any changes in mood, energy, or emotional awareness.
12. *Express gratitude:* Before leaving the space, take a moment to express gratitude for the dance. Appreciate the opportunity to connect with the self through movement and music, and acknowledge the freedom that came with letting go.
13. *(Optional) Rest in Savasana:* To close the practice, sit or lie down for a quiet period of rest. Lying down with face-up, arms on each side of the body to allow the body to relax completely, bringing a final moment of peace and calm.

Mindful free-expression dance invites participants to release the constraints of the mind and embrace the deep connection between the body and emotions. Martha Graham, a pioneering figure in modern dance, famously stated, "Dance is the hidden language of the soul" (Graham, 1985). Movement allows individuals to express their innermost feelings and releases stored energy, facilitating healing and self-discovery. This practice promotes authentic movement, creating space for personal exploration and emotional release.

11.6.7 Tonglen Practice (Sending and Receiving)

Tonglen is a meditation practice rooted in Tibetan Buddhism, focusing on compassion to alleviate suffering for oneself and others. The term *"Tonglen"* translates to "giving and taking" or "sending and receiving." This personal practice goes beyond formal meditation settings and can be practiced anywhere and in any situation—whether in hospital rooms, on buses, or other places when observing one's own or others' suffering.

The following exercises are inspired by the Tibetan *Tonglen* practice but are shared here with the religious aspects removed, which often involve prayers and connecting with deities and gurus. The basic practice of *Tonglen* includes these steps:

1. *Intention setting:* Begin the practice by setting clear intentions. Spiritual practitioners often incorporate prayers or visualize receiving empowerment from deities who symbolize specific qualities such as compassion, wisdom, or courage.
2. *Mindful breathing:* Sit comfortably with a straight spine, allowing the body to relax. Focus on the natural rhythm of the breath, gently observing each inhalation and exhalation without altering it.
3. *Visualization:* As breathing continues mindfully, visualize the suffering of others—this could be a specific person, a group, or all sentient beings. Embrace the pain and challenges.
4. *Taking in suffering:* On the in-breath, imagine inhaling others' suffering and negativity. Visualize this suffering as dark, smoky energy entering the body, where it becomes purified and transformed into transparent light.
5. *Transforming suffering:* As exhalation occurs, visualize sending out positive energy, love, and compassion. Picture transforming the suffering taken in into

healing light, energy, or an aura, directing this positivity back to the people suffering, visualizing their pain relieved.

6. *Expansion (optional):* Traditional practitioners also expand the focus to include all sentient beings, acknowledging the universality of suffering. With each inhale, take in the suffering of all beings; with each exhale, send out healing, love, and peace. Embrace the interconnectedness of existence and the shared experience of life.
7. *Tonglen prayer:* Seal the practice with a prayer, mantra, or positive affirmations. The famous Tonglen prayer is as follows:

   "May I and all beings be well;
   May I and all beings find peace and healing;
   May I and all beings be free from suffering;
   May I and all beings be free from pain;
   May I and all beings experience joy and happiness;
   May I and all beings find their true nature."

8. *Dissolution and oneness (optional):* In traditional Tibetan practice, the session may conclude by visualizing the dissolution of the deity and the self into the same pure, radiant light, symbolizing unity and oneness.

Tonglen can be a powerful practice that encourages embracing suffering rather than avoidance. It offers an opportunity to transform suffering into compassion, wisdom, and strength. This practice fosters the interconnectedness of all beings and nurtures an altruistic mindset often referred to as *"bodhicitta"* in the Buddhist context. *Bodhicitta* represents a commitment that seeks enlightenment not just for oneself but for all beings, driven by a deep sense of compassion and altruism (Palmo, 2022).

While Tonglen can be powerful, it may not be suit everyone, particularly those new to meditation or struggle with trauma or anxiety. A gradual approach can make the practice more accessible. For example, visualizing a purifying light or powerful energy can ease the anxiety of visualizing pain. Support from a qualified teacher can further deepen understanding and practice. Many renowned Buddhist teachers have offered guidance on Tonglen's practice. For example, Jetsunma Tenzin Palmo, recognized among the BBC's most influential women of 2023 for her advocacy and remarkable 12-year retreat in a Himalayan cave, provides profound insights into transforming suffering into compassion and cultivating altruism in her 2022 book *The Heroic Heart: Awakening Unbound Compassion* and through her teachings.

11.6.8 Guided Visualization and Yoga Nidra

Guided visualization, sometimes referred to as virtual dreams (Neimeyer et al., 2011) or guided imagery, is a technique where a facilitator or recorded audio guides individuals into deep relaxation through purposeful mental imagery. Drawing from meditation practices and contemplative exercises found in various cultures, guided visualization offers a wide range of psychological and physiological benefits, including stress reduction, enhanced athletic performance, goal achievement, and pain management.

Athletes and performers frequently use these visualization techniques to mentally rehearse movements and routines. In a study by Hall et al. (1990), athletes from different sports, such as football, gymnastics, and figure skating, were surveyed about their use of imagery. Interestingly, the findings showed that athletes use visualization more during competitions than in practice, particularly at higher competitive levels like national or international events. This suggests that athletes recognize mental imagery as a key component of performance preparation under high stress.

What is particularly noteworthy is that athletes use both visual and kinesthetic imagery, meaning they do not just picture their actions—they also attempt to *feel* the bodily sensations and movements as they mentally rehearse them. This mind-body connection draws upon the synergy between mental and physical engagement. Athletes also acknowledge how these techniques help them stay focused, manage stress, and boost motivation before important events. Stephen et al. (2022) supported these findings in their review, noting that visualization helps athletes sharpen their focus, improve their technique, and increase confidence, especially in high-pressure situations.

Beyond the physical and psychological benefits, guided visualization and meditation have been shown to positively impact the brain and immune function. Davidson et al. (2003) found that regular meditation practices lead to measurable changes in brain activity and immune responses, demonstrating how these techniques promote overall well-being.

One specific form of guided meditative visualization is *Yoga Nidra,* which induces deep relaxation while maintaining a state of awareness. Often referred to as "yogic sleep," Yoga Nidra promotes deep physical, mental, and emotional rest and reconstruct the subconscious mind. Many yogis use Yoga Nidra as a powerful tool for rest, healing, transformation, cultivating yogic powers, and making spiritual progress.

Structured guided visualization sessions can last anywhere from 10 min to an hour or longer, depending on the needs and goals of the individual. Short sessions of 5–10 min are ideal for grounding or positive affirmations, especially before training or teaching. In contrast, Yoga Nidra typically requires a minimum of 20 min to achieve deep relaxation, and with regular practice, the experience tends to deepen over time.

The following guidelines reflect insights from various traditions, drawing on established practices of contemplative traditions.[2] It is essential to adapt these prac-

[2] These guidelines integrate practices from Tibetan Buddhism and Indian yogic traditions, informed by Swami Satyananda Saraswati's classical text, *Yoga Nidra* (2013). Additionally, they are shaped by one of the authors, Dr. Yan Ciupak's training with respected meditation teachers, including Jetsunma Tenzin Palmo, Yongey Mingjur Rinpoche, Lama Karma Drodhul, and master yogis in India such as Swami Omkarananda, Upendra, and Vimal Sharma.

tices and symbolism to meet the unique strengths and preferences of each person. Facilitators are encouraged to adopt a humble attitude, viewing their role as one of creating a supportive and compassionate space where participants can explore their own experiences.

(1) *Preparation*

Guided visualization offers a simple and powerful way to achieve various goals. For best results, it should be conducted in a quiet, private space with good ventilation and a comfortable temperature. Interruptions should be minimized to maintain focus. The room's lighting can be dim, though not completely dark or overly bright. Practicing at the same time each day can enhance consistency and effectiveness. Classical Yoga Nidra, also known as conscious sleep, is especially beneficial when done early in the morning or just before bed, promoting deep and restful sleep. It is advisable to practice on an empty stomach to prevent discomfort or drowsiness.

Loose, comfortable clothing is ideal, and having a blanket or shawl nearby is recommended, as the body tends to cool down during the practice. When lying down, it is suggested not to use a pillow, although a thin folded blanket under the shoulders or neck can provide support. For lower back discomfort, a cushion or pillow can offer additional relief.

(2) *Position*

Guided visualization can be practiced in various positions, such as sitting, reclining, lying down in *shavasana* (on the back), or even standing. Yoga Nidra is performed in a lying down position without a pillow but can wrap a thin blanket to support the neck. Whichever position is chosen, maintaining a straight spine is essential. When lying down, a mat or blanket offers proper body support. The arms should remain slightly away from the body, with palms facing upward and fingers naturally relaxed. Legs should be placed slightly apart to avoid contact between the thighs.

(3) *The Procedure*

There are different ways to conduct guided visualization based on the goal, available time, and individualized needs. Adjustments can be made by adding or omitting elements, rather than altering the pace of instruction.

1. *Preparation and relaxation*: Start by getting the body and mind ready with some gentle relaxation.
2. *(Optional) Intention and resolve*: Set a clear, positive intention. It's best to focus on just one intention that speaks to the person's current needs.
3. *Awareness of breath*: After the body scan, shift attention to the natural breath without trying to control it—just stay aware of its flow.
4. *Rotation of consciousness/body scan*: Guide awareness through the body, quickly moving from one part to the next. Visualization of body parts is not necessary, but following a consistent sequence enhances the experience. Depending on the time available, a full-body scan may be conducted, or focus can be placed on central areas.

5. *(Optional) Feelings and sensations*: Gently guide the person to explore any emotions and/or bodily sensations. Let them experience and release emotions by noticing contrasts like heaviness and lightness, tension and ease, or joy and sadness.
6. *Visualization*: Introduce dynamic images with universal significance or personal resonance. Common imagery includes natural landscapes, symbols, or figures such as mountains, oceans, flowers, or sacred symbols. Customizing the imagery based on individual preferences while avoiding triggers identified in assessments.
7. *Ending the practice*: Wrap up the session with a peaceful image that brings a sense of calm. This is a good time to reinforce the positive affirmation or resolution set at the beginning. Make sure the transition back to waking awareness is gradual, so they don't feel disoriented or experience any discomfort.

11.6.9 Yoga Nidra (Complete Scheme)

This section provides a detailed 50-min yoga nidra sequence, along with two shorter variations in the subsequent sections. Each illustrates different approaches to body scans and relaxation techniques, offering flexibility in duration. Alternative visualizations are included to inspire customization. With permission, these scripts are adapted from transcripts of Swami Omkarananda's yoga nidra guidance. For further reading and additional scripts, refer to *Yoga Nidra* (2013) by Swami Satyananda Saraswati, published by the esteemed Bihar School of Yoga.

(Preparation) Get ready for yoga nidra. Lie down in shavasana and make yourself as comfortable as possible. Keep your feet apart and let them fall sideways; arms slightly away from the body with the palms of your hands upwards. (pause) Adjust your blanket, clothes and position, so that you can practice yoga nidra without moving and with no physical discomfort. Please close your eyes and keep them closed. (long pause) The practice of yoga nidra is the act of hearing and the act of feeling, these are the only important factors. (pause) In dreams you have no control, in yoga nidra you are the creator of the dream. (pause) Say to yourself mentally, "I will stay awake. I shall only listen to the voice"… Repeat to yourself, "I stay awake." (pause) Give yourself some time to become calm and steady… Take a deep breath and as you breathe in, feel calmness spreading throughout the body. (pause) As you are breathing out, say to yourself mentally, "R-e-l-a-x." (pause)

(Relaxation) Become aware of sounds in the distance…become aware of the most distant sounds that you can hear. (pause) Let your sense of hearing search out distant sounds and following them for a few seconds, without attempting to identify the source. (pause) Gradually bring your attention to closer sounds…to sounds outside this building… and then to sounds inside this building. (pause) Now develop your awareness of this room… without opening your eyes visualize the four walls, the ceiling, the floor, your body lying on the floor. See your body lying on the floor.

(pause) Become aware of the existence of our physical body lying on the floor…total awareness of your body lying in perfect stillness. (pause) Your body is lying on the floor… develop your awareness of all the physical meeting points between your body and the floor. (pause) Become aware of the natural breath, become aware of the deep, natural, spontaneous breath, do not concentrate too much. Know that you are breathing. (pause)

(Resolve) This is the time to set your intention/resolve. (pause) Simple intention/resolve… simple, clear, and use positive tense. Please state your resolve clearly with feelings and awareness three times. (pause)

(Rotation of Consciousness: Overview) Rotate your consciousness through the different centers of the body… as quickly as possible. Your awareness will jump from point to point. You may repeat mentally the name of each part after me, and simultaneously become aware of that part. The practice always begins with the right hand…

(Right Side) Right hand thumb, second finger, third finger, fourth finger, fifth finger; palm of the hand, back of the hand, wrist, lower arm, elbow, upper arm, shoulder, armpit, waist, hip, right thigh, knee, calf muscle, ankle, heel, sole, top of the foot, right big toe, second toe, third toe, fourth toe, fifth toe…

(Left Side) Left-hand thumb, second finger, third finger, fourth finger, fifth finger, palm of the left hand, back of the hand, wrist, lower arm, elbow, upper arm, shoulder, armpit, waist, hip, left thigh, knee, calf muscle, ankle, heel, sole, top of the foot, left big toe, second toe, third toe, fourth toe, fifth toe…

(Back) Right shoulder, left shoulder, right shoulder blade, left shoulder blade, right buttock, left buttock, the spine… the whole of the back together…

(Front) Top of the head, forehead, right eyebrow, left eyebrow, the eyebrow center, right eyelid, left eyelid, right eye, left eye, right ear, left ear, right cheek, left cheek, nose, tip of the nose, right nostril, left nostril, upper lip, lower lip, chin, jaw, throat, right collarbone, left collarbone, right chest, left chest, middle of the chest, naval, abdomen, lower abdomen…

(Major Parts) Whole of the right leg, whole of the left leg, both legs together… whole of the right arm, whole of the left arm, both arms together… whole of the back, whole of the front, whole of the head… together… legs, arms, back, front, head, together… the whole of the body together… the whole of the body together… the whole of the body together. (pause)

(Body/Floor Awareness) Develop awareness of the whole body… and become aware of the space occupied by the body. Become aware of the space occupied by the body. Become aware of the whole body and the floor and at the same time become aware of the meeting points of the body and the floor. (pause) Feel the meeting points between the back of your head and the floor… shoulder blades meeting the floor… the elbows and the floor… the back of the hands meeting the floor… the buttocks meeting the floor… the calves meeting the floor… the heels and the floor. (pause) Aware of all the meeting points between the body and the floor, the sensation of all points simultaneously, evenly. (pause) Go on feeling these points clearly and distinctly. Please do not sleep, continue. (Long pause) Notice the skin on our face. Switch your attention to the eyelids… feel the narrow line of meeting between the upper and lower eyelids. Intensify your awareness between the eyelids. (pause) and then the lips… center your attention on the line between the lips, the space between the lips.

(Breathing) From the lips we go to the breath, draw your attention to the natural ingoing and outgoing breath. (pause) Feel the breath moving along the passage between the naval and the throat; on exhalation, it descends from the throat to the navel. (pause) Be completely aware of your breath, naval to throat, throat to naval… do not try to force the breath, just awareness. (pause) Maintain your awareness and at the same time start counting your breath backwards from 51 to one. "51, I am breathing in. 51; I am breathing out. 50, I am breathing in; 50, I am breathing out, and so on from 51 to 1, or from 27 to 1. Count to yourself mentally as you follow the rise and fall of your breath from naval to throat and back again. (pause) Total awareness of the breathing and counting. (pause) The breathing is slow and relaxed… Please continue counting.

(Inner Space) Withdraw your mind and concentrate on the space in front of your closed eyes. (pause) Imagine before you a transparent screen through which you can see infinite space… a space that extends as far as the eyes can see. (pause) Concentrate on this space and become aware of any phenomena that manifest within it; whatever you see is the manifesting state of your mind. (pause) Continue your awareness of this space but do not become involved, practice detached awareness only. (long pause)

(Visualization: Healer's Hut) Picture yourself in a meadow as the sun is just starting to rise… (pause) The grass is soft and bouncy under your feet, and you can hear the birds singing their cheerful tunes. (pause) Take a moment to notice the vibrant flowers all around—roses in every color imaginable—yellow, pink, purple…each with a light morning dewdrop reflecting the sunlight. (pause) As you walk, feel the freshness of the morning air and the gentle warmth of the sun on your skin…Follow the sounds of a nearby stream. You can see the water gently flowing and fish swimming among the water lilies…Listen to the soothing sounds of the water and feel the coolness of the stream as you approach. (long pause)…Now, walk through the forest filled with tall, majestic trees… Notice the earthy scent of the trees and the softness of the grass beneath your feet… Find yourself in a clearing where a cozy hut stands, emitting a soft, inviting light. (pause) The door is open, and you walk into the hut.

You walk into the hut. The wise-looking healer in the room smiles warmly at you. (pause) Settle into a comfortable spot surrounded by cushions in soothing colors…So soft and comfortable, like clouds. You close your eyes and take in the aroma of the healing herbs… Experience the gentle presence of the healer, noticing warm and glowing healing energy flowing through you, renewing every cell of your body. (pause) The sounds outside the hut gradually fade away, leaving you in a peaceful and serene atmosphere… Take a moment to soak in this soothing energy, listen to the healer's words… Allow yourself to feel completely at ease in this sacred space. (long pause)

You stand up, saying bye and thank-you to the healer, knowing you could come back to the hut anytime.

(Inner Space) Bring your awareness back to the space you see in front of your closed eyes. (pause) Actually, this space can also be visualized in front of the forehead, so if you want to explore it a little you can shift your gaze slightly upwards…but do not strain. (pause) Watch the darkness that you see before you very carefully, with detachment, do not become involved. (pause) Rest your mind in this warm, friendly, and expansive space. If any subtle phenomena manifests, for example, colors or patterns, simply take note of these and continue with your awareness. (pause) If thoughts occur let them come and go but continue watching the dark space, continue this with detached awareness. (long pause)

(Intention/Revolve) Now remember your revolve (Sankalpa)/intention. Repeat the same revolve/intention you made at the beginning of the practice in the same words and with the same attitude. Repeat your resolve/intention three times clearly, with feeling and emphasis. (pause)

(Finish) Become aware of your breathing, become aware of your natural breathing. (pause) Awareness of breathing… and awareness of relaxation. (pause) Develop awareness of your arms, legs, and body lying stretched out on the floor. Become aware of meeting points between your body and the floor. (Pause) Develop awareness of the room. Start moving your body and stretch yourself… please take your time. (Pause) When you are ready, sit up slowly and open your eyes.

11.6.10 Short Relaxation Script 1

Make yourself comfortable and take three deep breaths. When you are ready, slowly close your eyes…Take in a nice, big, deep breath, and as you exhale, allow yourself to let go of any tensions you may be experiencing… Take another deep breath, feeling the muscles in your body relax and soften. (pause) As you exhale, release all anxiety and frustration… Now, take one more deep breath, fill your body, and as you exhale, feel your body heavier and heavier, sinking onto the floor or your seating/lighter and lighter, almost floating... Noticing how good it feels just to relax. (pause)

Then gently exhale once again and begin to allow yourself to let go fully. Bring awareness to the rhythm of your breathing… Notice your belly rising, falling, and softening with each breath…Allow this softening and relaxation to expand to your entire body, from the toes to the head and head to the toes. (pause) Relax and drift away with my words in and out of your awareness. Just allow your body to sink into a totally relaxed state.

11.6.11 Short Body Scan and Relaxation Script 2

Find a comfortable position to sit or lie down. Gently close down your eyes. Take a moment to focus on your breathing. Breathing deeply in and out… Feeling a wave of relaxation flowing down your body. Feeling your head relaxing… Your face. Feel the flow of relaxation. Soften all the muscles in your face and around your eyes. (pause) Feeling your throat and neck relaxing. Feel your shoulders relaxing. Imagine the wave of relaxation flowing down your body, gently softening your muscles, and moving any tension down your body and down out of your toes.

Feel your chest and stomach relaxing. Feel your back relaxing… Feeling the wave of relaxation moving down your legs, allowing any tension or stress to flow out of your body and dissipate into the vast universe. Feel the relaxation wave flowing through your feet and toes. Letting go… Relaxing…

Breathe deeply, in and out… Bring your awareness back to your body… Feel your hands and feet. Slowly wiggle your fingers and toes. Know that your vision is live within you. Knowing this creation and healing energy is within you, always. Gently open your eyes. Thank you.

11.6.12 Guided Mediation: Self-Inquiry

Take your attention to the space between your eyebrows… Allowing your attention to pour into this space. Feel your awareness going inside your head, behind your eyes… Focusing on this space. breathing into the space. (pause) Now, gently turn your attention around… Slowly feel your awareness, which is usually looking through your eyes outwards. Now, gently turn around 180 degrees so that you are looking into this space between your eyebrows, becoming the observer…Now, you're looking inward from the spirit's perspective. In your mind's eye, take a step back so that you are standing slightly away from your physical body, and watch your body sitting or lying down in front of you… Ask yourself, am I the body? Feel the senses. Am I the senses? Look at your thoughts. Am I the thought, the mind? (pause) Bring your awareness to your breath. Now bring awareness to the rising and falling of your naval area as you breathe… Now, bring your awareness to your chest area…Bring your awareness back to the third eye. Now, turn the awareness to watch the awareness itself. Who is aware? Who is watching? Be aware that you are aware;

be conscious that you are conscious. Look at this witnessing consciousness itself. (pause) Now, drop all inquiry and simply rest in this state of mind, vast, tranquil, and luminous.

11.6.13 Guided Visualization: On Peace

Gently focus on the word "relax." Relax... Relax... Relax…

Shift your focus to the word "peace." Peace... Peace... Peace...

Visualize the most peaceful location you can imagine… Picture a serene place. What does it look like?... Look in all directions at this peaceful place...Relax in this tranquil setting…

Now, with your eyes still closed, imagine the most pleasant smell you can think of… Breathe in this serene fragrance… Relax as you inhale this calming scent…

Next, picture the most soothing taste you can imagine… Savor this pleasant taste… Relax as you experience this peaceful flavor…

Move on to imagine the most relaxing touch you can think of…Picture being caressed and held with a comforting touch, embraced by someone you love dearly… Relax as you are gently touched by this loved one…

Relax as you visualize your peaceful scene, smell that soothing fragrance, taste that pleasing flavor, and feel the caress of a peaceful touch…Relax... You are at peace... You can relax... Peace... Peace... Peace...

11.7 Concluding Reflection

The search for meaning facing death or loss is a profound journey influenced by relationships, culture, and community. Holistic psychosocial care emphasizes the critical role of spiritual care in supporting individuals through terminal illness and grief. It offers pathways to meaning-making, connection, and resilience. This practice is grounded in cultural humility and celebration of diverse spiritual resources. Collaborating with spiritual leaders, comprehensive training of professionals, and integrating spiritual care into holistic plans foster an environment where dying and grieving persons may experience healing and growth.

As Sogyal Rinpoche aptly stated: "Do we not all have a right, not only to have our bodies treated with respect, but also, and perhaps even more important, our spirits? Spiritual care is not a luxury for a few; it is the essential right of every human being, as essential as political liberty, medical assistance, and equality of opportunity" (Sogyal, 1994, p. 438). His words highlight that spiritual care is a fundamental right, not an optional luxury.

References

Attig, T. (2011). *How we grieve: Relearning the world.* Oxford University Press.

Barks, C. (Trans.). (2004). *The Essential Rumi* (Expanded ed.). HarperOne.

Berger, P. L. (1969). *The sacred canopy: Elements of a sociological theory of religion.* Anchor Books.

Breitbart, W., Rosenfeld, B., Gibson, C., Pessin, H., Poppito, S., Nelson, C., et al. (2010). Meaning-centered group psychotherapy for patients with advanced cancer: A pilot randomized controlled trial. *Psychooncology, 19*(1), 21–28.

Bushfield, S. (2010). Use of spiritual life maps in a hospice setting. *Journal of Religion, Spirituality & Aging, 22*(4), 254–270.

Buxbaum, Y. (1999). *Jewish spiritual practices.* Jason Aronson.

Calhoun, L. G., & Tedeschi, R. G. (2014). The foundations of posttraumatic growth: An expanded framework. In *Handbook of posttraumatic growth* (pp. 3–23). Routledge.

Chakraborty, R., El-Jawahri, A. R., Litzow, M. R., Syrjala, K. L., Parnes, A. D., & Hashmi, S. K. (2017). A systematic review of religious beliefs about major end-of-life issues in the five major world religions. *Palliative and Supportive Care, 15*(5), 609–622. https://doi.org/10.1017/S1478951516001061

Chödrön, P. (2018). *The wisdom of no escape and the path of loving-kindness.* Shambhala Library.

Creswell, J. D. (2017). Mindfulness interventions. *Annual Review of Psychology, 68*, 491–516. https://doi.org/10.1146/annurev-psych-042716-051139

Davidson, R. J., Kabat-Zinn, J., Schumacher, J., Rosenkranz, M., Muller, D., Santorelli, S. F., et al. (2003). Alterations in brain and immune function produced by mindfulness meditation. *Psychosomatic Medicine, 65*(4), 564–570.

Dunphy, K., Federman, D., Fischman, D., Gray, A., Puxeddu, V., Zhou, T. Y., & Dumaresq, E. (2021). Dance therapy today: An overview of the profession and its practice around the world. *Creativity in Arts Education and Therapy (CAET), 7*(2), 158–186. https://doi.org/10.15212/CAET/2021/7/13

Frankl, V. E. (2006). *Man's search for ultimate meaning.* Beacon Press.

Graham, M. (1985, March 31). Martha Graham reflects on her art and a life in dance. *The New York Times.* https://archive.nytimes.com/www.nytimes.com/library/arts/033185graham.html?scp=4&sq=Dance%2520is%2520the%2520hidden%2520language%2520of%2520the%2520soul&st=cse

Guo, H. (Ed.). (1252). *Wu deng hui yuan* [Compendium of the Five Lamps]. Chinese Text Project. https://ctext.org/wiki.pl?if=gb&res=8127&remap=gb

Hall, C. R., Rodgers, W. M., & Barr, K. A. (1990). The use of imagery by athletes in selected sports. *The Sport Psychologist, 4*(1), 1–10.

Hodge, D. R. (2005). Spiritual lifemaps: A client-centered pictorial instrument for spiritual assessment, planning, and intervention. *Social Work, 50*(1), 77–87.

James, M., Carrette, J., James, W., & Taylor, E. (2003). *The varieties of religious experience: A study in human nature.* Routledge.

Janoff-Bulman. (1992). *Shattered assumptions: Towards a new psychology of trauma* (pp. 174–175). Maxwell Macmillan International.

Kabat-Zinn, J. (2013). Some reflections on the origins of MBSR, skillful means, and the trouble with maps. In *Mindfulness* (pp. 281–306). Routledge.

Klass, M. (2018). *Ordered Universes: Approaches to the anthropology of religion.* Routledge.

Kreinheder, A. (1991). *Body and soul: The other side of illness.* Inner City Books.

Linley, P. A., & Joseph, S. (2004). Positive change following trauma and adversity: A review. *Journal of Traumatic Stress, 17*(1), 11–21. https://doi.org/10.1023/B:JOTS.0000014671.27856.7e

Maslow, A. H. (1971). *The farther reaches of human nature.* Arkana/Penguin Books.

Neimeyer, R. A., Torres, C., & Smith, D. C. (2011). The virtual dream: Rewriting stories of loss and grief. *Death Studies, 35*(7), 646–672.
Nityaswarupananda, S. (Trans.). (1935/2001). *The heart of awareness: A translation of the Ashtavakra Gita*. National Geographic Books.
Nouwen, H. J. M. (2014). *The wounded healer: Ministry in contemporary society*. Image Books.
Ornish, D. (2006). Foreword. In R. N. Remen (Ed.), *Kitchen table wisdom: Stories that heal* (10th Anniversary ed., pp. xxvii–xxx). Riverhead Books.
Paramananda, S. (1923). *Self-mastery*. Vedanta Centre.
Pessoa, R. F., Neves, C. M., & Ferreira, M. E. C. (2019). Dance therapy in aging: A systematic review. *Journal of Physical Education and Sport, 19*(2), 1180–1187.
Ponlop, D. (2006). *Mind beyond death*. Snow Lion.
Puchalski, C. M., Ferrell, B., Virani, R., Otis-Green, S., Baird, P., Bull, J., et al. (2009). Improving the quality of spiritual care as a dimension of palliative care: The report of the Consensus Conference. *Journal of Palliative Medicine, 12*(10), 885–904.
Ramakrishna, S. (1999). *The gospel of Sri Ramakrishna*. (S. Nikhilananda, Trans.). Ramakrishna-Vivekananda Center. (Original work published 1942).
Roberts, K. A., & Yamane, D. (2020). *Religion in sociological perspective* (7th ed.). Sage.
Rogers, C. R. (1995). *On becoming a person: A therapist's view of psychotherapy* (1st ed.). HarperCollins.
Saraswati, S. (2013). *Yoga Nidra*. Bihar School of Yoga.
Sogyal, R. (1994). In P. Gaffney & A. Harvey (Eds.), *The Tibetan book of living and dying*. Harper.
Stephen, F. A., Ermalyn, L. P., Mangorsi, B. Y., Louise, L. J., & Juvenmile, T. B. (2022). A voyage into the visualization of athletic performances: A review. *American Journal of Multidisciplinary Research and Innovation, 1*(3), 105–109.
Stroebe, M., & Schut, H. (1999). The dual process model of coping with bereavement: Rationale and description. *Death Studies, 23*(3), 197–224. https://doi.org/10.1080/074811899201046
Talmud Bavli, Berakhot 5a. (n.d.). In *The Talmud*.
Palmo, T. (2022). *The heroic heart: Awakening unbound compassion*. Shambhala.
Wachholtz, A. B., & Pargament, K. I. (2005). Is spirituality a critical ingredient of meditation? Comparing the effects of spiritual meditation, secular meditation, and relaxation on spiritual, psychological, cardiac, and pain outcomes. *Journal of Behavioral Medicine, 28*, 369–384.
Wegela, K. K. (2010). *What really helps: Using mindfulness and compassionate presence to help, support, and encourage others*. Shambhala.
Willemse, S., Smeets, W., Van Leeuwen, E., Nielen-Rosier, T., Janssen, L., & Foudraine, N. (2020). Spiritual care in the intensive care unit: An integrative literature research. *Journal of Critical Care, 57*, 55–78.
World Health Organization. (n.d.). *Palliative care*. https://www.who.int/health-topics/palliative-care

Chapter 12
Spiritual Care for End-of-Life Transition

12.1 Introduction

Spiritual care for dying individuals traces its roots back to ancient civilizations, where the integration of spiritual and medical care was a fundamental aspect of supporting individuals facing illness and death. In these early cultures, rituals, prayers, and ceremonies were routinely employed to provide solace and address the profound spiritual needs of those in the final stages of life. As societies progressed into the Middle Ages, religious institutions and orders assumed a significant role in caring for the sick and dying persons (Marty & Vaux, 1982).

The twentieth century's hospice movement transformed healthcare and spiritual care. In 1967, British nurse Dame Cicely Saunders founded St. Christopher's Hospice, which laid the foundation for a holistic, person-centered and compassion-based approach to end-of-life care. Palliative care emerged as a specialized field, with an increasing recognition of the importance of spiritual care in improving the quality of life for people with life-limiting illnesses.

Despite the long-standing link between medical and spiritual care (Koenig et al., 2012), it is only in recent decades that this dialogue has gained prominence in both practice and research literature in the search for research-informed practices. Research on spiritual care for the terminally ill has explored its impact on the overall quality of life,[1] integration into palliative care,[2] and the efficacy of various specific assessments, interventions, or models of care.

The investigation into spiritual care for those confronting terminal illnesses is intricately intertwined with the broader landscape of healthcare, religion, and

[1] For a systematic review on this subject, see Chen et al. (2018) for the effects of spiritual care on quality of life among patients with terminal illness.

[2] For a systematic review on spiritual care in palliative care in the European literature, refer to Gijsberts et al. (2019).

Y. Z. Ciupak, D. C. Smith, *Death, Dying, and Grief*,
https://doi.org/10.1007/978-3-031-88467-2_12

philosophy within the cultural and temporal context. Notably, most research has been conducted in Western countries, particularly the United States, often without due consideration of cultural or ethical lenses. Recognizing this early limitation, the past decade has witnessed an encouraging surge in research that accounts for cultural and ethnic diversity. The evolution of spiritual care for the terminally ill mirrors shifts in societal attitudes and a heightened awareness of diversity and individuality as people approach the end of life. This historical progression demonstrates the dynamic interplay between cultural, philosophical, and medical dimensions. This chapter discusses contemporary initiatives, challenges, and research-informed best practices. It further provides practical tools and real-life examples drawing on multicultural resources, a testament that cultural diversity not only presents challenges but also serves as a valuable collective source.

In addition to these academic and practical approaches, this chapter also features a collection of poems in the form of prayers and transcendental conversations inspired by diverse spiritual traditions. These poems provide a contemplative pause and invite a more personal connection to the themes under discussion. Readers are encouraged to use these poems to engage with diverse perspectives, foster introspection and inspiration, and perhaps inspired to develop their own spiritual expressions. Together, this chapter reflects the Holistic Psychosocial Care (HPC) model and the 4A4C framework, providing strength-based, whole-person care to support persons through their end-of-life transitions.

12.2 Importance and Challenges

The spiritual dimension has become widely acknowledged as essential to quality end-of-life care. However, implementing spiritual care in clinical practices remains complex. This section examines both the significance of spirituality in palliative care and the challenges across diverse contexts.

12.2.1 Significance of Spiritual Dimension in EOL Care

By the first decade of this millennium, the importance of the spiritual dimension in quality end-of-life care has been widely recognized across professional,[3] national,[4] and international levels. Notably, the World Health Organization (2018) has included

---

[3] For example, American Nurses Association, 2015.

[4] For example, National Palliative and End of Life Partnership, 2015. In the United Kingdom, the National Health Service (NHS) Scotland has taken the lead in creating informational and training materials for spiritual care designed for all NHS healthcare professionals. Similarly, in Germany, the International Society for Health and Spirituality (IGGS) was established in 2011 with the aim of fostering an understanding of spirituality and spiritual care among healthcare professionals in

spiritual, physical, psychological, and social dimensions as the four key areas that palliative care addresses. It defines *Palliative Care* as a comprehensive approach that aims to prevent and alleviate suffering in these four areas through early identification, accurate assessment, and appropriate treatment.

Numerous international initiatives, such as the Spiritual Care Taskforce initiated in 2010 by the European Association for Palliative Care (EAPC) members, have shaped international understandings and standards on quality practices (Nolan et al., 2011). The European Association for Palliative Care (EAPC) task force provided an encompassing definition based on existing research of spirituality, defining *spirituality* as related to a person's experience, expression, and seeking meaning, purpose, and transcendence and the way they connect to the moment, individuals, nature, and the sacred. This task force is committed to advancing evidence-based spiritual care by developing a research agenda, improving staff expertise and confidence, and ultimately enhancing patient and caregiver outcomes. The Global Network for Spirituality and Health (GNSAH) was established in the United States in 2013, comprising clinicians, researchers, educators, policymakers, religious/spiritual leaders, and health organizations. GNSAH aims to "bring together resources, advocacy, and reach to influence more compassionate systems of health for all human beings (GNSAH, n.d.)." In addition to conducting robust research, GNSAH provides interprofessional spiritual care training.

In 2009, a Consensus Conference was convened among 40 representative national leaders, including physicians, nurses, psychologists, social workers, chaplains, clergy, and other spiritual care providers, and health care administrators, resulting in a foundational document known as the Consensus Report (Puchalski et al., 2009).The report urges that "spiritual care should be integral to any compassionate and patient-centered health care system model of care" (p.891). The historical convention provided guidelines and recommendations in seven key areas of spiritual care for palliative care settings.

12.2.2 Challenges

As spiritual care gains recognition as a vital aspect of supporting individuals at the end of life, its implementation continues to face significant challenges. These difficulties reflect the nuanced nature of spirituality, the variability in professional preparation, and the influence of cultural and individual diversity.

(1) *Conceptual Challenges*

Considerable confusion and inconsistency remain in defining spirituality and religion, determining the scope of "spiritual care," and clarifying the roles of

---

German-speaking countries. See the details in Gijsberts, M. J. H., Liefbroer, A. I., Otten, R., & Olsman, E. (2019). Spiritual care in palliative care: a systematic review of the recent European literature. *Medical Sciences*, *7*(2), 25.

various professionals. For instance, Taylor et al. (2023) observe that around the world, nurses are increasingly taught and expected to provide spiritual care. However, the definition and delivery of spiritual care are often vague and vary in frequency. Similarly, studies found significant differences between patients' and healthcare providers' perspectives on spirituality (Selby et al., 2017). While patients tended to offer rich, detailed descriptions of spirituality and spiritual distress, healthcare providers struggled to define these concepts and often focused on task-oriented aspects of spiritual care. This disconnect highlights the potential for healthcare providers to "miss the moment" in offering meaningful spiritual care by failing to fully engage with the patient's understanding of spirituality.

(2) *Clinical Challenges*

In clinical practice, nurses frequently take on roles as case managers responsible for providing spiritual care to end-of-life patients. However, a recent comprehensive literature review notes that many nurses report feeling inadequately prepared to assess or address spiritual needs, leading to spiritual care often being neglected or relegated to chaplains (Batstone et al., 2020). This result is confirmed by research on patients and family caregivers, who report prevalent spiritual distress in advanced disease but are often neglected or inadequately addressed, resulting in unnecessary suffering (Selman et al., 2018). Their research highlights the critical need for comprehensive spiritual care training and interdisciplinary collaboration to enhance competency and attention related to spiritual care at the end of life.

(3) *Challenges Posed by Cultural Diversity*

Significant cultural differences across borders or within multicultural societies complicate delivering effective spiritual care (Selman et al., 2018). For instance, numerous studies on spiritual care in palliative settings are conducted in the United States, where "spiritual" is commonly equated with factors more likely to be termed 'religious' in the UK (Gijsberts et al., 2019). In addition, gender, race, ethnicity, and spiritual identity also contribute to variations in spirituality as coping mechanisms.

Even within the same religious affiliations, there is notable diversity in practices. For example, among Muslims, prayers serve as a common source of solace, yet the approaches to prayer can vary significantly. Similarly, within Christianity, individuals may turn to prayer, scripture, confessions, or communal worship. In Hinduism, rituals, personal mantras, and devotion to personal deities can be sources of strength. While Buddhists share a common identity, there is diversity in practices, ranging from meditation to deity devotion and mantra recitation. This internal diversity within a single religious affiliation highlights the intricate and individualized nature of spiritual expressions. It emphasizes the crucial need for not just cultural competency but cultural humility—an openness to learning from the person and a willingness to follow their lead. (See Chap. 2: Culture in End-of-Life and Grief Support for further discussion on cultural competency, humility, and sensitivity for helping professionals.)

12.3 End-of-Life Spiritual Care Guidelines

Spiritual care has become an essential component of palliative care programs globally. Organizations and institutions have formulated guidelines and standards, ensuring the seamless integration of spiritual care into comprehensive patient care plans. The 2009 Consensus Conference made recommendations in seven areas:

1. Spiritual Care Models.
2. Spiritual Assessment.
3. Spiritual Treatment/Care Plans.
4. Interprofessional Team.
5. Training/Certification.
6. Personal and Professional Development.
7. Quality Improvement.

Subsequent conferences in 2012 and 2013 built upon their predecessors, producing a set of standards and recommending strategies for integrating spiritual care across the entire healthcare continuum, extending beyond palliative care. These standards continue to shape policies, protocols, and practices, contributing to an enriched and holistic well-being for terminally ill patients and their families across diverse healthcare settings.

12.3.1 Consensus Report Model and Implementation

The 2009 conference presented an interprofessional spiritual care model described as a "relational model in which the patient and clinicians work together in a process of discovery, collaborative dialogue, treatment and ongoing evaluation, and follow-up" (Puchalski et al., 2009, p. 890). The models involve conducting a spiritual history of the patient upon admission to the clinical setting. By analyzing the information from the spiritual history, clinicians can identify the presence of spiritual issues, whether it be spiritual distress or spiritual resources and strengths. Subsequently, appropriate referrals are made, directing patients to chaplains or other suitable spiritual care providers in outpatient settings. Clinicians need to identity psychosocial issues, spiritual matters, or a combination of any, ensuring the referral aligns with the specific needs presented. This model operates on a generalist–specialist care framework, where board-certified chaplains function as trained spiritual care specialists. These chaplains not only directly address spiritual concerns but also act as a valuable resource for identifying other suitable spiritual care providers for the patient.

12.3.2 Formulation of a Spiritual Care Plan

Incorporating spiritual care into the treatment plan entails (1) identifying spiritual concerns, (2) establishing spiritual goals (if relevant), and subsequently (3) implementing, and (4) evaluating spiritual interventions.

12.3.3 Primary Spiritual Concerns at End of Life

At the end of life, individuals may encounter a spectrum of spiritual concerns that manifest in diverse ways, reflecting the broad range of personal beliefs and experiences. The 2009 Consensus Report (Puchalski et al., 2009) identifies the following spiritual concerns:

Existential concerns are common, with individuals often pondering the meaning of their existence and legacy. Statements are: "I find myself asking, 'What have I accomplished?' every night," and, "Is there something beyond, or is this all there is?" These questions highlight such deep introspection.

A sense of abandonment by God or others also emerges as a poignant issue. Feelings of isolation might be articulated through expressions like, "It feels like everyone, even God, has left me to face this alone," and, "The silence from my friends is louder than the pain." Such sentiments illustrate the profound loneliness that can accompany end-of-life stages.

Anger at God or others frequently arises from unresolved grief or perceived lack of support, captured in statements such as, "I can't understand why I'm suffering like this—it's just not fair," and, "All my prayers seem unanswered; why bother anymore?" These reactions underscore the emotional turmoil involved.

Relationships with the divine often become *conflicted* or *challenged*, leading to questions like, "How can I reconcile my faith with the decision to stop treatment?" and doubts such as, "I struggle with the belief that this suffering must have a purpose." These reveal the dissonance between prior beliefs and current realities.

Despair and hopelessness may dominate, leaving individuals feeling devoid of direction. "What's the point of fighting when the outcome is inevitable?" and, "I just don't see any light at the end of this tunnel," are expressions of profound despair.

Feelings of *guilt and shame* often surface as patients reflect on their lives, evident in comments like, "I regret so many things, and now it's too late to make them right," and, "I feel guilty for the burden I've become to my family." These illustrate internal conflicts related to past actions and present dependencies.

Despite these challenges, many seek *reconciliation* and resolution, expressing desires to mend relationships with statements such as, "I wish to mend fences, but don't know where to start or if I have the time," and seeking self-forgiveness: "Forgiving myself has been harder than forgiving others."

Isolation exacerbates these issues, particularly as physical health declines. This disconnection extends to spiritual life, with some facing significant *religious struggles*: "I've always believed, but now I question everything," and "Praying doesn't bring the solace it used to."

These varied responses not only demonstrate the wide range of spiritual concerns faced by individuals at the end of life but also highlight the need for compassionate spiritual care that is responsive to this diversity. Importantly, not everyone will experience all these concerns, and some may experience several simultaneously, suggesting the need for personalized approaches to spiritual care.

12.4 Research-Informed End-of-Life Spiritual Care

As the field is robustly evolving, research and various organizational guidelines have identified some of the best practices and interventions for end-of-life spiritual care:

1. Appropriate spiritual assessment:

It is important to conduct screening and thorough spiritual assessment to understand the individual's beliefs and values and identify spiritual concerns. The 2009 Consensus Report outlines three pivotal communication and assessment stages in palliative care concerning spiritual dimensions:

1. An initial screening for potential spiritual concerns,
2. A detailed spiritual history conducted by trained care providers, and
3. A comprehensive spiritual assessment is performed by a board-certified chaplain.

To enhance the quality of care, the report advocates for the training of all healthcare professionals in conducting routine spiritual screenings as part of patient evaluations. Thorough assessment helps formulate a tailored spiritual care plan aligned with the individual's unique spiritual concerns and values. Many different assessment tools have been developed. Please refer to the chapter on spiritual assessment tools that can be used for the grieving and dying individuals.

2. Interdisciplinary collaboration:

   - Collaboration among healthcare professionals, including chaplains, social workers, nurses, and physicians, is crucial for holistic spiritual care.
   - Multidisciplinary teams can address diverse aspects of an individual's well-being.
   - Spiritual screenings, histories, and assessments should be communicated and documented in patient records to facilitate professional coordination.
   - According to the Consensus Report's advice, board-certified chaplains should function as spiritual care coordinators, facilitating referrals to other spiritual care providers or therapies, such as meditation training, when necessary. Though the chaplain's key role is highlighted, most research suggests the training, communication, and coordination of all involved professionals in spiritual care.

3. Communication skills:
    - Compassionate presence.
    - Active and reflective listening, queries about important life events.
    - Identify and support the patient's sources of spiritual strength (beliefs, values, and practices).
    - Life review, listening to the patient's story.
    - Follow the lead of the client.
4. Mindfulness-based interventions:
    - Mindfulness-based and contemplative practices have shown promise in reducing distress and enhancing spiritual well-being.
    - Mindfulness interventions can be integrated into palliative care programs.
    - Somatic therapy and mind-body connection practices, such as yoga and Tai Chi.
5. Existential and meaning-reconstruction psychotherapy:
    - Existential psychotherapy can be beneficial for addressing existential concerns and promoting a sense of meaning and purpose.
    - Meaning-centered therapy, Aligned Therapy, and other therapeutic approaches explore and help construct the coherence of life's meaning and autobiography (Breitbart et al., 2010).
6. Rituals and symbolic practices:
    - Incorporating rituals and symbolic practices aligned with an individual's beliefs can provide comfort and foster a sense of continuity.
    - Personalized rituals, symbols, and personal mantras contribute to spiritual and emotional well-being.
7. Education and training:
    - Ongoing education and training for healthcare providers enhance their competence in addressing spiritual needs.
    - The Consensus Report recommends that all palliative care team members should be trained in spiritual care.
    - Team members should have training in self-care, self-reflection, contemplative practice, and spiritual self-care.
8. Patient and Family-Centered Care:
    - Involving patients and their families in decision-making and care planning respects their autonomy and individualized spiritual preferences.
    - Family support is integral to the spiritual well-being of the terminally ill.
9. Cultural Competency and Humility:
    - Recognizing and respecting the cultural diversity of spiritual beliefs is essential for providing culturally competent care.

- Willing to learn (refer to Chap. 2 for more discussions on culture).

In conclusion, ongoing research and clinical experiences have enriched and advanced the progress of spiritual care for terminally ill individuals. Existing studies highlight the importance of a compassionate, holistic, and culturally sensitive approach that acknowledges diverse spiritual needs in the face of terminal illnesses or impending death. By integrating spiritual assessments into routine care, fostering multidisciplinary collaboration, and applying therapeutic communication, healthcare professionals can establish a supportive environment that aligns with the patients' beliefs and practices. Continuing education and a commitment to updated research and evaluation will further refine and enhance the delivery of compassionate spiritual care.

12.5 Tools for End-of-Life Spiritual Exploration and Support

This section provides various tools to address spiritual needs at the end of life, grounded in the principles outlined in the Consensus Report (Puchalski et al., 2009).

The core of spiritual care involves *therapeutic communication* such as compassionate presence and reflective listening, which allow caregivers to query about significant life events and support the person's spiritual strengths. These practices are complemented by direct inquiries about spiritual beliefs, values, and life stories, ensuring that care is both personalized and deeply respectful of each person's unique journey.

Techniques such as guided visualization for alleviating distress, progressive relaxation, and meaning-oriented therapy help patients navigate their feelings and find peace amidst suffering. Storytelling and dignity-conserving therapy are also vital, offering patients a chance to recount their experiences and affirm their worth during their final days.

Self-care methods are equally important, promoting holistic well-being and independence. This includes traditional practices like massage and yoga, as well as more introspective activities like meditation, sacred readings, and personalized rituals. Art therapy, including music, dance, and visual arts, provides a creative outlet for expression and coping, while journaling offers a private space for reflection and emotional processing.

The interplay of these interventions helps construct a comprehensive care framework that supports not only the dying persons but also their families. By integrating these therapeutic communications, therapies, and self-care practices into routine care, healthcare professionals can provide a compassionate and supportive environment that resonates with the patients' beliefs and practices.

The following section includes examples of spiritual storytelling, guided visualization, contemplative/meditative exercises, and prayers/transcendental writing to provide spiritual support during the end of life.

12.5.1 Spiritual Storytelling: My Spiritual Travelogue

Journaling offers profound benefits for individuals navigating life's complexities. It creates a safe space for emotions, thoughts, and spiritual reflections, helping individuals process difficult feelings and find a sense of peace. Research consistently supports its therapeutic value, with expressive writing shown to reduce stress and anxiety—benefits that can last long after the writing ends. As Wiggins (2011) highlights, spiritual journaling can help individuals explore their belief systems, deepen their connection to the sacred, process grief, and come to terms with mortality. It allows individuals to integrate their spiritual life with other aspects of their experience, providing a holistic approach to personal healing.

For someone facing the end of life or dealing with loss, journaling becomes a tool for self-discovery. It's more than just writing down thoughts—it's about understanding them, gaining clarity, and often finding comfort. The journal becomes a mirror for deep, unspoken emotions, which can be incredibly healing when expressed. Tan et al. (2023) found that even just 7 days of mindful gratitude journaling significantly reduced psychological distress and suffering in individuals with advanced cancer, improving their overall quality of life. This shows that even short periods of intentional reflection can foster resilience and emotional balance in those nearing the end of life.

Encouraging individuals to share their journaling with a trusted counselor, family member, or caregiver can deepen the experience. These reflections open up opportunities for meaningful conversations and insights into their spiritual journey. Whether they are reflecting on their beliefs, contemplating the afterlife, or exploring personal values, journaling gives them a space to honor their story. For professionals, suggesting journaling as part of spiritual care can open new pathways for emotional and spiritual support, guiding individuals toward a sense of peace as they approach their final days.

Free-style unprohibited writing allows the free flow of thoughts and emotions. The following provides a more structured journaling method to inspire deeper reflection:

1. Begin with a bound book of blank pages divided into three sections.
    - "Contemplations on the Divine" or "Reflections on a Greater Reality"
    - "Reflections on My Worth, Values, and Who I Am," and
    - "Thoughts about the Afterlife."
2. Journal your reflections and/or inspirations from readings, conversations, and other resources, making dated entries in at least one of the sections.
3. Regularly share your journaling insights with a trusted friend, family member, counselor, or caregiver to enrich your spiritual exploration and personal growth.

12.5.2 *Spiritual Life Map*

A spiritual life map offers a creative, reflective approach to exploring one's spiritual journey, values, and beliefs. This tool visually represents personal milestones and insights, helping to clarify spiritual purpose and navigate the complexities of inner life. Research demonstrates that spiritual life mapping empowers individuals and is a culturally sensitive way to assess and support spiritual well-being, especially in under-served diverse populations (Hodge & Limb, 2010).

Step 1: Gather Materials
Begin with a large sheet of paper, ideally 24″ × 36″, and assemble various drawing tools such as markers, pens, and colored pencils. Additional materials like cut-outs from magazines or scrapbooking elements can enhance the creative process, making the map a more personal reflection of one's journey. This is a process of exploration, not artistic perfection, and the focus remains on meaningful expression.

Step 2: Sketch the Chronological Path
The journey can be visualized as a path from birth to the present, with space for future growth or even thoughts about the afterlife. Symbols, designs, or personal representations can mark significant points along the way. Curves, zig-zags, or bridges can serve as metaphors for life's challenges, transitions, or transformations.

Step 3: Include Significant Life Events
Events like marriages, the birth of a child, or the loss of a loved one hold spiritual significance in many traditions. These life stages can be integrated into the map, acknowledging their impact on the development of one's beliefs and values over time.

Step 4: Reflect on Life Crises and Resources
The map can also illustrate challenges and the resources that helped overcome them. Symbols like storms, sunshine, or mountains offer a visual language for life's trials and triumphs. This step deepens the understanding of how resilience and strength have developed through adversity.

Step 5: Recognize Successful Strategies
By highlighting past strategies—whether rituals, practices, or supportive communities—the map becomes a tool for identifying ways to face current struggles. Successes and lessons learned can be visualized, recognizing the progress made and the possibilities for continued growth.

12.5.3 Dream Journal

Dream journals provide a safe, reflective space for exploring topics that may be difficult to address in daily conversations, such as fears, faith, mortality, and other deeply personal experiences. They offer insight into the subconscious and can be especially helpful when shared with a counselor. Through this sharing, counselors can help uncover underlying emotions, desires, or unresolved issues, facilitating deeper conversations and healing.

It is important to recognize that while dreams may provide valuable nourishment to the dreamer, they hold personal meaning. Rather than interpreting a dream through one's own lens, it's essential to support individuals in discovering the comfort and nourishment that resonate within their own beliefs and traditions. What nourishes one person may not be appropriate for another, so the process of reflection should remain personal and patient-centered.

Begin by documenting any memorable dreams, particularly those involving themes of mortality, transitions, or existential concerns. After recording the dream, take time to reflect using the following questions:

(A) *What is the dream revealing about the past?*

Is there an unresolved issue, a person to reconnect with, or something left unfinished? This reflection can highlight opportunities for reconciliation or closure.

(B) *How does the dream relate to the present?*

Is there a message about the current situation—something that needs attention, a change to be made, or a shift in perspective?

(C) *What does the dream suggest about the future?*

Does it offer any guidance on priorities, future choices, or actions to consider moving forward?

By regularly engaging with dream journals, individuals can explore deeper layers of their spiritual and emotional selves, gaining insight into their past, present, and future while fostering personal growth and healing.

12.5.4 A Worthy Self/Fulfilled Life Letter

For those who have received a terminal diagnosis, connecting with a sense of personal value and purpose can become more pressing, especially in moments of despair or doubt. An evaluation of one's life and fulfillment may arise during this period of time. Baumann and Ruch (2022) conceptualize "Fulfillment in life" as a cognitive-affective experience. Based on their research of predominantly German-speaking 40 to 89-year-old participants, they identified three critical criteria that participants use to evaluate their fulfillment and worthiness: a sense of wholeness, fit, and value toward the self, one's life, and one's impact.

It is important to note that, in modern industrial society, there is a significant emphasis on functionality, performance, and "doing" rather than simply "being." This can create additional emotional challenges for individuals who, due to physical constraints or illness, may feel that their worth is diminished because they are no longer able to "perform" in the way society values. Therefore, it is essential to recognize that a life's inherent value is not dependent on their abilities or productivity.

Philosopher Immanuel Kant's moral philosophy emphasizes the principle to "always treat humanity, whether in your own person or in the person of any other, never merely as a means, but always at the same time as an end." This principle highlights the inherent worth of every person, regardless of physical condition or societal performance. It calls for respect and recognition of each person's intrinsic value and dignity.

Drawing on Kant's philosophical insight and the research by Baumann and Ruch (2022) on the fulfillment in life (FiL) model, this activity invites reflection on the legacy of one's accomplishments and the intentions that have shaped those contributions. It serves as a reminder of the enduring value of one's life, regardless of external circumstances

1. *Compiling affirmations, achievements, and intentions:*

   Gather compliments or words of appreciation from family, friends, and colleagues. In addition, reflect on cherished accomplishments—moments where contributions and efforts felt particularly meaningful. Equally important are the underlying intentions—the motivations and values that guided actions, even when outcomes weren't immediately visible. Pay special attention to accomplishments and intentions that highlight

   - *Wholeness*: Living in a way that honors personal authenticity.
   - *Fit*: Aligning intentions with deeper values and a sense of purpose.
   - *Value*: Creating positive impacts through intentional actions or achievements.

2. *Reflect through Kant's lens:*

   In reflecting on these affirmations and accomplishments, Kant's wisdom offers insight: individuals are never merely a means to an end, but always an end in themselves. This reflection reinforces that worth transcends what is "done"—it is rooted in who one is and the respect shown for humanity, both in oneself and others. Intentions, regardless of their outcomes, reveal personal values and demonstrate respect for life.

3. *Compose a personal letter:*

   Drawing from these reflections, a letter can be composed to acknowledge not only accomplishments but also the positive intentions that have shaped life. This letter could emphasize how these actions align with Kant's principle of treating humanity as an end, and how they resonate with the FiL model's components of wholeness, fit, and value. Signing the letter "Yours truly" adds a deeply personal touch.

4. *Prepare and store the letter:*

   Once written, the letter can be placed in an envelope, with the recipient's name clearly marked on the outside. It serves as a reminder of the meaningful journey and the inherent worth carried throughout life.

5. *Use the letter:*

   Consider entrusting the letter to a trusted family member or friend, providing instructions for it to be delivered during moments of doubt or feelings of worthlessness. Alternatively, the letter can be kept in a visible place as a constant reminder of personal value. It may also serve as a living document, with ongoing reflections and additions as life continues to unfold.

This letter serves as a tangible reminder of life's inherent value, affirming both the achievements and intentions that have guided the journey. It reflects the understanding that true worth isn't just about accomplishments, but about how life is lived—with respect, dignity, and compassion toward oneself and others.

It is easy to focus on shortcomings—the mind naturally tends to lean toward the negative. On top of that, modesty often prevents people from reflecting on or acknowledging their own accomplishments. But taking the time to recognize both what's been done and the intentions behind it is an essential step toward embracing personal value. Engaging in this practice can bring clarity and self-compassion, offering reassurance even in the most difficult moments.

12.5.5 Meditation Exercises

Mindfulness practices, including meditation, offer significant health benefits (Davidson et al., 2003), as outlined in previous chapters. Prevost et al. (2024) emphasize that shared meditation practices—engaging cancer patients, caregivers, and healthcare professionals—can foster resilience and enhance well-being. These practices alleviate stress, promote emotional stability, and improve quality of life by addressing both psychological and social dimensions of care. For individuals with advanced cancer, mindfulness techniques have been particularly effective in reducing feelings of isolation and strengthening coping mechanisms, creating a supportive environment for holistic healing. The following sections introduce essential meditation methods, each grounded in spiritual or secular traditions, to support ongoing development and well-being.

12.5.5.1 Object-Abiding Meditation

Buddha Shakyamuni's principal instruction centers around "one-pointed object-abiding" meditation, with the breath often serving as the focal point. This form of meditation, closely associated with concentration and mindfulness, has shown to encourage a peaceful mind and improve cognitive abilities (Creswell, 2017). Object meditation, such as the well-known practice of focusing on a raisin, is a technique used in Mindfulness-Based Stress Reduction (MBSR) programs (Santorelli et al., 2017). For those unable to focus on the breath due to conditions like chronic obstructive pulmonary disease (COPD), amyotrophic lateral sclerosis (ALS), or lung cancer, alternative objects like sound or visual aids can also be helpful.

The steps outlined below provide guidance on how to practice "object-abiding" meditation:

1. *Find a quiet space*:
   Meditation can be practiced anywhere, though choosing a calm and comfortable space without distractions can be helpful, particularly in the beginning. It may be indoors or outdoors, depending on preference, but the goal is to establish a space that allows for peace and focus.
2. *Assume a comfortable posture*:
   Sitting in a relaxed yet alert posture is important. Sitting on the floor with a cushion or in a chair with feet grounded helps create a stable base. Ensure the spine remains straight while hands rest comfortably on the thighs or form a mudra of choice.
3. *Focus on the breath*:
   Attention can be drawn to the natural flow of breathing—at the nostrils, chest, or abdomen. Notice the sensations and observe the transitions between inhalation and exhalation. This allows awareness to deepen and distractions to fade. Be curious and nonjudgmental.
4. *Cultivate single-pointed concentration*:
   Bringing attention to a single point of focus, such as the breath or another object, allows the mind to settle. Distractions, like random thoughts, can be treated as passing clouds in the vast sky of the mind or floating leaves in a stream—acknowledged but not engaged.
5. *Gentle redirecting of the mind*:
   It's natural for the mind to wander. When this happens, the focus is gently returned to the chosen object, whether it is the breath or something else.
6. *Staying present*:
   Staying present is at the heart of meditation. Just as individuals in Indian and Japanese cultures leave their shoes at the door before entering a room, meditation calls for leaving behind social roles and distractions before entering a meditative state. The Himalayan meditation tradition, for example, encourages visualizing three rays of light forming a protective barrier that blocks distractions and negativity from entering the meditative sphere. Experiment with different ways to reduce distraction, cherishing this opportunity as a moment carved out solely for inner connection and peace.
7. *Gradual lengthening of sessions*:
   Beginning with shorter meditation sessions and gradually extending their length helps build consistency. Mingyur Rinpoche's advice of "short time, many

times" is a valuable way to establish a steady practice (Rinpoche & Swanson, 2008).

8. *Cultivate acceptance and compassion*:

   Approaching meditation with acceptance and compassion toward the natural tendencies of the mind is essential. The five senses habitually seek external stimulation, and part of the practice is turning that awareness inward, observing thoughts without judgment.

9. *Observe changes in awareness*:

   With consistent practice, subtle changes in awareness and focus may emerge. Over time, greater clarity, calmness, and focus can become more apparent.

While these instructions focus on the breath as the object of meditation, other objects that offer comfort can serve just as well. Some examples include:

- A crucifix
- A Buddha statue
- A mandala
- A menorah
- A flower
- A family photograph
- A stone
- A candle

Spending 10–15 min centering attention on an object of comfort can be deeply grounding. If distractions arise, gently closing the eyes and refocusing on the object may help. Peaceful music can also be played softly in the background to further support concentration.

12.5.5.2 God's Breath Meditation

The words for the following breath meditation come from a hymn found in many Christian hymnals. The meditation could be used with people of the Jewish and Hindu faiths, as well as other faiths, because of the natural association between "breath" and "spirit" in many languages. The out-breath phrases could be said aloud or silently. Change the word "God" to "universe" or other terms relevant to the care-recipient.

In-breath: (silence)
Out-breath: "Breathe on me, Breath of God."
In-breath: (silence)
Out-breath: "Fill me with life anew."
In-breath: (silence)
Out-breath: "That I may love what Thou dost love."
In-breath: (silence)
Out-breath: "And do what Thou wouldst do."
(repeat for as long as it feels good)

12.5.6 Guided Visualization/Imagery Exercises

Guided visualization, also known as virtual dreams or guided imagery (Neimeyer et al., 2011), is a technique where individuals are led into deep relaxation through purposeful mental imagery. Rooted in meditation and contemplative traditions from various cultures, this practice offers numerous benefits, from stress reduction to enhanced focus and even pain management. It is a technique often used by athletes to mentally rehearse before competitions, with studies showing that visualization helps sharpen focus, improve technique, and boost confidence in high-pressure moments (Stephen et al., 2022).

Tibetan Buddhists have been practicing deity visualization for thousands of years, particularly within Vajrayana practices. Here, the visualization unfolds in two stages: the *generation stage*, where one visualizes becoming a deity, embodying the characteristics of that deity, such as wisdom, compassion, purity, and strength, and the *dissolution stage*, where the deity dissolves into emptiness, symbolizing the impermanence of all things and oneness of all (Palmo, 2023).

Guided visualizations provide a deeply personal space for strength, healing, and spiritual connection. These practices can be adapted to fit one's own beliefs and traditions—names, deities, or symbols can be replaced with those that resonate personally. As Sogyal Rinpoche (2002) points out, people do not want to be "rescued" through the beliefs of others. The goal is not conversion, but rather supporting someone who connects with their inner strength, confidence, and spirituality in a way that works for them. Whether visualizing the presence of Jesus, Buddha, tree of life, or another spiritual guide, the heart of the practice remains the same: to cultivate inner peace, wisdom, and a deeper connection to the divine or one's higher self.

Moreover, it is important to approach these practices with humility and openness. As Confucius wisely stated, "Real knowledge is to know the extent of one's ignorance" (Confucius, trans. Dawson, 2008, 2:17). This reminder encourages cultural humility and an inclusive approach, allowing people of all faiths and backgrounds to embrace the practice in a way that honors their unique spiritual journey.

12.5.6.1 Guided Visualization: A Christian Conversation

Close your eyes and imagine that you are being transported to Gethsemane .... You see Jesus all alone, kneeling and praying .... You see his power. You also see his vulnerability. You see all of his internal struggles. No one understands him. He feels alone. He feels unloved... You quietly walk over to his side and kneel next to him. You kneel there in silence... After a short while, Jesus turns to you with love in his eyes and asks, "What can I do for you?"... You look Jesus in the eyes and say, "Please tell me how you feel when facing death." Listen to Jesus talk about death while he is in Gethsemane.... Imagine his words, his tone of voice, his facial expressions... What does Jesus say about death while he is in the garden of Gethsemane?... How does that make you feel?

Now imagine that you are being transported to the foot of the cross… You see Jesus hanging alone on that cross. He is in great pain. He feels completely deserted... After a while, Jesus sees you standing below him. With love in his eyes, he asks, "What can I do for you?"… You look Jesus in the eyes and say, "Please tell me how you feel as you are dying." Imagine how Jesus talks about death as he is hanging on the cross… What does he say about death while he is hanging on that cross?... How does that make you feel?

Now, imagine that you are being transported to the throne of the resurrected Jesus. You see Jesus relieved of all his pain, basking in the glory of God… You quietly approach the throne. You kneel in silence… After a while, Jesus turns to you with love in his eyes and asks, "What can I do for you?" … You look Jesus in the eyes and say, "Please tell me how you feel after you have died." Imagine how Jesus talks about death after he has experienced the resurrection… What does Jesus say about death after the resurrection?... How does that make you feel?

12.5.6.2 Guided Visualization: A Jewish Conversation

Close your eyes and imagine that you are going back to the time of Moses. You are going to be with Moses beside him in his life's journey… You are with Moses as he stands before the burning bush. He is receiving God's call and promises… Moses claims to be a nobody. Yet God says he will empower Moses; he will comfort him and strengthen him. God says he will pour out blessings upon Moses… After receiving all of God's blessings and promises, Moses turns and sees you and asks, "What can I do for you?"... You look at Moses and say, "Please tell me how you feel at this time in your life." Imagine how Moses would describe his life now after receiving all of God's blessings and promises... Notice how that makes you feel…

Now imagine yourself with Moses later in his life. Imagine yourself with Moses in the desert after he has witnessed the idolatry of Israel. Although Moses still has faith in God, he now feels despair and little hope for himself and his people … This despairing Moses now turns to you and asks, "What can I do for you?" … You look at him and say, "Please tell me how you feel about life now." Imagine how Moses describes life at this point in his journey... Notice how that makes you feel…

Now, imagine yourself meeting Moses at the very end of his life. He realizes that God will deliver all his promises even though his people have been unfaithful. He realizes that God can even feed people in the desert... Look upon Moses at this point in his journey… Moses turns to you and asks, "What can I do for you?" … You say, "Please tell me how you view life now at the end of your life"… What does Moses say? ... Notice how that makes you feel …

12.5.6.3 Guided Visualization: A Buddhist Conversation

Close your eyes and imagine yourself meeting Gautama in his youth before he had ever witnessed suffering before he had ever witnessed death. Imagine him in his protected environment, removed from all hardships and pain, isolated within his wealthy family's compound .... Look upon this protected, innocent youth named Gautama … This young man turns to you and asks, "What can I do for you?" … You look at him in all his innocence and say, "Please tell me how you feel at this time in your life." Imagine how Gautama would describe this time of his life … Notice how that makes you feel …

Now, imagine yourself meeting Gautama when he first discovers suffering and death. Imagine his feelings discovering suffering for the very first time … Look upon this shocked and disturbed young man, this man whose protected world has just been dramatically shattered by the existence of pain and death … This now disturbed young man turns to you and asks, "What can I do for you?" … You look at him and say, "Please tell me how you feel at this time in your life." Imagine how Gautama would describe his discovery of suffering and death … Notice how that makes you feel …

Now imagine yourself meeting the Buddha just as he has gotten up from sitting under the bodhi tree. Imagine his whole being aglow with the realization of enlightenment … Look upon the Buddha, this man who has now become aware of the way to overcome suffering, the way to transcend all the pain and death … The Buddha turns to you and asks, "What can I do for you?" … You look at the Buddha in the glow of his enlightenment and say, "Please tell me how you see death." Imagine how the Buddha would describe his enlightened perspective of death … Notice how that makes you feel …

12.5.6.4 Guided Visualization: A Naturalist Conversation

Close your eyes and imagine yourself standing before a majestic oak tree during the peak of the Summer season. This great oak tree towers before you with its deep, strong roots and its branches reaching out in all directions, each branch lavishly decorated with thousands of vibrant green leaves … Take a moment to look with wonder upon this mighty, richly decorated oak tree. You see that this tree has survived for many generations and has witnessed the passage of time … After you have examined this oak tree for a little while, a gentle voice emanates from the center of its massive trunk, asking, "What can I do for you?" … You look at this marvelous oak tree and say, "Please tell me how you feel in the midst of this Summer." Imagine how this oak tree would describe its summer state … Notice how that makes you feel …

Now, picture yourself standing before the same mighty oak tree during the Autumn season. Its leaves display a breathtaking array of glorious colors, with many clinging to the branches and others falling to the ground … Look at this tree at the height of its beauty and at the waning of its vitality ... After you have examined this oak tree in this transition stage, a beautiful voice arises from the center of its trunk, asking, "What can I do for you?" ... You look at this great oak tree and say, "Please tell me how you feel in the midst of the Fall." Imagine how this oak tree would describe its Fall condition .... Notice how that makes you feel …

Now, imagine that you are standing before this mighty oak tree in the heart of Winter. Its branches are bare; there are no more leaves. Several branches have been broken by an ice storm and lie scattered on the ground beneath the tree .... Look at this tree that has been stripped of all its beauty, standing in all of its vulnerability, shivering in the harsh winter wind ... After you have examined this oak tree in this stage of devastation, a quivering voice comes from the center of its trunk, asking, "What can I do for you?" ... You look at this great oak tree and say, "Please tell me how you feel in the midst of this Winter." Imagine how this oak tree would describe its Winter condition ... Notice how that makes you feel …

Finally, picture yourself standing before this mighty oak tree in early Spring. Buds are emerging all over its branches. Singing birds have returned to its branches and greet the tree with encouraging melodies each morning … Look at this tree amidst the renewal of life around it, upon it, and within it … After you have examined this oak tree in this rebirth stage, an excited voice emanates from the center of its trunk, asking, "What can I do for you?" ... You look at this great oak tree and say, "Please tell me how you feel in the midst of the Spring." Imagine how this oak tree would describe its Spring condition... Notice how that makes you feel …

12.5.6.5 Guided Visualization/Imagery: Family Reunion

Close your eyes. Picture yourself standing alone … Imagine your mother walking up to you … Picture her standing in front of you … Listen to your mother as she says, "I love you for all that you have been."… "I love you for all you have been." … Listen to your mother saying, "I love you for all that you are." … "I love you for all that you for all that you are." … Hear her saying, "I love you for all that you will be." "I love you for all that you will be." ...

Listen to your mother's request: "Forgive me for anything I have done to hurt you." ... "Forgive me for anything I have done to hurt you." ... Hear your mother saying, "I forgive you for anything that you have done to hurt me." ..."I forgive you for anything that you have done to hurt me." …

Listen to her say, "I love you; I always have; I always will." "I love you; I always have; I always will."... Notice how it feels when your mother wraps her arms around you and holds you ... Feel her holding you now ... Know she will always hold you… Know she will always hold you because she loves you. Know she really does love you ...

Picture yourself standing completely alone again …

Imagine your father walking up to you ... Picture your father standing in front of you… Listen to your father say, "I love you for all that you have been."... "I love you for all that you have been."... Listen to your father saying to you, "I love you for all that you are."… "I love you for all that you are."... Hear your father saying "I love you for all that you will be."... "I love you for all that you will be."…

Listen to your father's request: "Forgive me for anything I have done to hurt you."... "Forgive me for anything I have done to hurt you."... Listen to your father saying, "I forgive you for anything you have done to hurt me."… "I forgive you for anything you have done to hurt me."…

Hear your father saying, "I love you; I always have; I always will"… "I love you; I always have; I always will."… Notice how it feels when your father wraps his arms around you and holds you… Feel him holding you now… Know he will always hold you… Know he will always hold you because he loves you. Know he really does love you…

Now open your eyes knowing that your mother loves you and your father loves you…

12.5.7 Prayers and Transcendental Conversations

Prayers can be viewed as transcendental conversations with a higher power or any force that extends beyond a sense of limited self. Spiritual practices, including prayer, have been shown to improve emotional well-being, offering psychological comfort and fostering a deeper connection with higher powers. For instance, a study among cancer patients found that prayer helped ease emotional burdens and served as a powerful coping tool (Cheng et al., 2019). Furthermore, a systematic review has highlighted the role of spiritual care, including prayer, in enhancing both quality of life and spiritual well-being for those facing terminal illness (Chen et al., 2018).

The impact of prayer is shaped by various factors such as demographics, belief systems, and the broader social and psychological context in which it occurs. Among diverse social groups—such as Muslims and African American women—prayer has long been recognized as a significant coping mechanism. Beyond religious affiliations, those who identify as spiritual, agnostic, or secular also turn to prayer for comfort. This practice creates a space for mindfulness, self-reflection, and connection to a higher power or one's inner self. When done within a community or for others, prayer not only promotes a sense of belonging but also offers perceived social support, which is known to be a key factor in fostering resilience. Research has shown that for patients in hospice care, particularly those with terminal cancer, prayer often strengthens beliefs in an afterlife and contributes to improved psychological adjustment during difficult times (Bovero et al., 2016).

Though deeply personal, many religious and spiritual traditions offer collections of well-established prayers that provide comfort and reassurance. Whether practiced individually or in a group, and whether offered for oneself or others, these prayers hold significant psychological and social value.

For those who do not follow a specific religious tradition, creating a personalized form of conversation with the higher self, force of life, nature, etc., can still offer profound benefits. Drawing from principles of positive psychology and practices grounded in spirituality, the included guidelines can help shape these conversations in ways that nurture well-being and inner peace.

Guidelines for Transcendental Conversations

1. *Cultivate a sacred space.* Transcendental conversations can take place anywhere, but a peaceful environment—either internally or externally—can support the process. Whether it's through finding a quiet room or cultivating a calm mental space, fostering tranquility allows for a deeper connection with the inner self or a higher power.
2. *Reflect on intentions.* Before getting started, it is helpful to consider the purpose and intension of the prayer or conversation. Whether it is expressing gratitude, seeking guidance, or reaching out for connection, clarifying intentions can enrich the practice.
3. *Evoke positive feelings.* Engaging with emotions such as peace, love, or hope can deepen the experience.
4. *Incorporate gratitude.* Gratitude is a powerful element, whether at the start or the end of a conversation. Acknowledging the blessings or experiences that have brought joy can foster a sense of abundance and contentment.
5. *Use symbolic language.* Incorporating metaphors or symbols that resonate with spiritual beliefs can add depth and personal significance to the prayer.
6. *Include affirmations.* Positive affirmations reinforce intentions and promote a sense of empowerment. Using statements that align with personal or spiritual growth goals can instill a feeling of strength and possibility.
7. *Use present tense.* Framing intentions in the present tense creates a sense of immediacy. Speaking as though prayers or intentions are already being realized nurtures trust and confidence in the process.
8. *Express trust and let go.* Conclude with a sense of surrender and trust allows for releasing concerns. This step fosters a sense of peace, rooted in faith in the wisdom of life's processes.

The following section includes a collection of prayers and poems mainly composed by Dr. Yan Ciupak, drawing inspiration from multiple cultures and spiritual traditions. They reflect universal themes—love, peace, and the cosmos—while embracing the diverse ways different cultures engage with spirituality. Readers are encouraged to use these tools to find personal meaning and connection or create their own reflections.

Peace, Comfort, Strength, and Courage

May my mind filled with peace.
May my lungs breathe with ease.
May my heart beat with strength.
May my blood flow with courage.

Peace, Ease, Strength, and Courage

May they be mine to hold.
May they come to me.
May I share them freely.
May I live them fully.

May My Last Be My Best
May my last chapter shine brightest.
May my closing season be the finest.
May my ultimate act stand tallest.
May my final breath echo the sweetest.

A Prayer of Surrender
Lead me from individuality to collectivity.
Lead me from despair to hope, from fear to trust.
Lead me from death to life.
Lead me from myself to You.

A Prayer for Forgiveness
All that is precious in my life is fading away.
I look back, and for forgiveness, I pray.
May I be forgiven for the hearts I have wounded.
May I be forgiven for the time I have squandered.
May I be forgiven for the love I withheld.

In the remaining time bestowed upon me,
May I live fully, with joy and intention.
May I love freely, without hesitation.
May I listen deeply, with my heart wide open.
And may compassion and joy flow from you,
through me, into the world, without reservation.

A Prayer for Strength
I pray for a death free from pain.
But if the pain comes, may I face it with grace.
I pray for a death with grace,
But if grace slips, let me accept it with courage.
I pray for courage as the transition approaches.
But if courage falters, may I find peace.
And through it all, may I find strength in holding onto You.

A Prayer for Company
Please, stay with me through the night,
when shadows gather, and fears rise.
In the storms of life, be my stillness.
Let me see you; let me feel your presence.

When I'm lost in the unknown, reach for me,
hold me and lift me, give me strength.
Take my burdens, draw comfort near,
ease my soul, quiet my fear.

In your arms, I find rest,
like a spring meadow in soft sunlight.

With all that I am, I ask:
be with me, and let me be free.

A Sassy Conversation
Oh, mighty Almighty, up there on high,
Why'd you pick now to bid me goodbye?
I've got some ducks to put in a row,
and a few monkeys chirping hungry at home.

Your ways are mysterious, that much I know,
But couldn't you give me a heads-up before I go?
I've got suitcases full of unresolved issues
And a bag of half-baked projects and promises.

Your plan's all laid out, like a script on the floor,
But did you have to usher me out of the door?
I've still got Netflix shows to binge-watch,
And my cat's gearing up for a hairball rematch!

I'm not ready to go, I've still got some sass,
Half a dozen jokes to share,
and try some new hairdos.

I know you work in mysterious ways,
But why me, why now, and why somehow?
I'm finally learning to love, a big mystery to unravel.
The whole world awaits; an adventure to travel.

There are recipes to try, mountains to climb,
And a whole lot of mischief I've yet to prime.
And I'm not ready, what am I supposed to do?
Will I see the white light and a better place to pursue?

I've laughed, I've cried. I've had my drill,
Yet dreams linger on, waiting still.
So cut me some slack, strike a deal,
Hit pause, and I promise I'll be good and real.

But if not, well, I'll still hold a grudge,
As I shuffle off this mortal coil with a nudge.
But know this, Big Guy, when I take my last breath,
I'll meet you upstairs, and we'll chat and settle, even after death.

Note A transcendental conversation doesn't always have to be very serious. Express yourself genuinely, including frustrations, disappointments, or anger.

A Final Plea
As my time here fades and life slips away,
the things I once held dear begin to fray.

My heart, worn and tired, longs for rest,
my mind, once sharp, now foggy and tested.
This body that carried me now feels thin,
like an "old, worn-out garment" I'm ready to shed.

I look back on my days, feeling their weight,
seeking peace for the chances I didn't take.
Please, forgive me for any hurt I've caused,
for missed moments and love that was lost.
I hope for peace for words left unsaid,
as regrets rest heavy on my heart and head.

In whatever time remains, I make this plea:
let me bring no harm; let kindness flow from me.
With the moments left, however few,
let love be my guide in all I do.

And when the final curtain falls,
may I find peace beyond these walls.
Let forgiveness mend and make me whole,
so I leave this world with a lighter soul.

Note The metaphor of shedding an "old, worn-out garment" is inspired by Mahatma Gandhi, who said, *"To be afraid of death is like being afraid of discarding an old and worn-out garment"* (Gandhi, 1932/2024).

A Zen Prayer for Clarity

Buddha said we are never born
Therefore, never die.
Never gone, as we never came.
We are not the name, nor the form.
Never increasing, nor diminishing.

If there is no becoming,
let me arise in simply being.
If there is truth beyond thoughts,
let it reveal itself in silence.

This body, frail and fleeting,
this mind, restless and stubborn.
Clouds in the sky drifting.
Let me rest in the space between.

Fill the moment with peace,
Let it be as is.
Feel the breath with ease,
Blanket of awareness, revealing.

I seek no answers, only truth.
I seek no path, only a way home.
If there is nothing more, let it be enough.
If there is everything, let me awaken to it.

In stillness, let me see.
In seeing, let me be.

A Prayer
Please guide me and hold me,

as I embark this journey of transition.

Be ever present with me—

awake, dreaming, and deep sleeping.

Stand with me, beside me,

as I draw in the last, most precious breath.

A Buddhism-Inspired Prayer
In the sacred realms of boundless peace,
May I find myself in your loving embrace.
My lotus emerging in your radiant land,
Where Dharma whispers the sweetest tunes as petals open.

Note: Inspire by the Buddhist Pure land school.

A Prayer Amid Loneliness
I long for a kind word, a listening ear,
Craving love's caress, dispelling fear.
Yearning for the grace of a warm embrace,
A gentle kiss, a tender touch.

Fill this void, heavy and dark,
Release the tension that grips my heart.
Let me feel the warmth from deep within,
A gentle light wrapping, where shadows thin.

As breath becomes life-giving air,
And air breathes life's zest so dare.
My body, a vessel floating in space,
Each breath is a reunion, a sacred communion.

Hold me in my longings, ease this ache,
In my loneliness, a connection to make.
Let not solitude press on me,
Let your compassion set me free.

I believe in the Source, my life force,
The companion within, where truth runs its course.

Boundless fullness, a soothing grin,
Let it be, whatever may be,
In the divine companion.

So, I long for solace, in words unspoken.
A gentle touch that mends what's broken.
Embraced by a lover never apart,
In the still cave of the heart,
The soul finds its rest at last.

Note In Vedantic teachings, the "cave of the heart" symbolizes the innermost spiritual center where the Self (Atman, soul) resides. The Chandogya Upanishad (8.1.1) beautifully describes this: "In the city of Brahman, which is the body, there is a small lotus-like dwelling, within it is a small space. That which is to be sought after, that indeed, is what is to be realized" (Chandogya Upanishad, 8.1.1, Easwaran, 2007). This sacred space within the heart is where one realizes their divine essence and unity with Brahman through meditation and introspection.

I Give Thanks for Perceiving the Wonderful
I give thanks for perceiving the wonderful.
I look up into the heavens and see
a vast array of planets and stars,
and I know the world is wonderfully made,
held in the embrace of Your love.

I marvel at the intricacies of a single snowflake,
The strength of spring bulbs breaking the ground.
And I know the world is wonderfully made,
and the subject of Your love.

Thank you for sunsets painting the sky,
for the whispers of wind when it's time to say goodbye.
For memories gathered—both sweet and hard—
and for love that lifted me when I felt scarred.

My heart is weak,
my muscles and mind grow weary,
I know that I am fearfully and wonderfully made,
and the creation of Your boundless love.

Note Inspired by Psalm 139:14, *"I praise you, for I am fearfully and wonderfully made."*

Returning to the Land
I hear whispers of my ancestors
In the soft rustle of leaves
In the breath of the wind
In the earth, crumbling between my fingers.

They say:
You belong to this land
You are part of her pulse
In the depth of her flesh
Dance with the rhythm of her heartbeats.

I walk where they walked
Footprints fading into dust
And when my body tires
I will return—

I will be the soil
I will be the rain
I will push the sprouts to break the ground
And kiss the soft petals to bloom.

And my spirit will drift with the rivers
Flowing to the ocean, with an ancient tune, singing.

Note Inspired by indigenous reverence for the land, ancestors, and the cycles of life and death.

12.6 Real-Life Cases

The following offer real-life examples that highlight the unique challenges and spiritual journeys of patients and their families. The cases allow a glimpse into how spirituality can create moments of peace, resolve lingering questions, and foster meaningful connections between individuals, their families, and more. Each case demonstrates the healing power of presence, compassion, and spiritual awareness during life's transition.

12.6.1 Case Example: New Assignments

A 104-year-old woman lay in her home, surrounded by several generations of her family. Throughout her extensive life, she was an active matriarch, involved in numerous family projects, and consistently addressed the needs of her many relatives. She always finds fulfillment in knowing she is needed.

As her time drew near, the family gathered around her. Each family member took turns entering her room, sharing cherished memories, and bidding their final farewells.

Among the visitors was a 60-year-old granddaughter who had experienced the heartbreaking loss of a child many years ago. She spoke to her grandmother with a profound sense of certainty, "Grandma, I have always believed you are destined for heaven. Will you do something for me when you get there? I need you to watch over someone: my son, Jeremy. He has never been great at looking after himself, but you have always excelled at caring for many. Grandma, could you please keep an eye on Jeremy?" These words brought a radiant, big smile to the 104-year-old woman's face, thankful she had something more she could do for the family.

12.6.2 Case Example: Jean[5]'s Unveiling Perspective

Jean grew up in Atlanta during an era of ingrained discrimination and harbored many prejudices toward black people. As she approached the end of her life, her perceptions took a peculiar turn.

During the final 4 days, she consistently experienced vivid "hallucinations," claiming the presence of deceased relatives, including her husband and friends. On the day before her passing, she described seeing around 20 black individuals around her bed, engaged in singing and dancing. She said, "They told me I'm invited to a special party. They said they'd teach me how to sing and dance. And gracious me, do they know how to sing and dance!... And you know something else: they also told me that God loves them just as much as me. Can you believe that? ... You know, I think I believe them! I was totally convinced!"

Her children were convinced that she was hallucinating, but the authenticity of Jean's experience remains open to interpretation.

12.6.3 Case Example: A Special Visitor

Although just an adolescent, Tanya had come to terms with her impending death and embraced it without resistance. But Tanya's mother urged her to fight, saying that it was not God's will for Tanya to depart so soon. Tanya reluctantly followed her mother's suggestions and tried various difficult treatments at hospitals. But Tanya would still periodically, as best she could try to tell her mother that she thought that it was the right time and she was ready for it.

One day, Tanya told her mother that one of the hospital employees, a man she thought was a very caring person, was telling her that it was really okay for her to die. Tanya said that this caring man would often enter Tanya's room as soon as her mother finished her visit.

Tanya's mother, needless to say, was furious; she wanted to track down this hospital employee to confront him. So, she asked Tanya what the man's name was. Tanya said she didn't know. So, Tanya's mother asked for a description of this man,

---

[5] All names in this text are pseudonyms to protect the confidentiality of individuals. Exceptions are the authors and those that gave permission, such as Swami Omkarananda.

the man who had the audacity to sneak into the room immediately after her visits and tell her daughter that it was okay to die.

Tanya's description was very detailed. She said the man was about 6 ft tall, had a white goatee, had a twitch in his right eye, spoke in a loud whisper, and always wore a black shirt and black boots. As Tanya was describing the man, her mother started crying. Tanya had just described her mother's father, who had died 3 years before Tanya was even born.

Tanya's mother then knew it was indeed "God's will" that Tanya goes soon.

12.6.4 Case Example: My Body Is Sick, But I Am Well

I (Yan Ciupak) had the honor of video chatting with Anara Maa, mother of Swami Omkarananda, 2 weeks before her passing. Her story was already familiar to me. According to Swami Omkarananda, over three decades ago, his 7-year-old sister passed away in their home in Southern India. Inspired by her last words, their mother stopped eating solid food and spent the next 11 years living solely on water and chai tea. Though she lost a significant amount of weight, she managed to maintain remarkable health, fulfill household duties, and engage in intense spiritual practices. Her story drew attention from the medical community, local administration, and the media, giving her an honorable nickname "Anara Maa" (meaning "the mother who does not eat") by the media.

During those 11 years, Anara Maa frequently dreamed of her daughter with two monks in various villages. Despite facing ridicule and judgment from others, she insisted on searching for those places. All the details of her dreams were eventually verified, except for the girl's.

Deeply puzzled yet inspired by his mother's faith, Swami Omkarananda left his promising engineering career to embark on a journey to the Himalayas. His goal was to learn the ancient techniques to identify people's reincarnations. He promised his mother that he would find her daughter's reincarnation before either of them took their last breath. Three decades passed. He studied under multiple accomplished masters, eventually becoming a revered monk himself, earning the title of Swami Omkarananda. He traveled to 67 countries and helped thousands of people. Through his training, along with some extraordinary gifts by birth, he was able to perceive people's life forms and subtle energies transforming between different existences. The veil between life and death became increasingly transparent to him.

One day, quite unexpectedly, he encountered his sister's reincarnation during a counseling session in the United States. This reunion brought many tears and laughter through video calls between mother and daughter. However, just a month later, Anara Maa suddenly fell ill with a brain tumor.

During our video call, Anara Maa appeared frail as she leaned her head gently on Swami Omkarananda's shoulder. Her voice was soft yet carried a peaceful strength. Looking at me with a smile, she said, "Everything you've heard is true. I always knew I would find my daughter. Now that I have found her, I am ready to leave this world."

I gently asked her, "How are you feeling?"

With a serene smile, she replied, "My legs can't move, and my body is sick, but *I am well*."

Note: The above is based on the December 23 video call between Dr. Yan Ciupak and Anara Maa and interviews with Swami Omkarananda in November 2023 and November 2024. The story of Swami Omkarananda and his mother is currently in production as a documentary and is also being developed into a book.

12.6.5 Case Example: Doug's Growing Awareness

(Personal email communication from Doug Smith to Yan Ciupak, March 4, 2024)

The condition of my congestive heart failure is changing. Up until recently, I would merely have waves of symptoms: occasional heart arrhythmia and struggles for breath, periods of tiredness, unpredictable episodes of kidney pain, intermittent losses of balance, irregular bodily functions, and sporadic brain fog. Recently, the symptoms have become steadily and progressively worse: frequent arrhythmia and breathlessness, constant tiredness, persistent kidney pain, always careful with my balance, regular irregularity in my bowels, and increasing brain fog.

Yet, mysteriously coupled with the intensifying deterioration of my earthly being, there is another aspect of my being that seems to be growing (expanding, maturing). The growing aspect is an increasingly clear Awareness of what is happening to me, an Awareness like no awareness I have ever had. It feels like an omniscient, vigilant Observer encircling my body and mind with a consciousness of all that is within me and around me. This Awareness—this Observer—sees and transcends everything from a non-temporal, nonphysical perspective, comprehensively seeing from a place of peace and contentment, a peace and contentment not found in this temporal, physical world. And this Awareness (this painless Awareness of my pain), this Observer (this clarifying Observer of my unclarity), is just as much—and even more—amalgamated to me as my earthly trials and tribulations. However, those trials and tribulations often feel as though they are overpowering all of what I have previously labeled "me." Yet, despite the seeming sensation of overpowering, I still have a comprehensive Awareness of that seeming sensation; I still am the omniscient, vigilant Observer who can somehow see with peace and contentment, unperturbed by the temporal and physical.

I anticipate that eventually, the earthly aspects of me will become so overpowered with trials and tribulations and pain and confusion, that I will not be able to communicate to those encapsulated in this earthly plain anything about my Awareness or the Observer, even though the Awareness is ever-expanding, and the Observer is omniscient and ever-advancing—me eventually coming to a place where one of my two aspects (my earthly aspect) will completely disappear. Then, I will enter a reality where One is mysteriously and undeniably greater than two.

Reflection The co-author of this book, Doug, shared the above reflections with Yan a few months before his passing. Though Doug was a long-time Christian priest devoted to his faith, his language strikingly resonates with Buddhist and Vedantic traditions. His description of an observing consciousness closely parallels teachings in non-dualistic philosophies. Remarkably, Doug used this language and these ideas without prior familiarity or preconceived notions of these concepts.

Doug's reflections demonstrate that profound spiritual experiences can lead to similar insights across religious frameworks. While honoring diverse expressions, his insights highlight a universal humanity that transcends religious and cultural boundaries.

12.7 Concluding Reflection

Facing mortality often prompts existential questions and spiritual reflection. Spiritual care at the end of life is more than a responsibility—it is an act of profound respect for the human spirit. As Sogyal Rinpoche emphasized in his talk at the 1st International Spiritual Care Conference (as cited in Kangataran, 2009), spiritual care is not a luxury for a few but an essential right for every individual, as crucial as political liberty and medical care. This concept highlights the role of spirituality in helping individuals navigate one of life's most challenging transitions. By addressing spiritual dimensions, professionals can nurture the whole person—mind, body, and spirit—when holistic support is most needed.

The real challenge, however, lies in the delivery of spiritual support and care. Competing demands, time constraints, diversity of cultures, and individual needs all create a complex landscape that requires patience, humility, and compassion toward the self as well as those receiving care. As this chapter highlights, the essence of spiritual care is not about fixing or solving but about being present, deeply listening, and validating each unique spiritual journey. This was echoed at the First International Spiritual Care Conference, themed "Compassion and Presence" where it was emphasized that a kind heart is as valuable as medical expertise (Kangataran, 2009). Kindness can promote healing even when medicine cannot, reflecting Thomas Moore's notion that "our work would change remarkably if we thought about it as ongoing care rather than a quest for a cure" (Moore, 2009, p. 19).

The tools shared in this chapter invite reflection and connection, allowing professionals and caregivers to facilitate peace and resilience at the end of life. Healing is always accessible, even when curing is not.

References

Baumann, D., & Ruch, W. (2022). Measuring what counts in life: The development and initial validation of the Fulfilled Life Scale (FLS). *Frontiers in Psychology, 12*, 795931. https://doi.org/10.3389/fpsyg.2021.795931

Batstone, E., Bailey, C., & Hallett, N. (2020). Spiritual care provision to end-of-life patients: A systematic literature review. *Journal of Clinical Nursing, 29*(19–20), 3609–3624. https://doi.org/10.1111/jocn.15411

Bovero, A., Leombruni, P., Miniotti, M., & Rocca, G. (2016). Spirituality, quality of life, psychological adjustment in terminal cancer patients in hospice. *European Journal of Cancer Care*. https://onlinelibrary.wiley.com/doi/abs/10.1111/ecc.12360

Breitbart, W., Rosenfeld, B., Gibson, C., Pessin, H., Poppito, S., Nelson, C., et al. (2010). Meaning-centered group psychotherapy for patients with advanced cancer: A pilot randomized controlled trial. *Psychooncology, 19*(1), 21–28.

Chandogya Upanishad. (2007). *The Upanishads* (E. Easwaran, Trans.). Nilgiri Press.

Chen, J., Lin, Y., Yan, J., Wu, Y., & Hu, R. (2018). The effects of spiritual care on quality of life and spiritual well-being among patients with terminal illness: A systematic review. *Palliative Medicine, 32*(7), 1167–1179.

Cheng, Q., Liu, X., Li, X., Wang, Y., Mao, T., & Chen, Y. (2019). Improving spiritual well-being among cancer patients: Implications for clinical care. *Supportive Care in Cancer*. https://link.springer.com/article/10.1007/s00520-019-4636-4

Confucius. (2008). *The Analects* (R. Dawson, Trans.). Oxford University Press.

Creswell, J. D. (2017). Mindfulness interventions. *Annual Review of Psychology, 68*, 491–516. https://doi.org/10.1146/annurev-psych-042716-051139

Davidson, R. J., Kabat-Zinn, J., Schumacher, J., Rosenkranz, M., Muller, D., Santorelli, S. F., et al. (2003). Alterations in brain and immune function produced by mindfulness meditation. *Psychosomatic Medicine, 65*(4), 564–570.

Gandhi, M. (1932/2004). *Selected letters*. Shambhala.

Gijsberts, M. J. H., Liefbroer, A. I., Otten, R., & Olsman, E. (2019). Spiritual care in palliative care: A systematic review of the recent European literature. *Medical Sciences, 7*(2), 25.

Global Network for Spirituality and Health (GNSAH). (n.d.). https://gwish.smhs.gwu.edu/programs/global-network-gnsah

Hodge, D. R., & Limb, G. E. (2010). A Native American perspective on spiritual assessment: The strengths and limitations of a complementary set of assessment tools. *Health & Social Work, 35*(2), 121–131.

Kangataran, M. (2009, April 28). *Conference review: 1st International Spiritual Care Conference, Dzogchen Beara Retreat Centre, Beara Peninsula, Co. Cork.* Irish Association of Humanistic and Integrative Psychotherapy. https://iahip.org/page-1075877

Koenig, H. G., King, D., & Carson, V. B. (2012). *Handbook of Religion and Health*. OUP USA.

Marty, M., & Vaux, K. (Eds.). (1982). *Health/medicine and the faith traditions: An inquiry into religion and medicine*. Fortress Press.

Moore, T. (2009). *Care of the Soul: A Guide for Cultivating Depth and Sacredness in Everyday Life*. HarperCollins.

Neimeyer, R. A., Torres, C., & Smith, D. C. (2011). The virtual dream: Rewriting stories of loss and grief. *Death Studies, 35*(7), 646–672.

Nolan, S., Saltmarsh, P., & Leget, C. J. W. (2011). Spiritual care in palliative care: Working towards an EAPC task force. *European Journal of Palliative Care, 18*, 86–89.

Palmo, J. T. (2023). *Reflections on a mountain lake: Teachings on practical Buddhism*. Shambhala.

Prevost, V., Tran, T., Leconte, A., Lequesne, J., & Fernette, M. (2024). The potential added value of shared meditation involving people with cancer, health professionals, and third persons compared to meditation conducted with patients. *BMC Cancer*. https://link.springer.com/article/10.1186/s12885-024-12521-1

Puchalski, C., Ferrell, B., Virani, R., Otis-Green, S., Baird, P., Bull, J., et al. (2009). Improving the quality of spiritual care as a dimension of palliative care: the report of the consensus conference. *Journal of Palliative Medicine, 12*(10), 885–904.

Rinpoche, Y. M., & Swanson, H. (2008). T*he Joy of Living: Unlocking the Secret and Science of Happiness.* Harmony Books.

Santorelli, S. F., Kabat-Zinn, J., Blacker, M., Meleo-Meyer, F., & Koerbel, L. (2017). *Mindfulness-based stress reduction (MBSR) authorized curriculum guide.* Center for mindfulness in medicine, health care, and society (CFM). University of Massachusetts Medical School.

Selby, D., Seccaraccia, D., Huth, J., Kurppa, K., & Fitch, M. (2017). Patient versus health care provider perspectives on spirituality and spiritual care: The potential to miss the moment. *Annals of Palliative Medicine, 6*(2), 14352–14152.

Selman, L. E., Brighton, L. J., Sinclair, S., Karvinen, I., Egan, R., Speck, P., et al. (2018). Patients' and caregivers' needs, experiences, preferences, and research priorities in spiritual care: A focus group study across nine countries. *Palliative Medicine, 32*(1), 216–230. https://doi.org/10.1177/0269216317734954

Sogyal, R. (2002). *The Tibetan book of living and dying.* HarperCollins.

Stephen, F. A., Ermalyn, L. P., Mangorsi, B. Y., Louise, L. J., & Juvenmile, T. B. (2022). A voyage into the visualization of athletic performances: A review. *American Journal of Multidisciplinary Research and Innovation, 1*(3), 105–109.

Tan, T. T., Tan, M. P., Lam, C. L., Loh, E. C., Capelle, D. P., Zainuddin, S. I., et al. (2023). Mindful gratitude journaling: Psychological distress, quality of life, and suffering in advanced cancer: A randomised controlled trial. *BMJ Supportive & Palliative Care, 13*(e2), e389–e396. https://doi.org/10.1136/bmjspcare-2022-003729

Taylor, E. J., Pariñas, S., Mamier, I., Atarhim, M. A., Angeles, L., Aslan, H., Aktürk, Ü., Ercİ, B., Soriano, G., Sinaga, J., Chen, Y.-H., Merati-Fashi, F., Odonel, G., Neathery, M., Permatasari, W., Ricci-Allegra, P., Foith, J., Caldeira, S., & Dehom, S. (2023). Frequency of nurse-provided spiritual care: an international comparison. *Journal of Clinical Nursing, 32*(3–4), 597–609. https://doi.org/10.1111/jocn.16497

Wiggins, M. I. (2011). Spiritual journaling. In J. D. Aten, M. R. McMinn, & E. L. Worthington Jr. (Eds.), *Spiritually oriented interventions for counseling and psychotherapy* (pp. 303–321). American Psychological Association. https://doi.org/10.1037/12313-012

World Health Organization. (2018). *WHO definition of palliative care.* https://www.who.int/news-room/fact-sheets/detail/palliative-care

Chapter 13
Spiritual Support Tools for Grieving

13.1 Spirituality and Religiosity

Spirituality and religiosity are two concepts that can sometimes be confusing. The *Handbook of Religion and Health* (Koenig et al., 2001) outlines the distinction between them. Religion is described as community-focused, observable, measurable, and objective, characterized by formal, orthodox, and organized practices with an outward behavioral orientation and elements of authority. In contrast, spirituality is portrayed as more individualistic, less visible, and subjective. It tends to be less formal and systematic, more emotionally oriented, inwardly focused, nonauthoritarian, and unifying rather than bound by doctrine. While this distinction provides valuable insights, there is still little universal consensus among scholars or communities regarding the relationship and distinctions between spirituality and religion.

Within the care setting, spirituality is often defined through three basic elements: "connectedness," "meaning and purpose of one's life," and "transcendence" (Willemse et al., 2020). These dimensions align with Puchalski's widely accepted definition of spirituality:

> Spirituality is a dynamic and intrinsic aspect of humanity that refers to the way individuals seek and express meaning, purpose, and transcendence, and is often tied with the feeling of connectedness to the moment, self, family, others, community, society, nature, and the significant or sacred. Spirituality is expressed through beliefs, values, traditions, and practices.
> —Puchalski, M. and Ferrell, B. (2010, p.25)

Spirituality and religiosity are not mutually exclusive, and significant individual variation exists even within the same religious affiliation. Therefore, spiritual care requires cultural humility while embracing spiritual diversity.

Y. Z. Ciupak, D. C. Smith, *Death, Dying, and Grief*,
https://doi.org/10.1007/978-3-031-88467-2_13

13.2 Spirituality in Grieving and Healing

Spirituality can play a supportive role as people navigate loss and grief. It provides a lens through which grieving persons interpret their experiences and make sense of their emotions and actions. Traumatic loss, in particular, can trigger intense emotional pain and cognitive challenges, often shaking a person's core beliefs and leading to what is known as a spiritual crisis or complicated spiritual grief (Burke & Neimeyer, 2014; Janoff-Bulman, 1992).

In response to loss, some may distance themselves from their prior religious beliefs, feeling anger or disillusionment toward a higher power, while others may find new spiritual paths or deepen their existing religious practices. Čepulienė and Skruibis's (2022) qualitative study on spirituality during suicide bereavement found that spirituality, when personally meaningful and supported by others, can be a valuable resource for post-traumatic growth. This study highlights the importance of the cultural and social frameworks that shape grief and spiritual coping mechanisms, suggesting that the effectiveness of spiritual resources may depend on their alignment with the individual's social and cultural context. Conversely, when spiritual practices are stigmatized or when there is an absence of meaningful traditions, bereaved individuals may experience greater distress. Spiritual experiences and questions often become deeply entwined with the grieving process, shaped by broader social and cultural factors.

Research consistently shows that spiritual beliefs and practices promote peace and acceptance, aiding people in reconciling with their loss. Spiritual practices have been shown to enhance emotional regulation and foster a sense of meaning and agency during grief (Burke & Neimeyer, 2012). Religious coping has also been associated with mitigating the negative impacts of grief while encouraging resilience and personal growth (Park & Halifax, 2021).

The relationship between religiosity and mental health is evident in findings showing that religious involvement contributes to better emotional adjustment, especially during stressful or medically challenging times (Koenig, 2008). Regular participation in religious communities often strengthens social support networks, providing critical support during life's challenges. Furthermore, recent studies have highlighted how spirituality serves as a protective factor in coping with loss and trauma. For instance, spirituality played a vital role in helping individuals cope with the trauma of losing loved ones during the COVID-19 pandemic in Italy, with funeral rites offering social-emotional support and facilitating healthy grieving (Biancalani et al., 2022).

13.3 Rituals and Other Spiritual Practices in Grief Therapy

Spiritual practices, such as prayer, meditation, rituals, and community worship, have also been shown to positively influence the grieving process and outcomes (Park & Halifax, 2021). Engaging in these practices not only brings comfort but also aids in healing by nurturing a sense of continuity, connection, and purpose. Prayer and meditation connect individuals with a higher power or their innermost self, potentially inducing an empowering "identity fusion" (Whitehouse & Lanman, 2014). Cultural rituals foster cohesion and activate the "motivational systems and cognitive processes present in humans for evolutionary reasons" (Boyer & Liénard, 2006, p. 825). Additionally, creating personal sacred spaces or altars with meaningful symbols can serve as focal points for remembrance and healing.

In therapeutic settings, there has been an increasing incorporation of symbolic and ritual communications drawn from different traditions, particularly in the treatment of prolonged or traumatic grief. Various types of grief rituals have been identified in the therapy literature, such as (1) honoring rituals, (2) letting-go rituals, farewell ceremonies, or reconciliation rituals focusing on asking for or extending forgiveness, and (3) self-transformation rituals (Doka, 2012; Sas & Coman, 2016). Wojtkowiak et al. (2021) broadly define rituals in therapeutic interventions as "sensory, attentive, and intentional acts that are performed in a structured, imaginative, or aesthetic way and make use of symbols, symbolic language, and symbolic action" (p. 2). In their scope review of 22 studies, they found that rituals in therapeutic interventions can mitigate the adverse effects of grief, reducing prolonged grief disorder symptoms.

These structured, tangible approaches to grieving provide a channel for emotional expression and connection through symbolically meaningful embodied forms, such as lighting candles, writing letters, or holding commemorative ceremonies. The emotional intensity experienced during these modalities is contained within a safe framework, allowing for deep expression without overwhelming the individual. The symbolic reality and behavioral engagements offer an emotional anchor while providing space for authentic expression, thus aiding in emotional regulation and fostering a sense of agency and connectedness.

When incorporating these tools into therapy, care providers must remain attuned to cultural sensitivity (Wojtkowiak et al., 2021). For practitioners working with clients from diverse cultural backgrounds, it is essential to conduct a thorough cultural assessment of bereavement and grief to ensure that treatments are aligned and effective. The Bereavement and Grief Cultural Formulation Interview (BGCFI), an extension of the Diagnostic and Statistical Manual of Mental Disorders, 5th edition (DSM-5) Cultural Formulation Interview, offers brief, open-ended, person-centered questions that explore cultural traditions surrounding death, mourning, and coping. By using these tools, practitioners can gain insights and deliver culturally sensitive care.

The following sections offer examples of tools that can be applied in various settings, including remembrance practices, rituals, meditation, prayers, dream journaling, and the creation of altars. Many of these practices, inspired by various spiritual and cultural traditions, have been adapted for a wider audience and can be further customized to meet the specific needs of those receiving care. These tools reflect the richness and diversity in cultural heritages, showcasing humanity's innate capacity for healing and transcendence.

13.4 Remembrance

Remembrance allows those who are grieving to honor the lives of their loved ones in deeply personal and meaningful ways. Whether through intimate gatherings or private acts of reflection, these practices offer comfort and help maintain a sense of connection to the deceased. From private services to marking anniversaries or finding ways to remember from afar, these rituals provide moments of healing, support, and continuity in the midst of loss.

13.4.1 Private Service of Remembrance

In addition to the public funeral service, mourners may find solace in holding a special, intimate service at their home. This can be scheduled for the same day as the public service, the following weekend, or on the 1-month anniversary. This service is designed for close family and friends, providing a personal space to remember and honor the deceased. The following provides some examples for inspiration and customization:

A. *Theme-centered service*: Selecting a theme that reflects the personality or life of the loved one can create a unique and meaningful atmosphere. The theme could be celebratory, reflective, humorous, or solemn, helping guide the tone and activities of the service.
B. *Sharing a meal*: Sharing a meal before or after the service can offer comfort and foster a sense of community. Food has a special way of bringing people together, nourishing both body and spirit in times of grief.
C. *Personal contributions*: Encouraging attendees to share something personal—whether it be a eulogy, a favorite reading, a poem, or music—adds depth to the service and allows for meaningful expression.
D. *Memories on display*: Filling the space with photos and mementos of the loved one invites stories and conversations. These tangible reminders help everyone celebrate the life lived and connect through shared memories.

13.4.2 Anniversary Service of Remembrance

A year after the loss, many find it healing to hold a special memorial service to honor the deceased and reflect on the journey of grief and healing over the past year.

A. *Readings, prayers, and music*: Choosing readings, prayers, and music that resonate with the deceased's personality and beliefs can offer comfort and continuity.
B. *Involvement of loved ones*: Inviting family and friends to participate in specific parts of the service adds significance and fosters a deeper connection by involving those closest to the deceased.
C. *Reflecting on change*: Structuring the service to reflect on changes over the past year—how grief has been navigated and how healing has progressed—can honor both the past and the journey ahead.
D. *Activity of closure*: Ending the service with a symbolic act, such as releasing balloons, planting a tree, or creating a memory quilt, provides a meaningful way to close the ceremony while continuing to honor the deceased.
E. *Sharing stories*: Including a time for attendees to share memories and stories can foster a sense of community and keep the loved one's memory alive. This can be done through an open mic or a more structured format.
F. *Digital tributes and virtual gatherings*: For those who are unable to attend in person, an online memorial page or a virtual service allows distant friends and family to share in the remembrance.
G. *Charity donations*: Organizing a fundraiser in memory of the deceased can be a meaningful way to honor their legacy, supporting causes that were important to them and turning the anniversary into a moment of positive action.

13.4.3 Remembrance from Afar

When circumstances prevent someone from attending a funeral service in person, there are still many meaningful ways to honor the deceased from afar:

A. *Prayer or liturgy*: Saying a prayer or reading a funeral liturgy at the same time as the actual service can create a sense of connection, participating in spirit even from a distance.
B. *Lighting a candle*: Lighting a candle at home or in a place of worship is a simple but powerful act of remembrance, symbolizing the light the deceased brought into the lives of others.
C. *Reflecting with a photograph*: Spending time with a photograph of the deceased and reflecting on memories can help process emotions and provide a personal moment of connection and closure.
D. *Writing a letter*: Writing a letter to the deceased can be a therapeutic exercise, offering a way to express what remains unsaid and maintain a connection with their memory.

E. *Planting in memory*: Planting a tree, flower, or shrub in a meaningful location creates a living tribute, offering comfort as it grows and becomes a lasting reminder of the loved one's life.
F. *Digital memorials*: Contributing to an online memorial page allows others to share memories, photos, and messages, creating a communal space for remembrance and connection.
G. *Virtual gatherings*: Organizing a virtual memorial or remembrance gathering brings together friends and family who cannot attend in person, providing a space to share memories and offer support.
H. *Digital scrapbooks or videos*: Compiling a digital scrapbook or video montage with contributions from family and friends serves as a lasting tribute, something that can be shared and revisited.
I. *Charitable donations or fundraisers*: Setting up a digital fundraiser or making charitable donations in memory of the deceased offers a meaningful way to honor their legacy and support causes that were important to them.

13.5 Personal Spaces and Altars

Personal spaces for remembrance offer the bereaved a tangible and meaningful way to honor their loved ones. Through altars, memory jars, or other setups, these spaces serve as reminders of the deceased's presence, providing a place for reflection and connection. They can be adapted to reflect the unique personality, culture, and life of the person being remembered.

13.5.1 Altar of Remembrance

An "Altar of Remembrance" at home can provide a comforting space for reflection and connection with a loved one. This space—whether a coffee table, end table, or dresser—can be personalized to gently remind the bereaved of the ongoing influence of the deceased. Here are a few ideas to help create and customize this space:

A. *Altar cloth and personal items*: An altar cloth made from the deceased's clothing, such as a favorite scarf or piece of fabric from an outfit, can add a personal touch. Personal items like jewelry (rings, watches) or objects related to hobbies (a model train car, a kitchen utensil, a golf ball, or a favorite book) can further personalize the space.
B. *Photographs and documents*: Display photos from different stages of the loved one's life, creating a visual timeline of their journey. A digital photo frame could offer a more interactive experience with a rotating slideshow. Framed certificates of achievement or a laminated obituary can also be included.

C. *Memorabilia and writings*: Adding favorite quotes, meaningful passages from scripture, or letters and notes that were written by or to the deceased can create a deep emotional connection. These reminders can provide moments of reflection and comfort.
D. *Candles, incense, and aromatics*: A candle on the altar can be lit on special occasions—birthdays, anniversaries, or holidays—as a way to honor and remember the loved one. Incense or essential oils can also be added to create a soothing atmosphere and evoke pleasant memories tied to specific scents.
E. *Natural elements and seasonal items*: Incorporating natural elements like flowers or plants can bring a sense of life to the altar. Changing the decorations to reflect the seasons, holidays, or significant dates keeps the altar dynamic and evolving, much like the ongoing process of grief and remembrance.
F. *Cultural and artistic items*: Including cultural or religious symbols, statues, or artifacts can reflect the loved one's beliefs and background. Artwork or crafts created by the deceased can also be displayed, adding another layer of personal significance to the space.

13.5.2 Memory Jar

A Memory Jar is a simple yet deeply meaningful way for families to remember and honor a loved one. To create one, start with a beautiful clear jar or container. Next to it, place a basket filled with colorful paper or sticky notes, pens, and a small decorative item like a pebble or silk flower petal. A picture of the deceased can be placed on or beside the jar as a focal point.

Whenever someone feels the need to express their thoughts, share a memory, or simply reflect on the loved one, they can write it on one of the papers, fold it, and place it in the jar, along with the small decorative token. This practice encourages everyone, including children, to openly share their feelings and memories, fostering a sense of emotional connection and healing within the family.

Over time, the jar becomes filled with notes and tokens, creating a tangible collection of cherished memories and sentiments. Reading these notes together can serve as a comforting family activity, bringing the family closer through shared remembrance. Alternatively, a small fire ritual or puja can be held where the notes are burned, symbolically sending blessings and wishes through the flame and smoke, offering a moment of release and peace.

13.6 Rituals and Symbolic Actions

Ritual provides a symbolic and tangible tool for individuals and communities to work through grief. It offers a structured way to engage with emotions, grounding them in concrete actions that create a sense of control amid overwhelming loss. For many, rituals serve as a bridge between personal mourning and collective experience, allowing grief to be shared and supported within a community.

Across cultures, rituals have been used for centuries to help people navigate the pain of loss. These shared practices—whether religious ceremonies, memorial services, or simple acts of remembrance—provide a space where grief can be expressed, processed, and ultimately transformed. The act of lighting candles, offering prayers, or even preparing a meal in honor of the deceased creates a moment where grief is held and recognized.

For example, *Día de los Muertos* in Mexican culture gathers families and communities to honor their loved ones by building altars, offering food, and sharing memories. This ritual helps keep the memory of the deceased alive and fosters a sense of connection among the living. Similarly, in Buddhist traditions, the chanting of prayers over several days not only guides the deceased's spirit but also supports the bereaved through their communal mourning.

These rituals, whether elaborate or simple, allow people to step into a shared cultural framework, offering both emotional release and a sense of continuity. They remind us that grief, while deeply personal, is also something that can be carried together. The following sections provide a few examples of rituals inspired by various cultures.

13.6.1 *The Ancient Stone Ceremony*

The Ancient Stone Ceremony provides a structured and symbolic approach to honor and remember the deceased, integrating elements of reflection, gratitude, and meditation. It draws inspiration from various cultural and spiritual traditions, such as Native American, Celtic, and African indigenous practices, all of which employ stones and nature to connect with the spiritual realm.

Native American rituals often involve the use of circles, cardinal directions, and natural elements like stones to create sacred spaces for spiritual connection. These traditions emphasize harmony with nature and the significance of the four directions, which are believed to represent different aspects of life and spirituality. Similarly, Celtic traditions, with their stone circles and megalithic structures like Stonehenge, use stones to mark significant spiritual sites and perform rituals that honor the cycles of life and death. African indigenous practices also incorporate natural elements and symbolic objects in rituals to connect with ancestors and the spiritual world, honoring the ongoing relationship between the living and the deceased. In addition, the circle could also be viewed as the "circle of life" in Tibetan Buddhism.

1. Go to a place with many stones and draw a 6-ft-wide circle in the dirt.
2. Stand in the center of the circle and invoke the presence of the deceased, inviting them to stand beside you. Spend time feeling the presence of the departed within the circle.

3. Leave the circle to find four stones, placing each on the edge of the circle in one of the four cardinal directions: south, west, north, and east.
4. From the center of the circle, face the stone on the southern edge. While facing this stone, bring to mind the childhood and childlike qualities of the deceased. Approach the stone, touch it, and verbalize appreciation for the child in the deceased.
5. Return to the center, then face the stone on the western edge. Reflect on the deceased's bravery and courage. Approach the stone, touch it, and express appreciation for its bravery and courage.
6. Next, face the stone on the northern edge, recalling the deceased's skills and talents. Approach, touch the stone, and verbalize appreciation for these qualities.
7. Face the stone on the eastern edge and think about the deceased's visions and dreams. Approach, touch the stone, and express gratitude for the deceased's visions and dreams.
8. Sit in the center of the circle, thanking the deceased for all their contributions. Meditate on the gifts received from the deceased.
9. When ready to leave, return the stones to their original places, erase the circle, and restore the area to its original state. During this process, meditate on two important realities:

    - *Acceptance of reality:* From one point of view, we cannot change time or place. What has happened has happened. Reality is what reality is. When someone has died they are no longer here and will not return.
    - *Continued presence:* From another point of view, no thing or person is completely confined to a particular time or place. I can now carry that person with me wherever I go. That person can now be embodied in me and in everything I witness and experience.

13.6.2 A Farewell Ceremony

Farewell ceremonies or letting-go rituals are meaningful and structured activities designed to help the bereaved process their grief and find a sense of closure. This ritual combines physical actions with emotional reflection, which can be particularly effective in the grieving process. It is important to understand that letting go does not mean letting go of the relationship. Death ends a body, but not love or the bond shared. Letting go or farewell is about accepting the change while integrating the deceased into a continuing bond.

1. First, the bereaved individuals choose a meaningful item that symbolizes the deceased, such as clothing, a photograph, or another cherished possession.
2. They then bring this object to a place of significance shared with the deceased, enhancing the ritual's personal significance.
3. Depending on the chosen method, a pit is dug or a fire pit is prepared for a ceremonial burial or respectful burning of the object. Safety and environmental

considerations are crucial, with options like using biodegradable materials for burning.

4. Before burying or burning the object, the bereaved engages in a brief meditation, possibly jotting down thoughts to focus their reflection.
5. The object is then laid to rest in the earth or consumed by flames. Alternatively, if burial or burning is not preferred, consider other symbolic actions like casting the object into water.
6. Afterward, the bereaved individuals meditate on releasing both the object and their connection to the departed. Symbolic acts, such as lighting and extinguishing a candle, signify the transition from holding on to letting go.
7. Finally, the ritual concludes with a positive gesture, like planting a flower or tree in the same spot, symbolizing renewal and hope. Continuing activities like journaling, creating a memory book, or joining support groups can further aid in the healing process.

Notes: Additional Considerations

1. While a solitary ritual can be powerful, inviting close friends or family members to participate or witness the ceremony can provide additional support and a sense of communal grieving. Additionally, a farewell ceremony could be conducted in a group setting or at the end of a treatment, with the option of inviting family, friends, or other loved ones to attend.
2. Encourage the bereaved individuals to customize the ritual with elements that are personally significant, such as specific prayers, readings, or songs that are meaningful to the deceased or the bereaved.
3. Consider the environmental impact of the ritual method chosen. Opt for eco-friendly practices where possible.

13.6.3 River of Life

The "River of Life" ritual is a serene and reflective activity designed to help the bereaved process their grief and find a sense of peace and continuity. This ritual involves a natural waterway and a symbolic object, creating a metaphor for the journey of life and the enduring connection with the deceased.

1. Locate a quiet stream or meandering river where you can sit quietly and undisturbed.
2. Choose or create an object that symbolizes your relationship with the departed loved one.
3. Hold the object in your hand while meditating upon the stream and your relationship with the deceased.
4. When you are ready, drop the object into the stream or river.
5. Watch the object's movement along with the river's current.

6. Notice the obstacles it encounters as it passes along the waterway, symbolizing the challenges faced in life.
7. Notice the beauty of its free-flowing movement as it slips further out of sight, representing the natural progression of life and letting go.
8. Meditate upon the eventual destination of the object as it takes nature's course, symbolizing the continued journey and integration of the deceased's memory into the broader stream of life.

13.7 Guided Visualization

Guided visualization, also known as virtual dreams (Neimeyer et al., 2011) or guided imagery, is a practice where a facilitator leads individuals into deep relaxation through focused mental imagery. Rooted in meditation and contemplative traditions from various cultures, it has shown broad psychological and physiological benefits, such as stress reduction, improved performance, and effective pain management. Beyond these immediate effects, research highlights that mindfulness techniques like guided visualization can positively impact brain function and immune health. Davidson et al. (2003) found that regular meditation leads to observable changes in brain activity and immune response, showcasing how these practices support overall well-being.

13.7.1 Guided Visualization: Releasing Your Loved One

The following guided visualization/imagery can be read to the individual or recorded for their use.

Close your eyes and feel the coolness of each breath that you inhale. Feel the coolness in your lungs. Notice the freshness of the air. Feel the freshness as you inhale. Notice how the cool freshness soon turns to warm heaviness. Feel the warmth of the air in your lungs. Feel the heaviness as you exhale. Feel the warmth and heaviness of the air as you exhale. Feel the cool freshness coming in and the warm heaviness going out.

Picture in your mind the most loving person or divine being you can imagine. Picture this most loving being standing in front of you. Imagine this person's arms stretched out toward you.

Imagine hundreds of people standing in a line behind this loving person. The line extends far into the distance and disappears into the glow of a warm and peaceful light. You see this long line of hundreds of people disappear into that warm and peaceful light.

In your arms, you are carrying someone who has died, someone with whom you have shared great love. The body hardly has any weight at all. You're looking at this person in your arms, this person who has died, this person you have loved. You are reminded of some special moments you had with this person. Picture in your mind a few of those special moments. Look once again at this person in your arms. Remember, give your thanks, and say goodbye.

Now you carry the body you are holding over to the loving person with outstretched arms. Then gently place the body into their outstretched arms. Notice how the loving person/divine being turns and places the body in the arms of the next person in the line, and you watch the body being passed along the line of people from one to another toward the glowing, warm, and peaceful light. The body is carefully passed from one person to another to another. The body is finally passed into that glowing light. You see the light become brighter and warmer and more peaceful as the body enters the light. You know that the body is now safe, very safe, and relaxed.

You look once again at the loving being across from you. That being shares a warm and accepting smile and says, "Thank you. Your friend is safe now, very safe. So, it is okay for you to go now."

You turn around and begin walking away from this special place. As you are leaving, you once again become aware of your breathing. Feel the coolness and freshness of each breath that you inhale. Feel the warmth and heaviness of each breath that you exhale. Feel the freshness come in and the heaviness goes out. Your friend is safe. You are experiencing great relief. Your friend is safe. You feel peaceful. Your friend is safe. You are relieved.

13.7.2 Guided Visualization: Healing the Heart

Find a quiet and comfortable place where you won't be disturbed. Sit or lie down in a relaxed position. Make sure your spine is straight, and your body feels at ease. Make any adjustments you need to be comfortable. When you are ready, close your eyes gently. Take a few deep, calming breaths, and sigh out if you'd like to. Feel your body relaxing and settling in.

Take a deep breath through your nose, feeling your lungs fill completely. Hold your breath for a moment, then slowly exhale through your mouth, releasing any tension. Repeat this process three times, each time becoming more relaxed.

Bring your awareness to the top of your head, slowly scanning down through your forehead, eyes, cheeks, and jaw. With each exhalation, release any tension you might be holding in these areas. Continue scanning down through your neck, shoulders, and arms, softening any tightness with each breath out.

Move your focus to your chest. As you inhale, feel your chest expanding, filling with warmth and light. With each exhalation, imagine the area around your heart softening and becoming more expansive. Feel the sensation of relaxation spreading throughout your chest, releasing any pain or tightness you may be holding there. Continue and we will stay here for 3 min.

Continue the body scan down through your solar plexus, abdomen, hips, legs, and feet. With each breath, allow your body to become more relaxed and heavier and heavier. Notice any sensations that arise, gently breathing into them and releasing tension with each exhalation.

Bring your focus back to your heart. Visualize a warm, glowing light in the center of your chest. With each inhalation, imagine this light growing brighter and more vibrant. As you exhale, feel the light spreading throughout your chest, softening and healing any areas of pain or discomfort.

Imagine this light expanding beyond your chest, filling your entire body with warmth and healing energy. With each breath, feel the sensation of peace and comfort growing stronger. Allow yourself to fully immerse in this feeling of healing and love.

Spend a few moments in this state of deep relaxation and healing, breathing in the warmth and light, and exhaling any remaining tension or pain.

When you are ready to come out of the visualization, slowly bring your awareness back to your breath. Take a few deep breaths, feeling the air entering and leaving your body. Gently wiggle your fingers and toes, and when you feel ready, open your eyes.

Take a moment to sit quietly and reflect on the experience, noticing any changes in your body or emotions. Allow yourself to carry this sense of healing and peace with you as you go about your day.

13.8 Affirmations and Journaling

Affirmations and journaling are powerful tools supporting the grieving process. When repeated regularly, affirmations help reconstruct neuron pathways and allow a shift from intruding negative thoughts. Journaling opens a reflective space for processing the multifaceted emotions and thoughts of grief, making it easier to track progress and gain deeper insights over time.

The therapeutic value of these tools is well supported by research. Borkin (2014) underscores the healing power of writing, noting that journaling can serve as a structured outlet for emotional expression. Similarly, Ullrich and Lutgendorf (2002) found that journaling, particularly when it includes both cognitive and emotional processing, enhances awareness of the positive aspects of stressful experiences.

13.8.1 A Bereaved Person's Spiritual Affirmations

A care provider could recommend that the individual repeat one or a couple of the following affirmations each day, verbally or internally:

A. I receive strength through the comfort of God. I receive comfort through the strength of God.

B. Although clouds of loss and despair might enter my world, I know that the light of the Divine can never disappear.
C. I will take a day at a time knowing that Universal Energy is with me when the sun rises and will not desert me when the sun sets.
D. God was with me yesterday. God is with me today. God will be with me tomorrow.
E. The Divine Mother's love is behind me. The Divine Mother's love is before me. The Divine Mother's love is in me.
F. May the wisdom and compassion of my Buddha nature shine upon me and radiate from within me.

The word "God" etc. can be substituted with "Jesus," "Krishna," "Brahman," "the Revered Buddha," "Allah," "the Goddess," "the Divine Spirit," "the Universe," or any other wording that resonates with you.

13.8.2 Grief Journaling

Unstructured writing, often known as "expressive writing," allows those who are grieving to process their emotions freely without inhibition. This type of journaling encourages a spontaneous flow of thoughts and feelings, creating a space where grief can be expressed without concern for judgment or structure. Research by Ullrich and Lutgendorf (2002) highlights the value of combining emotional expression with cognitive processing in journaling, showing that this approach can lead to greater insight and emotional relief.

A balanced journaling practice that incorporates both unstructured and structured prompts offers the best of both worlds—allowing for free emotional release while also fostering thoughtful reflection. Below are prompts inspired by this approach, designed to support emotional expression and cognitive processing:

- *Unspoken words:* Write directly to the loved one who has passed, expressing anything that remained unsaid—whether it is an apology, gratitude, or reflections on the relationship.
- *Manifestation of grief:* Noticing how grief manifests physically, cognitively, behaviorally, or spiritually, in addition to emotions. Validate the manifestations and extend compassion and patience toward the self.
- *Catch the ANTs (automatic negative thoughts):* During grief, automatic negative thoughts (ANTs) often arise, particularly those fueled by guilt. Common cognitive errors include "all or nothing" thinking ("I didn't do all I needed to do, so I failed my loved one"), overgeneralization ("I always let them down"), or personalizing ("It was my fault"). For example, a bereaved person might think, "I didn't do enough to help them, and now I've failed completely," disregarding all the supportive efforts they did provide. Catching and reframing these thoughts into more compassionate and realistic perspectives is crucial for healing.

- *Finding meaning:* Reflecting on the lessons or insights that have emerged from the grieving journey and considering how these insights might shape one's growth and path forward.
- *Continuing bond:* Reflect on the ways in which the loved one could live through personal actions, care for one's own well-being, and service to others. Carry the legacy on.

13.8.3 Dream Journal

A dream journal can serve as a meaningful tool for those processing grief, especially when dreams involve the departed loved one. By documenting and reflecting on these dreams, the bereaved person can explore deeper emotional and symbolic meanings. After recording each dream, the following questions may help guide the reflection:

A. Are there any regrets or unfinished business from the past apparent in this dream? What actions do I need to take regarding those regrets or unfinished business?
B. What does this dream suggest about what I need to do now to aid my recovery from this loss?
C. What insights does this dream provide about how I should interact with the loved ones who are still present in my life?

13.9 Holidays

The holidays following a loss can be particularly difficult, especially the ones with spiritual significance, which may appear bereft of their typical meanings. Through compassionate and thoughtful support, care providers can facilitate individuals and families' reintroduction of significance and new traditions to these occasions. Difficult times are thus transformed into opportunities for meaningful remembrance, growth, and strengthening family unity.

13.9.1 Alternative Holiday Rituals

Instead of replicating traditional routines that may bring sadness, consider starting new traditions. Here are some ideas:

1. *Movie marathon:* Spend the day watching a selection of movies featuring a favorite actress or actor.

2. *Day trip with a friend:* Plan a day trip with a friend who has also experienced a recent loss.
3. *Volunteer:* Serve a holiday meal at a soup kitchen or local charity, or donate to a cause your loved one cared about.
4. *Home project:* Embark on a home redecorating project to refresh your surroundings.
5. *Planting:* Plant a tree, flowers, or vegetables in memory of your loved one.
6. *Reading list:* Make a tradition of revisiting a favorite book each year, starting on the holiday itself.
7. *Words of the Year:* Choose "Words of the Year" as forward-looking affirmations.
8. *Memory sharing:* Start a conversation with family and friends to share significant memories of your loved one during the holidays. This can be a profound part of the grief recovery process.
9. *Letter writing:* Write a letter to your loved one expressing your feelings during the holidays. This can be a personal reflection or part of a group activity where letters are read aloud, kept as keepsakes, or burnt in a remembrance ritual.
10. *Evening gathering:* Host an evening gathering or memorial where you light a candle, prepare a special menu of your loved one's favorite dishes, or toast to their memory.
11. *Creative decorating:* Decorate with family, incorporating items that remind you of your loved one, such as creating a wreath or displaying pictures.
12. *Burning regrets:* Start a tradition of lighting a fire, writing down your regrets from the past year, and then throwing them into the fire to symbolize a fresh start.

13.9.2 The First Christmas After a Death

1. Each surviving family member reflects on a favorite gift, tangible or intangible, received from the departed person.
2. Each family member writes the name of the gift on a piece of paper, places it in a box, and wraps the box.
3. These special gifts are either the first or last gifts opened on Christmas morning.
4. Upon opening the gift, each family member reads aloud what they had written, elaborating on why that gift means so much to them.

13.9.3 The Holiday Tablecloth

During each holiday meal, all family members sign their names on a special tablecloth if they have not done so previously. These names can later be embroidered onto the tablecloth. Each time the tablecloth is brought out, it bears the signatures of those present and those who have previously sat at the table. Each meal begins with a silent meditation to remember those not currently at the table.

13.10 Prayers and Remembrance

Research has shown that prayers can provide significant emotional support and alleviate the distress resulting from grief (Wojtkowiak et al., 2021). They help individuals cope by offering a sense of control, reducing feelings of isolation, and promoting emotional healing. Furthermore, prayers and spiritual rituals are associated with positive emotions, which play a crucial role in regulating grief and promoting overall well-being. By incorporating prayers into their daily routine, grieving individuals can find solace and strength during their difficult times. The following prayers, which can be read as they are or adapted to fit personal beliefs, offer comfort to those in mourning.

Prayer of Mourning
I pray for all of us who mourn.
May we face each day with courage, strength, and hope.
May the gifts of love and connection remain unbroken.
May our memories shine brighter than the pain of loss.
May all the good of the past chase away the fear of the future.
May hope illuminate the shadow in our hearts.
May we find peace and stillness beneath life's turbulent waves.
I pray for all of us who mourn.

I Remember
As the dawn paints the sky in soft hues,
I remember your eyes,
Clear and gentle as the morning light,
A glimpse of you lingers in every beam of sun, so bright.
As the moon rises, cool and tender,
I feel your touch,
Soft as the breeze upon my cheeks,
A whisper of love that never fades.
With every passing moment,
In the stillness of night and warmth of day,
I hear you whisper love,
A quiet echo that always lives within me.

13.11 Inspirations from the World

Around the world, cultures have developed unique holidays and rituals to honor and remember loved ones who have passed away. Here are some examples that showcase these diverse practices:

13.11.1 Ngaben in Bali

In Bali, the Ngaben ceremony is a joyful event marking the soul's journey into reincarnation. Families consult spiritual advisors to determine an auspicious day for cremation. The body is placed in an elaborately crafted casket, often in the shape of an animal, and a procession with music and dance accompanies the cremation. The ashes are then scattered in the sea, which symbolizes a return to nature.

13.11.2 Qingming Festival in China

The Qingming Festival, also known as Tomb-Sweeping Day, is a traditional holiday for Chinese families to honor their ancestors. They visit gravesites to clean and maintain them, offer food and drinks, and burn incense. Willow branches are traditionally used to ward off evil spirits, and certain foods symbolizing memory and cleansing are eaten. Kites are flown to symbolize good luck and sending wishes.

13.11.3 Tibetans at Anniversaries

Buddhists from various schools, such as Tibetans and some Japanese schools, conduct prayers and rituals to support the deceased's journey through Bardo, the intermediate state between death and rebirth. Memorial services are held for 7 days after death and traditionally continue until the 49th day. Anniversary memorial services are observed on the 1st, 2nd, 7th, and 13th anniversaries, among others. Prayers are often recited, and donations are made to monasteries. The merits accumulated through these auspicious activities are dedicated to the deceased. These events often involve family, friends, and the community, providing an important way to strengthen the community fabric and facilitating healing and support.

13.11.4 Obon Festival in Japan

The Obon Festival in Japan is a 3-day event where families honor ancestral spirits. Lanterns are lit to guide the spirits back to their homes, and offerings of food and flowers are made at household altars and gravesites. Traditional dances and ceremonies celebrate the lives of the deceased and their continued presence in the family.

13.11.5 A Bowl for the Departed

In some East Asian societies, at holiday dinners, a bowl filled with the best food is prepared for the departed as if they will show up to enjoy the holiday meal with the rest of the family, with the chopsticks vertically inserted into the food. In some families, this is also done daily on an altar in front of a picture, indicating the presence of the protective ancestor.

13.12 Concluding Reflection

In the vast cycle of life and death, grief is the thread that weaves our hearts to those who have touched our lives and moved beyond. Just as the moon waxes and wanes, so does sorrow—ebbing and flowing in its rhythm, reminding us of the cycles of renewal and remembrance.

In humanity's shared vulnerability, there is solace in knowing that across the world, grieving hearts beat in unison. As loved ones are honored, so must the light and connection be remembered.

A contemplative prayer suggests, "Whatever is had will eventually be lost." But can one ever truly "*have*" another person? Human connection is not ownership but a shared journey. Loved ones, whether family or friends, walk alongside and accompany one another for a time, sharing the sacred dance of life. If they were never anyone's to possess, can we ever truly "lose" them? Coming from life, merging back into life; life flows continuously from one to another, vibrating tirelessly in every cell, every memory, and every heartbeat. Everyone is always part of that oneness of *life* itself.

No one chases away the darkness, but anyone can light a candle. In the flicker of the flame and the gentle tunes of the moon, may the tune of love gently whisper; in the silence of the mind and depth of the heart, may healing unfold.

In every act of remembrance—through prayer, ritual, shared embraces, and tears—love weaves between worlds. Emotions come and go; love endures. Death may end a body, but never a relationship.

References

Biancalani, G., Azzola, C., Sassu, R., Marogna, C., & Testoni, I. (2022). Spirituality for coping with the trauma of a loved one's death during the COVID-19 pandemic: An Italian qualitative study. *Pastoral Psychology, 71*(2), 173–185.

Borkin, S. (2014). *The healing power of writing: a therapist's guide to using journaling with clients*. WW Norton.

Boyer, P., & Liénard, P. (2006). Why ritualized behavior? Precaution systems and actions parsing in developmental, pathological and cultural rituals. *Behavioral and Brain Sciences, 29*(6), 595–650. https://doi.org/10.1017/S0140525X06009332

Burke, L. A., & Neimeyer, R. A. (2014). Complicated spiritual grief I: Relation to complicated grief symptomatology following violent death bereavement. *Death Studies, 38*(4), 259–267.

Burke, L. A., & Neimeyer, R. A. (2012). Spirituality and health: Meaning making in bereavement. In *The textbook on spirituality in healthcare* (pp. 127–133).

Čepulienė, A. A., & Skruibis, P. (2022). The role of spirituality during suicide bereavement: A qualitative study. *International Journal of Environmental Research and Public Health, 19*(14), 8740.

Davidson, R. J., Kabat-Zinn, J., Schumacher, J., Rosenkranz, M., Muller, D., Santorelli, S. F., et al. (2003). Alterations in brain and immune function produced by mindfulness meditation. *Psychosomatic Medicine, 65*(4), 564–570.

Doka, K. J. (2012). Therapeutic ritual. In R. A. Neimeyer (Ed.), *Techniques of grief therapy: Creative practices for counseling the bereaved* (1st ed., pp. 341–343). Routledge.

Janoff-Bulman, R. (1992). *Shattered assumptions*. Free Press.

Koenig, H. G. (2008). *Medicine, religion, and health: Where science and spirituality meet*. Templeton Foundation Press.

Koenig, H. G., McCullough, M. E., & Larson, D. B. (2001). *Handbook of religion and health*. Oxford University Press.

Neimeyer, R. A., Torres, C., & Smith, D. C. (2011). The virtual dream: Rewriting stories of loss and grief. *Death Studies, 35*(7), 646–672.

Park, C. L., & Halifax, R. J. (2021). Religion and spirituality in adjusting to bereavement: Grief as burden, grief as gift. In *Grief and bereavement in contemporary society* (pp. 355–363).

Puchalski, C. M., & Ferrell, B. (2010). *Making healthcare whole: Integrating spirituality into patient care*. Templeton Press.

Sas, C., & Coman, A. (2016). Designing personal grief rituals: An analysis of symbolic objects and actions. *Death Studies, 49*(5), 558–569. https://doi.org/10.1080/07481187.2016.1188868

Ullrich, P. M., & Lutgendorf, S. K. (2002). Journaling about stressful events: Effects of cognitive processing and emotional expression. *Annals of Behavioral Medicine, 24*(3), 244–250.

Whitehouse, H., & Lanman, J. A. (2014). The ties that bind us: Ritual, fusion, and identification. *Current Anthropology, 55*(6), 674–695. https://doi.org/10.1086/678698

Willemse, S., Smeets, W., Van Leeuwen, E., Nielen-Rosier, T., Janssen, L., & Foudraine, N. (2020). Spiritual care in the intensive care unit: An integrative literature research. *Journal of Critical Care, 57*, 55–78.

Wojtkowiak, J., Lind, J., & Smid, G. E. (2021). Ritual in therapy for prolonged grief: A scoping review of ritual elements in evidence-informed grief interventions. *Frontiers in Psychiatry, 11*, 623835.

Epilogue

When Yan and I decided to write this book, we wanted something that combined theories and practice. We wanted to write a "useful" text: something that would be "used" to understand the phenomenon of grieving and "used" to address the needs of dying and grieving individuals. The book needed to have time-honored research and time-tested praxis, something "useful" in the past, present, and future.

Experts in any field have come upon situations where, for one reason or another, their expertise has been completely forgotten, as if their knowledge and practical tools have suddenly disappeared—sometimes when that knowledge and tools are most needed. This has happened to me more than a couple of times. The occasion when this became most obvious to me occurred when my daughter, Maren, was dying in 2004.

Although by 2004 I had written a couple of books on grieving and had lectured around the country to grief counselors, the emotional impact of watching my daughter dying of neurofibromatosis seemed to completely erase all my supposed expertise—all my academic knowledge and my therapeutic tools had been completely forgotten. I felt totally confused and "useless."

I was in Maren's room at the Mayo Clinic during her final weeks of life when Maren turned to me and said, "Dad, there's a social worker here who has been doing some really helpful things for me. She says I'm going through something called 'anticipatory grief,' and she has helped me address some of that grief."

"What has she been doing, Maren?"

"She's been doing guided imagery with me, and it helps bring me a sense of pain relief and some peace. And I really need that now."

I responded, "That's nice. I'm glad she has been helpful."

Maren continued, "And Dad, she said she got the guided imagery from a book you wrote. How come you're not using guided imagery with me?"

In the emotional chaos of Maren's dying, I had forgotten how to "use" my knowledge and tools.

Y. Z. Ciupak, D. C. Smith, *Death, Dying, and Grief*,
https://doi.org/10.1007/978-3-031-88467-2

Yan and I wish to thank you for reading this book. Please "use" and "reuse" the knowledge and tools we have shared with you and try not to forget what you have learned (as I did), especially when that knowledge and those tools are most needed.

Thank you again.

Doug Smith

January 16, 2024

> We try to grasp ahold of so many things,
> failing to realize there is nothing we need to hold onto,
> for we are the ones who are being held,
> held in *being*,
> held in Love[1].
>
> —Douglas Corry Smith (1947–2024)

[1] Dated July 5, 2024, this was the co-author, Doug's final entries in his hospice diary. Doug described the process of writing the diary incredibly therapeutic. The diary is being edited by Dr. Yan Ciupak into a book powerfully entitled: *How I Choose to Die: A Hospice Expert's Final Diary.*

Index

A

Activities for terminally ill, 231, 245, 251, 258, 260
Advanced care planning, 135, 177
Affirmations, 150, 154, 156, 159, 160, 170, 205, 207, 208, 211, 221–223, 251, 271, 308, 315, 318, 319, 321, 341, 350, 375–378
Ambiguous loss, 16, 55, 58–60, 79
Anticipatory grief, 5, 13, 16, 56, 63–65, 79, 97, 98, 108, 204

B

Bereavement support, 10, 150
Bereavement therapy, 226

C

Care plans, 44, 60, 107–109, 114, 131, 132, 144, 156, 163, 175–201, 203–227, 234, 293, 333–335
Case studies, 6, 18, 36, 37, 41, 46, 189
Cognitive-behavioral grief support, 151, 206, 265, 266
Collective and cumulative grief, 70
Compassion fatigue prevention, 157, 161, 164–169
Compassionate care, 46, 100, 109, 115, 119, 132, 142, 151, 170, 183
Compassionate person-centered care, 135
Contemplative practices, 336
Continuing bonds, 23, 24, 78, 83, 89, 94–97, 102, 145, 158, 161, 204, 212, 214–215, 260, 371, 377
Cultural awareness, 34–36, 38, 43–44, 46, 47
Cultural competence, 13, 35, 37–44, 46, 133
Cultural humility, 11, 14, 35, 40–43, 45, 47, 160, 233, 290, 300, 326, 332, 345, 363
Culturally responsive practices, 36
Culturally sensitive practices, 80
Cultural sensitivity, 11, 13, 20, 35, 36, 44, 78, 130, 135, 155, 160, 163, 365
Culture, 4, 9, 11, 14, 29–47, 53, 54, 58, 69, 74, 83, 95, 143, 160, 167, 185, 266, 289, 290, 296, 318, 326, 329, 332, 337, 343, 345, 350, 360, 368, 370, 373, 379

D

Death and grief education, 7–9, 12–13, 25, 142
Death and grief in the digital age, 20, 22
Death attitudes, 14–16, 18, 54
Death awareness movement, 17–19
Death café, 21
Death studies, 15, 17–19
Death trajectory, 15, 16, 105, 107, 109
Depression, 22, 55–57, 64, 66, 71, 72, 76, 77, 79, 86, 91, 110, 165, 167, 175, 176, 188, 215, 221, 231, 232, 236, 266–268, 272, 292, 305, 307, 309, 310
Disenfranchised grief, 45, 55, 56, 58, 65–67, 79, 94, 148
Diversity, 19–22, 30–36, 38, 39, 41, 42, 44, 45, 47, 80, 187, 290, 295, 302, 330–332, 335, 336, 360, 363, 366
Dual process model, 83, 89–91, 102

Y. Z. Ciupak, D. C. Smith, *Death, Dying, and Grief*,
https://doi.org/10.1007/978-3-031-88467-2

E

Empowerment in end-of-life decision making, 20
End-of-life and grief assessment, 175
End-of-life care, 5, 10, 16, 18, 32, 33, 44, 46, 64, 105–135, 142, 151, 159, 177, 200, 231, 233, 238, 245, 256, 259, 291, 329, 330
End-of-life rituals, 329
End-of-life support, 151, 169
Ethical challenges in end-of-life care, 135
Ethical principles in bereavement care, 152, 159, 169

F

Forgiveness, 204, 206, 207, 209, 211–214, 220, 261, 268–270, 272, 273, 276, 278, 285, 351, 353, 365
4A4C competency framework, 142, 153–160, 170, 205
4A4C framework, 6, 154, 170, 203–205, 216, 330

G

Grief, 3, 31, 53, 83, 105, 141, 175, 203, 265, 289, 332, 364
Grief competency and training, 142
Grief coping tools, 266, 269–280
Grief counseling, 10, 13, 19, 107, 109, 142–152, 163, 177
Grief support, 6, 9–11, 13, 14, 23, 24, 29–47, 58, 80, 89, 141, 143–164, 169, 170, 177, 274, 285
Grief support and counseling, 175–201
Grief support and counseling principles, 142
Grief support techniques, 269–280
Grief theories, 83, 84, 102, 159
Grief therapy exercises, 266, 270
Grieving, 3, 31, 58, 83, 143, 179, 203, 266, 299, 335, 364
Grieving processes, 24, 32, 43, 56–58, 61, 63, 66, 67, 71, 83–102, 111, 144, 145, 147, 148, 150, 156, 158, 177, 182, 189, 205, 215, 216, 224, 226, 266–268, 364, 365, 371, 375
Grieving styles, 87, 89, 92, 93, 146, 186–187, 196
Guided visualization/imagenery, 10, 22, 147, 148, 166, 200–201, 253–255, 277–280, 291, 318–321, 326, 337, 345–349, 373–375
Guilt and forgiveness in grieving, 267–269

H

Holistic end-of-life care plans, 113–114
Holistic Psychosocial Care (HPC), 5, 6, 203–226, 266, 311, 326, 330
Holistic psychosocial care plans, 203–226
Hospice, 16, 18, 19, 32, 114–118, 120, 153, 165, 176, 180, 194, 238, 244, 246, 256, 260, 262, 329
Hospice care, 17, 18, 114–118, 151, 349

I

Interdisciplinary perspectives, 101, 116, 118

K

Kübler-Ross stage model, 83, 84, 86, 110, 111, 215, 238, 265

L

Legacy building, 231, 241–245
Loss and bereavement, 8

M

Meaning, 4, 39, 56, 84, 116, 144, 176, 205, 232, 265, 289, 331, 363
Meaning reconstruction, 15, 55, 59, 62, 84, 92–95, 102, 145, 149, 204, 268, 302, 336
Mindfulness, 7, 8, 22, 62, 69, 147, 149, 150, 164, 166, 167, 207, 292, 309, 336, 342, 349, 373
Mindfulness-based practices, 292, 336
Mindfulness practices, 150, 160, 161, 166, 342
Mindfulness tools, 377
Multicultural, 5, 36, 37, 40, 42, 47, 330, 332
Multicultural spirituality, 332

N

Nonfinite losses, 226

P

Palliative care, 19, 32, 44, 108, 109, 113–115, 118–120, 125, 126, 134, 151, 153, 176–177, 247, 260, 291–293, 329–331, 333, 335, 336
Personal and professional, 8–12, 159, 160, 169, 333

Person-centered approach, 10, 231, 232
Person-centered care, 20, 35, 45, 144, 151, 155, 175, 177, 189, 232, 262
Physician-assisted suicide (PAS), 122, 131, 132
Post-traumatic growth (PTG), 272, 273, 302, 303, 364
Professional self-care, 69, 141, 158–160, 164–169, 337
Prolonged grief disorder (PGD), 21, 56, 71–79, 84, 91, 177, 267, 365
Psychosocial grief tools, 269–280
Psychosocial support, 231–262, 265–285

R
Remembrance activities for bereavement, 276
Resilience and empowerment, 175
Rituals, 3, 30, 60, 90, 134, 148, 178, 205, 234, 268, 291, 329, 365

S
Secondary losses, 55–57, 79, 89, 97, 204, 216, 218, 219
Self as an instrument, 9–12, 141
Sociocultural impact on grief, 101
Spiral model of grieving and healing, 4, 6, 32, 33, 83, 101–102, 112, 203, 209, 224, 226, 265
Spiritual assessment tools, 335
Spiritual care, 45, 46, 114, 133–135, 167, 176, 291–293, 310, 326, 329–338, 349, 360, 363
Spirituality, 4, 40, 158, 161, 272, 289–291, 293–295, 302, 309–310, 330–332, 345, 350, 356, 360, 363, 364, 370
Spiritual support, 18, 114, 115, 291–292, 337, 338, 360, 364
Stage model of grieving, 86
Strength-based practices, 175

T
Tasks of mourning, 88, 90, 224
Thanatology, 6, 8, 17, 18, 152
Therapeutic alliance, 9–12, 144, 161, 163, 189, 291
Therapeutic rituals, 67, 150
Tools, 6, 60, 95, 106, 142, 175, 203, 231, 268, 292, 330, 365
Transcendence, 96, 290, 331, 363, 366
Traumatic losses, 20, 54, 55, 60–63, 76, 94, 97, 98, 364

The manufacturer's authorised representative in the EU is Springer Nature Customer Service Centre GmbH, Europaplatz 3, 69115 Heidelberg, Germany. If you have any concerns regarding our products, please contact ProductSafety@springernature.com

Printed and bound by CPI Group (UK) Ltd, Croydon, CR0 4YY

30/09/2026

02225569-0016